The Facial Nerve

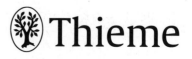

The Facial Nerve

William H. Slattery III, MD
Partner, House Clinic
Clinical Professor of Otolaryngology
University of Southern California Keck School of Medicine
Los Angeles, California

Babak Azizzadeh, MD, FACS
Director, Facial Paralysis Institute
Center for Advanced Facial Plastic Surgery
Beverly Hills, California
Associate Clinical Professor for the Division of Head and Neck Surgery
David Geffen School of Medicine, UCLA
Los Angeles, California

Thieme
New York • Stuttgart

Thieme Medical Publishers, Inc.
333 Seventh Ave.
New York, NY 10001

Executive Editor: Timothy Y. Hiscock
Managing Editor: J. Owen Zurhellen IV
Editorial Assistant: Heather Allen
Senior Vice President, Editorial and Electronic Product Development: Cornelia Schulze
Production Editor: Meredith Bechtle, Maryland Composition
Medical Illustrator: Peggy Firth
Front Cover Illustration: Karl Wesker
International Production Director: Andreas Schabert
Vice President, Finance and Accounts: Sarah Vanderbilt
President: Brian D. Scanlan
Compositor: Maryland Composition
Printer: Everbest Printing Co.

Library of Congress Cataloging-in-Publication Data
The facial nerve / [edited by] William H. Slattery III.
    p. ; cm.
Includes bibliographical references and index.
ISBN 978-1-60406-050-8 (hardcover) -- ISBN 978-1-60406-857-3 (ebook)
I. Slattery, William H., III, editor of compilation. II. Title.
[DNLM: 1. Facial Nerve. 2. Facial Nerve Diseases. 3. Facial Paralysis. WL 330]
RD523
617.1'56--dc23
                                                                                    2013022603

Important note: Medical knowledge is ever-changing. As new research and clinical experience broaden our knowledge, changes in treatment and drug therapy may be required. The authors and editors of the material herein have consulted sources believed to be reliable in their efforts to provide information that is complete and in accord with the standards accepted at the time of publication. However, in view of the possibility of human error by the authors, editors, or publisher of the work herein or changes in medical knowledge, neither the authors, editors, nor publisher, nor any other party who has been involved in the preparation of this work, warrants that the information contained herein is in every respect accurate or complete, and they are not responsible for any errors or omissions or for the results obtained from use of such information. Readers are encouraged to confirm the information contained herein with other sources. For example, readers are advised to check the product information sheet included in the package of each drug they plan to administer to be certain that the information contained in this publication is accurate and that changes have not been made in the recommended dose or in the contraindicationsfor administration. This recommendation is of particular importance in connection with new or infrequently used drugs.

Some of the product names, patents, and registered designs referred to in this book are in fact registered trademarks or proprietary names even though specific reference to this fact is not always made in the text. Therefore, the appearance of a name without designation as proprietary is not to be construed as a representation by the publisher that it is in the public domain.

Printed in China

ISBN 978-1-60406-050-8
eISBN 978-1-60406-857-3

MIX
Paper from
responsible sources
FSC® C021256

Contents

Preface

The facial nerve, 1 of 12 cranial nerves, controls the muscles that permit movement (and in particular those muscles which convey expressions) of the face. Diseases of or injuries to this nerve commonly result in an enhanced asymmetry of the face, a decrease in the patient's ability to communicate emotion, and may result in temporary or permanent paralysis. This book offers a concise and yet comprehensive review of facial nerve diseases and injuries, as well as the most up-to-date recommendations for medical and surgical treatments. Written with the busy clinician in mind, we do our best to cover all the relevant topics without being exhaustive in the nonessentials. We are fortunate to have a host of expert contributors who bring broad and multifarious perspectives from a wide range of acclaimed institutions. What is most exciting is that each contributor has paired his or her clinical practice with clinically relevant research offering an unparalleled textbook among current publications.

This book is divided into five major sections: overview, examination, disease processes, selected topics, and rehabilitation. The overview section includes an excellent chapter on the anatomy and physiology of the facial nerve. The corresponding illustrations make the complex and often difficult-to-navigate anatomy of the facial nerve tractable. The physiology chapter highlights general nerve physiology with specific reference to the facial nerve structure and function. The histopathology chapter will be particularly valuable for the resident who is preparing for board examinations.

The examination section is essentially an overview aimed at offering important observations from experienced clinicians that will assist both the novice and the not-so-novice in the evaluation of facial nerve disorders. No book on the facial nerve is complete without a discussion of the facial nerve "grading" systems, and herein we provide a thorough survey. The imaging chapter is comprehensive and includes images of rarer but observable facial nerve lesions that might otherwise be overlooked by an inexperienced practitioner.

With regard to the section called disease processes, we mean to equip the reader with a working knowledge and practical plan for a complete differential diagnosis. Because Bell palsy is the most common facial nerve disorder, this book takes an extensive look at both the surgical and medical management of this disease. We follow by undertaking an in-depth discussion of trauma, tumor, and lesser known diseases associated with facial paralysis. Facial nerve monitoring, which in recent years has become commonly practiced during skull base and parotid surgeries, as well as other otologic procedures, is evaluated. We cover indications for it and challenges to it, giving special reference to monitoring throughout the removal of an acoustic neuroma. Another highlight is the review of topics that are specific to improving outcomes in acoustic neuroma surgery.

The subject of the last section, Rehabilitation of Permanent Facial Nerve Paralysis, is of great importance to the patient. Patient satisfaction has always been at the forefront when considering the value of any treatment and reputation of any practitioner. As health care options become more limited, clinicians must remind themselves that a multidisciplinary approach is often the surest way to achieve that goal. Both surgical and nonsurgical techniques are presented here. Such things as eyelid springs and gold weights have shown promising results with regard to management of the eye in acute or chronic facial palsy. Options for the patient with a lower face paralysis may include slings or muscle transposition flaps. Botulinum neurotoxin therapy and traditional physical therapies help many patients with long-standing disorders, yet when surveyed, many clinicians still do not recommend further treatments or refer patients to specialists outside their own area of expertise. It is our hope that this book will allow those who treat one aspect of facial nerve disorders to offer a more fully comprehensive approach to the presenting patient.

A recent *The New York Times* article reported on the desperate need for a more integrated approach in medicine, ". . . where every patient's care is team based, preventative, and comprehensive." In an era of unmatched scrutiny of the way health care dollars are spent, it behooves us as health care providers to be ever more cognizant of the best practices and most current approaches for those who entrust their care to us. This book then, is both relevant and indispensable to otolaryngologists, facial plastic surgeons, ophthalmologists, neuroradiologists, neurologists, oromaxillofacial surgeons, dentists, nurses, physical therapists, and others who treat such diseases.

Certainly and perhaps as never before, it is only an unwavering and sincere passion to alleviate and when possible, heal another human being's suffering that motivates every trainee and long practicing provider. Commentator Peggy Noonan once said, "Sincerity and competence is a strong combination." She made that statement in reference to another discipline, but it most certainly applies to the art and science of medicine, and it's to that end that this book is written.

Contributors

Marcus D. Atlas, MBBS, FRACS
Winthrop Professor of Otolaryngology–Head & Neck
 Surgery
University of Western Australia
Director, Ear Science Institute Australia
Perth, Western Australia
Australia

Babak Azizzadeh, MD, FACS
Director, Facial Paralysis Institute
Center for Advanced Facial Plastic Surgery
Beverly Hills, California
Associate Clinical Professor for the Division of Head and
 Neck Surgery
David Geffen School of Medicine, UCLA
Los Angeles, California

Maurizio Barbara, MD, PhD
Professor of Otorhinolaryngology, NESMOS
Sapienza University
Sant'Andrea Hospital
Rome, Italy

Carien H.G. Beurskens, PhD
Department of Physiotherapy
University Medical Centre Nijmegen
Nijmegen, Netherlands

Derald E. Brackmann, MD
Associate, House Clinic
Clinical Professor of Otolaryngology–Head and Neck
 Surgery and Neurological Surgery
University of Southern California Keck School of Medicine
Los Angeles, California

Kevin D. Brown, MD
Assistant Professor of Otolaryngology–Head and
 Neck Surgery
Weill Cornell Medical College
New York, New York

Claire-Lise Curto Faïs, MD
Assistant of Otology and Head and Neck Surgery
CCU–AH service d'ORL
Hôpital Nord
Marseille, France

H. Jacqueline Diels
Department of Orthopedics and Rehabilitation
University of Wisconsin Hospital and Clinics
Madison, Wisconsin

Jose N. Fayad, MD
House Clinic
Los Angeles, California

Bruce J. Gantz, MD, FACS
Professor and Head, Department of Otolaryngology–Head
 and Neck Surgery
Brian F. McCabe Distinguished Chair in Otolaryngology–
 Head and Neck Surgery
Professor, Department of Neurosurgery
University of Iowa Carver College of Medicine
Iowa City, Iowa

Michael B. Gluth, MD
Assistant Professor and Director of The Comprehensive
 Listening Center
Section of Otolaryngology–Head & Neck Surgery
University of Chicago Medical Center
Chicago, Illinois

Ajay Gupta, MD
Assistant Professor of Radiology
NewYork-Presbyterian Hospital
Weill Cornell Medical College
New York, New York

Tessa A. Hadlock, MD
Associate Professor and Director of Facial Plastic and
 Reconstructive Surgery and Facial Nerve Center
Massachusetts Eye and Ear Infirmary
Harvard Medical School
Boston, Massachusetts

Douglas K. Henstrom, MD
Assistant Professor and Director of Facial Plastic Surgery
 and Nerve Center
University of Iowa
Iowa City, Iowa

Michael Hoa, MD
Assistant Professor of Otolaryngology—Head and
  Neck Surgery
Georgetown University Medical Center
Washington, DC
Medical Officer of NIH/NIDCD
Bethesda, Maryland

John W. House, MD
House Clinic
Clinical Professor
University of Southern California Keck School of Medicine
Los Angeles, California

Brandon Isaacson, MD
Associate Professor of Otolaryngology—Head and
  Neck Surgery
University of Texas Southwestern Medical Center
Dallas, Texas

Bradley W. Kesser, MD
Associate Professor of Otolaryngology—Head and
  Neck Surgery
University of Virginia Health System
Charlottesville, Virginia

Jonathan S. Kulbersh, MD
Carolina Facial Plastics
Charlotte, North Carolina

J. Walter Kutz Jr., MD
Assistant Professor of Otolaryngology
University of Texas Southwestern Medical Center
Dallas, Texas

Kimberly J. Lee, MD
Assistant Professor of Otolaryngology—Head and
  Neck Surgery
UCLA Medical Center
Director of Beverly Hills Facial Plastic Surgery Center
Beverly Hills, California

John P. Leonetti, MD
Professor and Vice Chairman of Otolaryngology—
  Head and Neck Surgery
Loyola University Medical Center
Maywood, Illinois

Robert E. Levine, MD
Clinical Professor of Ophthalmology
University of Southern California Keck School of Medicine
Los Angeles, California

Thomas E. Linder, MD
Assistant Professor and Chairman of Otolaryngology–Head
  and Neck Surgery
Luzerner Kantonsspital
Luzern, Switzerland

Fred H. Linthicum Jr., MD
Department of Histopathology
House Research Institute
Los Angeles, California

Mark Brandt Lorenz, MD
Department of Otolaryngology
Alaska Native Medical Center
Anchorage, Alaska

Jacques Magnan
Professor Emeritus and Head of ORL Department
University Aix-Marseille
Marseille, France

Sam J. Marzo, MD, FACS
Professor of Otolaryngology—Head and Neck Surgery
Loyola University Medical Center
Maywood, Illinois

Guy G. Massry, MD
Beverly Hills Ophthalmic Plastic Surgery
Beverly Hills, California

Sarah E. Mowry, MD
Assistant Professor of Otolaryngology
Georgia Regents University
Augusta, Georgia

Shingo Murakami, MD, PhD
Professor and Chairman of Otolaryngology—
  Head and Neck Surgery
Nagoya City University Medical School
Japan

J. Gail Neely, MD
Professor and Director of Otology/Neurotology/Base of
  Skull Surgery
Washington University School of Medicine
St. Louis, Missouri

Brendan P. O'Connell, MD
Department of Otolaryngology—Head and Neck Surgery
Medical University of South Carolina
Charleston, South Carolina

C. Douglas Phillips, MD, FACR
Professor of Radiology
Director of Head and Neck Imaging
NewYork-Presbyterian Hospital
Weill Cornell Medical College
New York, New York

Peter S. Roland, MD
Professor and Chairman of Otolaryngology
University of Texas Southwestern Medical Center
Dallas, Texas

Felipe Santos, MD
Instructor of Otology and Laryngology
Massachusetts Eye and Ear Infirmary
Harvard Medical School
Boston, Massachusetts

Barry M. Schaitkin, MD
Professor of Otolaryngology
University of Pittsburgh
Pittsburgh, Pennsylvania

Samuel H. Selesnick, MD
Professor and Vice Chairman of Otolaryngology—
   Head and Neck Surgery
Weill Cornell Medical College
New York, New York

Randolph Sherman, MD, FACS
Vice Chairman of Surgery
Cedars-Sinai Medical Center
Los Angeles, California

William H. Slattery III, MD
Partner, House Clinic
Clinical Professor of Otolaryngology
University of Southern California Keck School of Medicine
Los Angeles, California

Emily Z. Stucken, MD
Resident of Otolaryngology—Head and Neck Surgery
Weill Cornell Medical College
New York, New York

Jeffrey T. Vrabec, MD
Professor of Otolaryngology—Head and Neck Surgery
Baylor College of Medicine
Houston, Texas

Eric P. Wilkinson, MD, FACS
Partner, House Clinic
Los Angeles, California

Ronald M. Zuker, MD, FRCSC
Professor of Plastic and Reconstructive Surgery
University of Toronto
The Hospital for Sick Children
Toronto, Ontario
Canada

1 Anatomy of the Facial Nerve and Associated Structures

Bradley W. Kesser

The anatomy of the facial nerve beautifully illustrates the complexities of the human peripheral, central, and autonomic nervous systems. The facial nerve, the seventh cranial nerve, contains motor, general sensory, special sensory, and autonomic (visceral) components, all of which are reviewed in this chapter.

The course of the facial nerve as it runs intracranially, intratemporally, and extratemporally is perhaps one of the most intricate routes of any cranial nerve. The physician (otologic/neurotologic surgeon, head and neck surgeon, general otolaryngologist, neurosurgeon, and neurologist) must have comprehensive knowledge of the anatomy, physiology, and course of the facial nerve to diagnose and treat lesions and disorders of the nerve, to avoid surgical complications such as facial nerve injury, and to rehabilitate patients with facial nerve disorders. This chapter will details these elements as well as the anatomic path of the facial nerve and its branches as it emerges from the brainstem and takes its long, circuitous route to its targeted structures.

■ Embryology

This section describes an overview of the embryology of the facial nerve. Sataloff has written an entire textbook describing in depth the embryology of the facial nerve.[1] The facial nerve, the nerve of the second branchial arch, develops from a collection of neural crest cells in close caudal proximity to the otic placode, the facioacoustic primordium, first seen around the third week of gestation.[2] The primordium splits into a caudal main trunk and a rostral sensory (chorda tympani) trunk, which enters the first mandibular arch. By the sixth week, ganglia, including the geniculate ganglion, for the sensory cranial nerves are visible, the facial nerve is distinct from the vestibulocochlear nerve, and the nervus intermedius (see subsequent discussion) can be identified. The peripheral motor divisions appear by the eighth week when development of the second arch progresses to individual muscle groups. At this time, the horizontal and vertical portions of the facial nerve run anterior to the external auditory canal and have started to demarcate. The weeks following the eighth week are characterized by extensive arborization of the peripheral facial nerve and the corresponding development of the muscles of facial expression. By the 16th week, all connections are established, but the nerve itself still runs superficial and anterior to the ear canal with respect to its final position. The nerve finally exits the stylomastoid foramen in its usual position by week 30, but

it continues to lie superficial until the development of the mastoid tip between 1 and 3 years of age.

Gerhardt and Otto suggest that the final course of the facial nerve was influenced by two processes of motion of global development of the head with relation to the temporal bone.[3] The first is a shifting of the meninges, the labyrinth, and the proximal parts of the first (mandibular) branchial arch and the second (hyoidal) branchial arch in a rostral direction. The proximal facial nerve around the geniculate is tethered to the labyrinth and shifts anteriorly to form the first genu relative to the more distal portion of the nerve, which keeps its dorsoventral pathway along with the second branchial arch, whose most dorsal aspect is the stapes blastema. The second global movement is a rotation of the lateral temporal bone in the dorsal direction due to differentiation of the first branchial arch. As the mandible and mastoid develop, the nerve is pulled posteriorly and inferiorly. Gerhardt and Otto further suggest that when there is hypoplasia of the first mandibular arch, possibly due to early stapedial artery involution, the nerve becomes foreshortened. This foreshortening leads to a relative rostral overshifting of the hyoidal arch structures. The distal portion of the facial nerve as it makes its second genu is more anterior and inferior than normal. This anterior and inferior displacement can put the nerve at the level of the oval window thus interfering with the normal development of the stapes and its interaction with the otic capsule, as well as with the development of the incudostapedial joint.[3]

In congenital aural atresia, the facial nerve typically takes a slightly more anterior position at the second genu and mastoid segments. The tympanic segment is often dehiscent of bone. Children with aural atresia in the setting of Goldenhar or hemifacial microsomia (hypoplasia of first arch structures) can also have facial nerve weakness, most commonly in the marginal mandibular division. The greatest risk to the facial nerve during the surgical repair of aural atresia is during the canalplasty: drilling the new external auditory canal (**Fig. 1.1**).

The facial nerve can course laterally as the drilling proceeds inferiorly, interfering with access to and exposure of the stapes bone and mesotympanum. Hugging the tegmen superiorly and the glenoid fossa anteriorly to open into the middle ear at the level of the epitympanum will keep the atresia surgeon away from the facial nerve. Risk of injury to the facial nerve in atresia surgery has been estimated at 0.1%.[4] In congenital malformations of the middle ear with a patent ear canal and normal tympanic membrane, an aberrant facial nerve was found in 24% of patients.[5] While transposition of the facial nerve with drilling of the endochondral bone of the

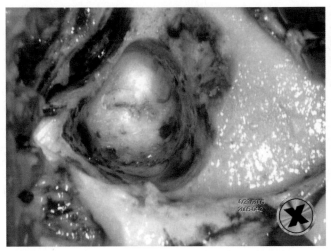
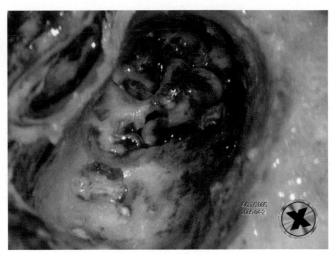

Fig. 1.1a, b (**a**) Aberrant course of the facial nerve in surgery for congenital aural atresia. The facial nerve courses laterally in the atretic bone. (**b**) Drilling was redirected anteriorly and superiorly to open into the epitympanum and find the ossicular complex.

otic capsule to create an oval window has been described,[6,7] enthusiasm for the oval window drillout has waned in recent years due to lack of stability of early hearing gains.[8,9]

■ Gross Anatomy

Intracranial–Intramedullary

The facial motor nucleus, located in the pontine tegmentum, receives input for voluntary facial expression from the motor cortex located in the precentral gyrus of the cerebral hemispheres. Fibers from the precentral gyrus project to the contralateral facial motor nucleus in the pons via the corticobulbar tract through the thalamus along the posterior limb of the internal capsule. Axons carrying motor output to the frontalis and upper part of the orbicularis oculi extend both to ipsilateral and contralateral facial motor nuclei. Thus, a facial paralysis that spares the upper face (frontalis) is caused by a central lesion, such as a tumor or stroke in the contralateral precentral gyrus. A complete facial paralysis, affecting all muscles of facial expression, is caused by a lesion of the lower motor neuron, anywhere from the facial motor nucleus to the stylomastoid foramen (**Fig. 1.2**).

These fibers from the precentral gyrus synapse in the facial motor nucleus; postsynaptic fibers initially travel dorsally toward the fourth ventricle where they become myelinated and loop around the motor nucleus of the abducens nerve. This loop, the internal genu, causes a slight bulge in the floor of the fourth ventricle called the facial colliculus. These fibers turn laterally and ventrally, and exit the ventrolateral aspect of the brainstem at the caudal border of the pons at the level of the middle cerebellar peduncle between the sixth and eighth cranial nerves, medial to the nervus intermedius (**Fig. 1.3**).

Sensory fibers of the facial nerve, traveling in the nervus intermedius, end in the nucleus of the tractus solitarius in the brainstem.

Intracranial–Extramedullary

The extramedullary portion of the facial nerve exits the inferior border of the pons in the recess between the olive and the inferior cerebellar peduncle, with the motor root medial, the vestibulocochlear nerve lateral, and the nervus intermedius between.[10] The facial nerve and nervus intermedius run in the cerebellopontine angle and join the vestibulocochlear nerve to enter the internal auditory canal at the porus acousticus.

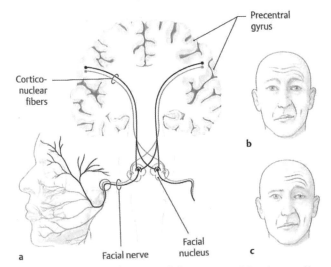

Fig. 1.2a–c Intracranial–intramedullary course of facial nerve fibers. (**a**) The *gray line* represents contralateral innervation of the mid and lower sections of the face. The *black line* shows both ipsilateral and contralateral innervation of the upper portion of the face. Corticonuclear (corticobulbar) fibers exit the motor cortex in the precentral gyrus and synapse in the facial nerve nucleus located in the pontine tegmentum. (**b**) Appearance of the face after an upper motor neuron lesion (e.g., stroke) in which upper facial nerve function is preserved due to bilateral innervation of the upper face. (**c**) Appearance of the face after a lower motor neuron lesion (e.g., Bell palsy; neoplasm of the facial nerve) with loss of function of all divisions of the facial nerve.

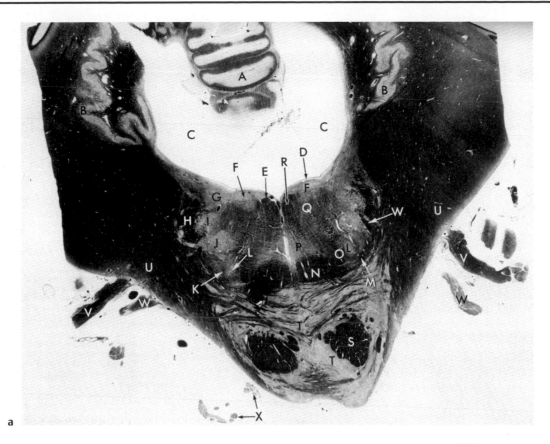

a

A. Nodulus of the cerebellar vermis
B. Dentate nucleus of the cerebellum
C. Fourth ventricle
D. Facial colliculus
E. Genu of facial nerve (VII)
F. Abducent nucleus
G. Lateral vestibular nucleus
H. Spinal tract of trigeminal nerve (V)
I. Nucleus of spinal tract of V
J. Facial nucleus
K. Lateral lemniscus
L. Superior olivary nucleus

M. Anterior and lateral spinothalamic tracts
N. Medial lemniscus
O. Central tegmental tract
P. Reticular formation
Q. Region of pontine center for horizontal gaze
R. Medial longitudinal fasciculus (MLF)
S. Pyramidal tract
T. Pontine nuclei
U. Middle cerebellar peduncle
V. Vestibulocochlear nerve (VIII)
W. Facial nerve (VII)
X. Fibers of the abducent nerve (VI)

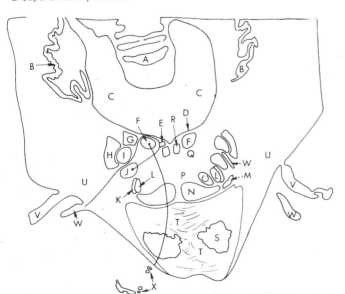

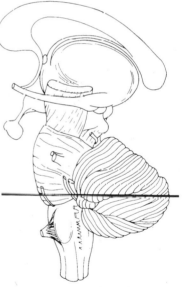

Fig. 1.3a, b Cross-sectional anatomy of the human brainstem at the level of the lower pons just above the junction with the medulla. [Used with permission from Watson C. *Basic Human Neuroanatomy: An Introductory Atlas, Third Edition.* Boston: Little, Brown and Company; 1985:166 (Figure 65).]

b

Intratemporal

The intratemporal facial nerve refers to the portion of the facial nerve that runs in the temporal bone in the fallopian canal (~30 cm in total length) and has been classically divided into segments based on location within the temporal bone: meatal, labyrinthine, tympanic (horizontal), and mastoid (vertical) before it exits the temporal bone through the stylomastoid foramen (**Fig. 1.4**).

Meatal

The meatal segment of the facial nerve, measuring ~1.5 cm— the length of the internal auditory canal (IAC)—enters the porus acousticus in an anterior, superior position. The nervus intermedius runs between the facial and vestibulocochlear nerves as they enter the porus. The facial nerve and nervus intermedius travel in the IAC adjacent to the superior vestibular nerve posteriorly and the cochlear nerve inferiorly (**Fig. 1.5**). The transverse (falciform) crest separates the facial nerve from the cochlear nerve inferiorly, and a small lateral ridge of bone, Bill bar, separates the facial nerve from the superior vestibular nerve posteriorly. The nerves of the IAC are surrounded by dura all the way to the fundus—a "meningeal glove finger."[11] A magnetic resonance imaging and cadaveric study showed the facial nerve to remain superior

and anterior to the vestibulocochlear nerve and to maintain a tubular shape throughout its course in the IAC.[12]

Labyrinthine

As the facial nerve exits the IAC at the fundus, it turns gently anteriorly and runs in the otic capsule bone for ~3 to 6 mm between the cochlea and superior semicircular canal (**Fig. 1.6**). The portion of the nerve as it exits the fundus of the IAC is the thinnest part of the facial nerve, and any decompression of the nerve (e.g., for idiopathic facial paralysis) should encompass this portion of the nerve (see Chapter 11).[13]

At the lateral end of the labyrinthine segment is a swelling of the nerve, the geniculate ganglion, containing the cell bodies of the pseudounipolar neurons carrying taste sensation to the anterior two-thirds of the tongue via the chorda tympani nerve, and some sensory fibers from the soft palate via the greater superficial petrosal nerve. The greater superficial petrosal nerve, carrying preganglionic parasympathetic innervation to the lacrimal gland and the glands of the nasal mucosa, is joined by the deep petrosal nerve from the carotid plexus carrying postganglionic sympathetic innervation (from the cervical sympathetic ganglion) to become the nerve of the pterygoid (Vidian) canal. This nerve

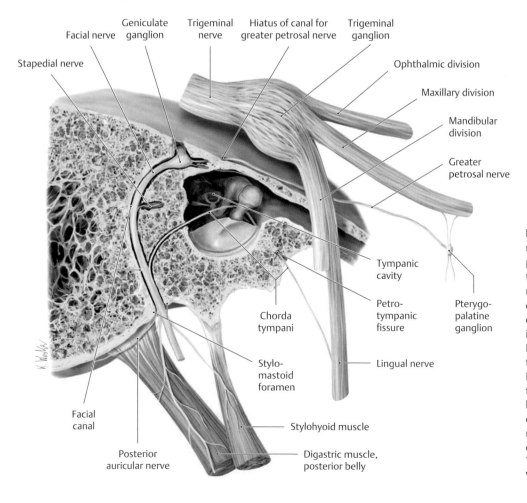

Fig. 1.4 Course of the intratemporal facial nerve. Note the greater superficial petrosal nerve exiting the temporal bone through its hiatus, running along the floor of the middle cranial fossa to send preganglionic parasympathetics to synapse in the pterygopalatine ganglion. Note the mastoid branches (nerve to stapedius and chorda tympani). Note the branches at the stylomastoid foramen (nerve to posterior belly of the digastric and stylohyoid muscles and posterior auricular nerve). (From Thieme Atlas of Anatomy, Head and Neuroanatomy, © Thieme 2007, Illustration by Karl Wesker.)

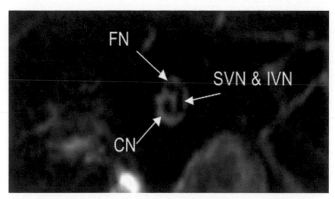

Fig. 1.5 Parasagittal cross section of the right internal auditory canal on magnetic resonance imaging constructive interference in steady state sequence showing the facial nerve (*FN*) superior and anterior in the internal auditory canal, with the cochlear nerve (*CN*) inferior and anterior, and the vestibular nerve components (superior [*SVN*] and inferior [*IVN*]) posterior. (Courtesy of Dr. Sugoto Mukherjee.)

enters the pterygopalatine (sphenopalatine) fossa where the parasympathetic fibers synapse in the pterygopalatine (sphenopalatine) ganglion and both postganglionic sympathetic and parasympathetic (visceral efferent; secretomotor) innervation continues to the minor salivary glands of the soft palate, mucus membrane of the nose, as well as to the lacrimal gland via branches of the trigeminal nerve (greater and lesser palatine branches to the soft palate, pharyngeal branch to the pharynx, posterior superior nasal branches to the nose, auriculotemporal to zygomaticotemporal then to lacrimal nerve to the lacrimal gland).

Tympanic (Horizontal)

At the geniculate ganglion, the nerve turns almost 180 degrees, runs parallel to the axis of the petrous pyramid, and enters the middle ear in the tympanic segment. This

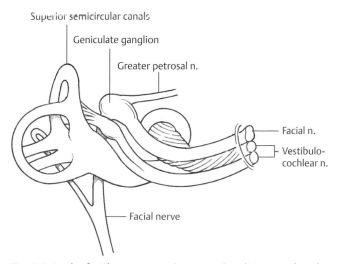

Fig. 1.6 As the facial nerve exits the internal auditory canal at the fundus, it turns gently anteriorly and runs in the otic capsule bone for ~3 to 6 mm between the cochlea and superior semicircular canal.

segment runs ~8 to 11 mm and courses just superior to the oval window where small dehiscences in the bony canal are often noted. In one study of patients undergoing chronic ear surgery, almost 20% of patients were found to have dehiscences in this segment, with 80% identified just above the oval window and 12% anterior to the cochleariform process.[14] There are no branches of the facial nerve in this segment.

Mastoid (Vertical)

As the facial nerve traverses the epitympanum and approaches the inferior face of the horizontal semicircular canal in the mastoid bone, it turns inferiorly in its mastoid segment and runs directly inferiorly to the stylomastoid foramen, a length of 9 to 18 mm. The nerve gives a motor branch to the stapedius muscle, which, when activated, tilts the suprastructure of the stapes bone posteriorly.

The chorda tympani nerve has a variable takeoff from the mastoid segment of the facial nerve and can come off anywhere from the stylomastoid foramen to the pyramid, but usually ~6 mm above the stylomastoid foramen.[10] The chorda tympani nerve courses superiorly, almost along the facial nerve, but angles anteriorly where it enters the mesotympanum through the iter chordae posterius. The chorda tympani passes between incus (below) and malleus (above), and exits the mesotympanum through the iter chorda anterius where it travels in the petrotympanic fissure (canal of Huguier) and exits the skull. It joins the lingual nerve where it conveys taste (special sensory) information from the anterior two-thirds of the tongue and supplies preganglionic parasympathetic (visceral efferent; secretomotor) innervation synapsing in the submandibular ganglion to the submandibular, lingual, and other minor salivary glands.

Within the facial nerve, nerve bundles do lie in some order: branches to the lower portion of the face and mouth lie on the anterior part of the nerve, toward the middle ear, whereas branches to the upper face, including the frontal branch, course posteriorly within the epineurium, toward the mastoid side.[11,15]

Extratemporal

The facial nerve exits the skull at the stylomastoid foramen enveloped in tough connective tissue (skull base fascia). The nerve runs anteriorly and pierces the parotid gland and runs in the gland where it branches into the temporofacial and cervicofacial branches at the pes anserinus to supply motor (somatic efferent) innervation to the muscles of facial expression. Prior to its terminal branches in the parotid gland, the facial nerve, at the stylomastoid foramen, gives off the posterior auricular nerve supplying general sensory innervation to the skin of the posterior ear canal and concha as well as motor innervation to the intrinsic muscles of the auricle and the occipitalis muscle. Patients with large acoustic neuromas can have hypesthesia of the posterior ear canal due to loss of this sensory innervation from tumor compression of the facial nerve/nervus intermedius (Hitselberger sign). The digastric branch supplies motor innervation to the posterior belly of the digastric muscle, and the stylohyoid branch innervates the stylohyoid muscle.

Classically, five terminal branches of the facial nerve supply the muscles of facial expression: temporal, zygomatic, buccal, mandibular, and cervical. In reality, the branching pattern of these terminal slips of nerve can be extremely variable with multiple anastomoses, arcades, and communications (for a scholarly review, see Tzafetta and Terzis[16]). The nerve itself runs deep to the facial fascia (superficial musculoaponeurotic system [SMAS]) and innervates the muscles of facial expression from the deep side. The facial soft-tissue architecture can be described as being arranged in a series of concentric layers: skin, subcutaneous fat, superficial fascia, mimetic muscle, deep facial fascia (SMAS), and the plane containing the facial nerve, parotid duct, and buccal fat pad.[17] The deep facial fascia (SMAS) represents a continuation of the deep cervical fascia cephalad into the face, the importance of which lies in the fact that the facial nerve branches within the cheek lie deep to the SMAS.[17]

■ Microscopic Anatomy

This review of the microscopic anatomy of the facial nerve is taken from an elegant anatomic study by Captier et al.[18] This histological study of the facial nerve throughout its course shows an absence of fascicular arrangement with no perineurium or epineurium from the brainstem to the geniculate ganglion. In this segment, groups of fibers without real organization are surrounded by an arachnoid sheath. Fascicular organization first appears at and just distal to the geniculate ganglion. Here, one or two fascicular bundles are identified, and as the nerve moves more distally, fascicles increase in number and decrease in size. By the mastoid segment of the nerve, the fascicles increase to as many as 16 (mean, 11). At the stylomastoid foramen, as many as 15 fascicular bundles can be counted. The temporofacial branch was larger (with a larger number of myelinated fibers) than the cervicofacial branch but contained fewer fascicles. The total number of myelinated fibers (~7,800) remained relatively stable from brainstem to mastoid segment.

From the horizontal segment distally, the nerve is surrounded by a thin connective tissue sheath (epineurium) throughout the fallopian canal. The epineurial sheath thickens as the nerve emerges from the stylomastoid foramen, most likely to add support and protection. Individual fascicles within the epineurium are also surrounded by a connective tissue sheath—the perineurium—and a connective tissue network resides inside the fascicle—the endoneurium—which surrounds each nerve fiber within the fascicle supporting the arterioles and capillaries supplying the nerve fiber.

Captier et al conclude,

The structural organization of the connective tissue in the facial nerve is extremely variable. From the ponto-cerebellar cistern to the geniculate ganglion, there is an absence of real fascicular organization without connective tissue. After the geniculate ganglion, the fascicular distribution and connective tissue appear, but the spatial organization of the fascicles is extremely heterogeneous. The number of fascicles varies in the different segments of the facial nerve, and the number of fascicles and their organization changes in each segment every 2 mm. The high number of nerve fibers and the spatial variability of the fascicle along the course of the facial nerve observed in this study could explain in part the difficulty of facial nerve repair.[18]

The spatial anatomy of the facial nerve in the temporal bone is, as noted, organized in such a fashion that the middle ear side of the facial nerve maps to the lower face whereas the mastoid side maps to the upper face. Site (or side) of facial nerve compression can therefore be inferred from the involved portions of the face. In the horizontal segment, the upper face has been reported to be lateral (or superficial), whereas motor neurons destined for the lower face and lower lip course in the medial (deep) and posterior fascicles.[15]

■ Function

As noted, the facial nerve contains somatic motor (efferent) innervation to the muscles of facial expression including buccinator and platysma, the posterior belly of the digastric muscle, intrinsic muscles of the auricle, the occipitalis, the stylohyoid, and the stapedius muscles.

Special sensory innervation (i.e., taste to the anterior two-thirds of the tongue, hard and soft palate) is mediated by the chorda tympani nerve, whose cell bodies are located in the geniculate ganglion and whose dendritic processes synapse in the nucleus of the tractus solitarius (**Fig. 1.7**).

The posterior auricular nerve supplies general sensory (somatic afferent) innervation to the skin of the concha, a small area of skin behind the ear, and posterior ear canal.

Visceral motor (efferent) neurons supply preganglionic parasympathetic innervation (secretomotor) to the mucus glands of the nose, hard, and soft palate, and lacrimal gland via the greater superficial petrosal nerve, which synapses in the pterygopalatine ganglion. Postganglionic fibers ride along branches of the trigeminal nerve to their varied destinations. The facial nerve also supplies visceral motor innervation to the submandibular, sublingual, and minor salivary glands via the chorda tympani nerve, whose preganglionic fibers synapse in the submandibular ganglion, and postganglionic fibers ride along the lingual nerve (branch of trigeminal nerve) (see **Fig. 1.7**). Both parasympathetic and sensory (special and general) functions of the facial nerve are mediated by the nervus intermedius.

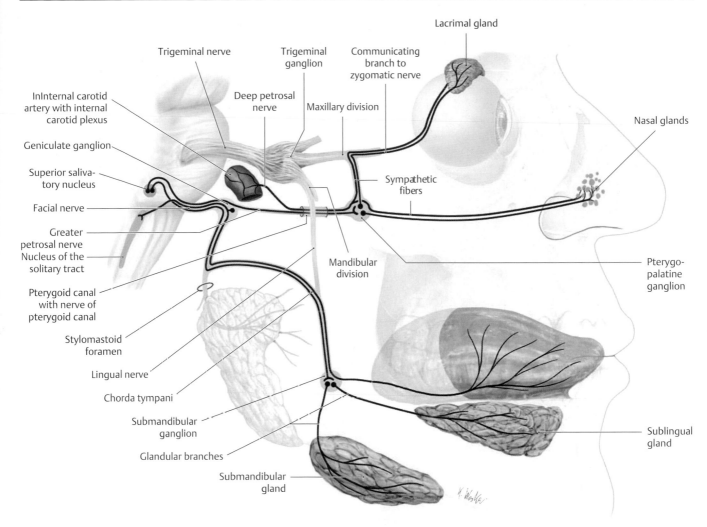

Fig. 1.7 The nervus intermedius supplies taste sensation to the anterior two-thirds of the tongue (chorda tympani nerve) and preganglionic parasympathetic innervation to the submandibular, sublingual, and minor salivary glands (chorda tympani nerve; via synapses in the submandibular ganglion) and preganglionic parasympathetic innervation to the nasal mucus glands and lacrimal glands (greater superficial petrosal nerve; via synapses in the pterygopalatine ganglion). (From Thieme Atlas of Anatomy, Head and Neuroanatomy, © Thieme 2007, Illustration by Karl Wesker.)

■ Vascular Supply

The arterial supply to the facial nerve consists of extensive collateralization and anastomoses from branches emanating from two main trunks: the vertebral system and the external carotid system (for an excellent review, see Anson et al[19]). The proximal (at the brainstem and cerebellopontine angle) facial nerve receives blood supply from branches of the anterior inferior cerebellar artery. In the IAC, the internal auditory (labyrinthine) artery (branch of anterior inferior cerebellar artery) provides vascular input. Through the fallopian canal, the nerve is fed through an arcade between petrosal branches of the middle meningeal artery (branch of the maxillary artery from the external carotid) and the stylomastoid branch of the posterior auricular artery (external carotid). If there is a "weak spot" in the arterial supply of the facial nerve, it would be in the labyrinthine segment proximal to the geniculate ganglion

where the anastomotic network between the external carotid system (petrosal branches of the middle meningieal) and vertebral system (labyrinthine branches) are not as robust.[11]

The extrinsic vascular network consists of one or two main arterial trunks with their venae comitantes that run in the space between the periosteum of the fallopian canal and the epineurial sheath of the nerve. An intrinsic vascular network exists within the epineurial sheath of the nerve and consists of small arterioles, capillaries, and venules variably arranged. Lymph vessels have not been identified in the neural compartment.[20] The extrinsic and intrinsic vascular systems support the facial nerve such that one of the major vessels can be ligated without effect on nerve function.[20] The vessels of the bony canal wall can also be severed as the nerve is lifted out of the fallopian canal in surgery to transpose the facial nerve without untoward effect on nerve function.[20]

◾ Muscles of Facial Expression

The striated facial (mimetic) muscles derive from the second branchial arch mesoderm and are innervated by the facial nerve. These muscles typically reside in the SMAS layer, and originate from the facial bones or deep fascia (periosteum) of the face; they insert into the skin to give the face an essentially unlimited array of expressions. Superiorly, this system of investing fascia and muscle is continuous with the galea aponeurotica, and inferiorly, with the platysma muscle, also innervated by the facial nerve. The facial muscles can be thought of in groups: the muscles of the scalp (occipitofrontalis, temporoparietalis), extrinsic muscles of the ear, muscles of the eyelid, muscles of the nose, and muscles of the mouth.[10]

Rather than presenting a narrative listing all the muscles of facial expression and their actions, they are shown in **Fig. 1.8** and **Table 1.1**.

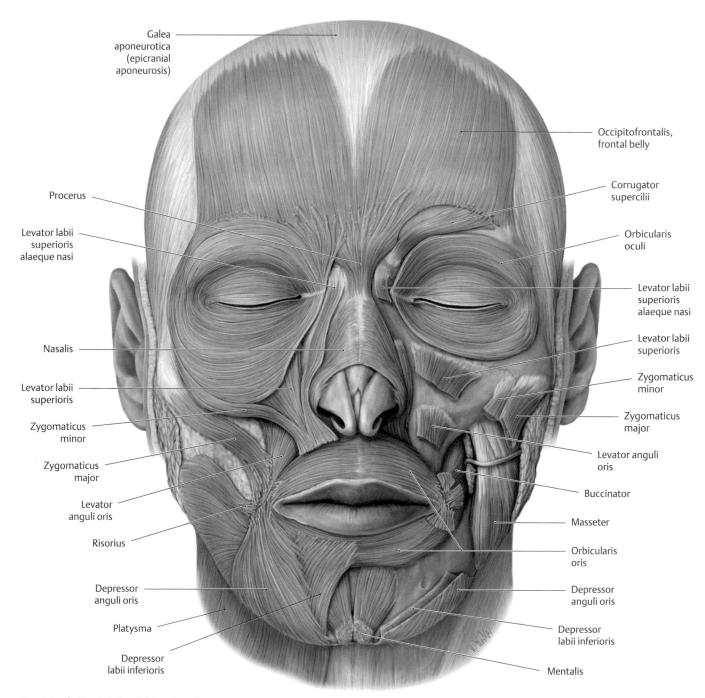

Fig. 1.8a, b Frontal view (**a**) (*continued*)

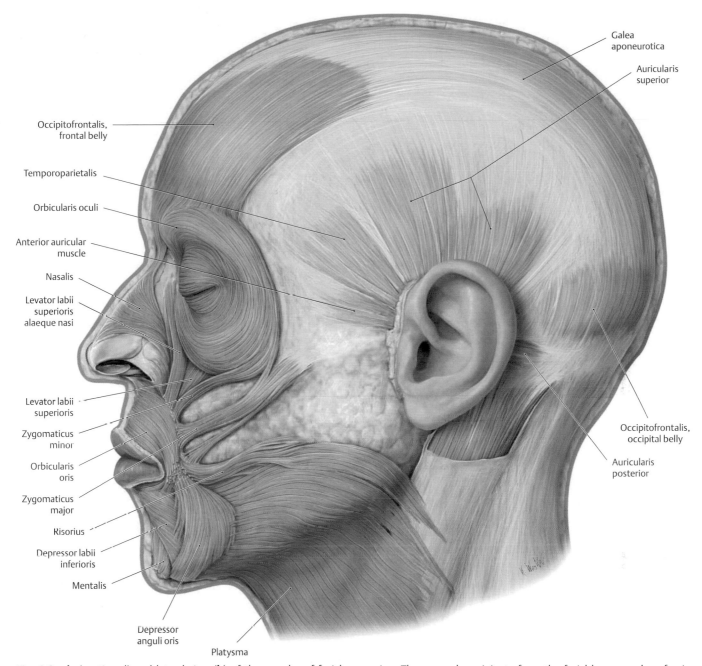

Occipitofrontalis, frontal belly

Temporoparietalis

Orbicularis oculi

Anterior auricular muscle

Nasalis

Levator labii superioris alaeque nasi

Levator labii superioris

Zygomaticus minor

Orbicularis oris

Zygomaticus major

Risorius

Depressor labii inferioris

Mentalis

Depressor anguli oris

Platysma

Galea aponeurotica

Auricularis superior

Occipitofrontalis, occipital belly

Auricularis posterior

Fig. 1.8a, b (*continued*) and lateral view (**b**) of the muscles of facial expression. These muscles originate from the facial bones or deep fascia (periosteum) and insert into the skin. They are invested in fascia to create the superficial musculoaponeurotic system. The facial nerve runs deep to the superficial musculoaponeurotic system layer. (From Thieme Atlas of Anatomy, Head and Neuroanatomy, © Thieme 2007, Illustration by Karl Wesker.)

■ Conclusion

The anatomy and physiology of the facial nerve elegantly depict the complexities of the human nervous system. The varied functions of the facial nerve are reflected in its targeted structures (gland, muscle, skin). Thorough knowledge of the course and actions of the facial nerve is critical for the neurologist, otolaryngologist, and otologist/neurotologist for diagnosis, avoidance of injury, and rehabilitation of injury. Future research will undoubtedly address facial nerve regeneration after injury, infection, or other process, as well as other means to rehabilitate the patient with loss of facial nerve function.

Table 1.1 The muscles of facial expression and their actions

Muscle	Action(s)
Muscles of the scalp	
Occipitofrontalis	Draws back scalp, raises eyebrows, wrinkles forehead (surprise)
Temporoparietalis (distinct from temporalis)	Tightens scalp, draws back skin of the temples, raises the auricles (fright, horror)
Extrinsic muscles of the ear	
Auricularis anterior	Draws the auricle forward and upward
Auricularis superior	Draws the auricle upward
Auricularis posterior	Draws the auricle backward
Muscles of the eyelids	
Levator palpebrae superioris	Raises upper eyelid; antagonist of orbicularis
Orbicularis oculi	Sphincter muscle of the eyelids (palpebral portion closes eye gently; orbital portion closes eye forcefully)
Corrugator supercilii	Draws the eyebrow downward and medial (frown; "muscle of suffering"; vertical forehead wrinkles)
Muscles of the nose	
Procerus	Draws down the medial angle of the eyebrow (anger; transverse wrinkles on the nose)
Nasalis	Transverse part: depresses the cartilaginous part of the nose and draws the ala toward the septum Alar part: enlarges the nasal aperture ("flares" the nostril)
Depressor septi	Draws the ala downward, constricts the aperture
Muscles of the mouth	
Levator labii superioris	Raises the upper lip
Levator labii superioris alaeque nasi	Raises the upper lip, dilates the nostril
Levator anguli oris	Elevates angle of mouth (smile)
Zygomaticus major	Draws angle of mouth upward and backward (laughing)
Zygomaticus minor	Draws the upper lip backward, upward, and outward (sad)
Risorius	Retracts the angle of the mouth (insincere smile)
Depressor labii inferioris	Draws the lower lip downward (depresses) and laterally (irony)
Depressor anguli oris	Depresses the angle of the mouth (frown)
Mentalis	Raises and protrudes lower lip, wrinkles skin of chin (pout)
Transversus menti	Pulls lower lip downward; tightens skin of the chin
Orbicularis oris	Closure of the lips, alters shape of mouth (speech, feeding, drinking)
Buccinator	Compresses/flattens the cheek (holds food under teeth)

References

1. Sataloff RT. Embryology of the facial nerve. In: Embryology and Anomalies of the Facial Nerve and their Surgical Implication. New York: Raven Press; 1991:3–91
2. Gasser R, May M. Embryonic development of the facial nerve. In: May M, ed. The Facial Nerve. New York: Thieme Stratton; 1987
3. Gerhardt HJ, Otto HD. The intratemporal course of the facial nerve and its influence on the development of the ossicular chain. Acta Otolaryngol 1981;91(5–6):567–573
4. Jahrsdoerfer RA, Lambert PR. Facial nerve injury in congenital aural atresia surgery. Am J Otol 1998;19(3):283–287
5. Jahrsdoerfer RA. The facial nerve in congenital middle ear malformations. Laryngoscope 1981;91(8):1217–1225
6. Jahrsdoerfer RA. Transposition of the facial nerve in congenital aural atresia. Am J Otol 1995;16(3):290–294
7. Jahrsdoerfer RA. Congenital absence of the oval window. Trans Sect Otolaryngol Am Acad Ophthalmol Otolaryngol 1977;84(5): ORL904–ORL914
8. Lambert PR. Congenital absence of the oval window. Laryngoscope 1990;100(1):37–40
9. de Alarcon A, Jahrsdoerfer RA, Kesser BW. Congenital absence of the oval window: diagnosis, surgery, and audiometric outcomes. Otol Neurotol 2008;29(1):23–28
10. Gray H. The peripheral nervous system: Cranial nerves. In: Clemente CD, ed. Anatomy of the Human Body. 29th ed. Philadelphia: Lea and Febiger; 1985
11. Miehlke A. The anatomy of the facial nerve. In: Miehlke A, ed. Surgery of the Facial Nerve. second ed. Philadelphia: WB Saunders Company; 1973:7–21
12. Rubinstein D, Sandberg EJ, Cajade-Law AG. Anatomy of the facial and vestibulocochlear nerves in the internal auditory canal. AJNR Am J Neuroradiol 1996;17(6):1099–1105
13. Gantz BJ, Rubinstein JT, Gidley P, Woodworth GG. Surgical management of Bell's palsy. Laryngoscope 1999;109(8):1177–1188
14. Moody MW, Lambert PR. Incidence of dehiscence of the facial nerve in 416 cases of cholesteatoma. Otol Neurotol 2007;28(3):400–404
15. May M. Anatomy of cross section of facial nerve in the tmeporal bone: Clinical application. In: Fisch U, ed. Facial Nerve Surgery. Amstelveen, The Netherlands: Kugley Medical Publications, B.V.; 1977:40–46

16. Tzafetta K, Terzis JK. Essays on the facial nerve: Part I. Microanatomy. Plast Reconstr Surg 2010;125(3):879–889
17. Stuzin JM, Baker TJ, Gordon HL. The relationship of the superficial and deep facial fascias: relevance to rhytidectomy and aging. Plast Reconstr Surg 1992;89(3):441–449, discussion 450–451
18. Captier G, Canovas F, Bonnel F, Seignarbieux F. Organization and microscopic anatomy of the adult human facial nerve: anatomical and histological basis for surgery. Plast Reconstr Surg 2005;115(6):1457–1465
19. Anson BJ, Warpeha RL, Donaldson JA, Rensink MJ. The facial nerve, sheath and blood supply in relation to the surgery of decompression. Ann Otol Rhinol Laryngol 1970;79(4): 710–727
20. Bagger-Sjoback D, Graham MD, Thomander L. The intratemporal vascular supply of the facial nerve: A light and electron microscopic study. In: Graham MD, House WF, eds. Disorders of the Facial Nerve: Anatomy, Diagnosis, and Management. New York: Raven Press; 1982:17–31

2 Physiology of the Facial Nerve

Felipe Santos and William H. Slattery III

The facial nerve is the motor nerve of the face, scalp, auricle, and neck via the platysma. Mastication and swallowing are in part driven by facial nerve innervation of the posterior belly of the digastric and the stylohyoid muscles. The facial nerve is also the sensory supply to the external auditory canal and the taste buds of the anterior two-thirds of the tongue, and it provides parasympathetic contributions to the submandibular, sublingual, and intralingual salivary glands. Involuntary mimetic function and involuntary motor reflexes are also mediated by the facial nerve; these include the corneal reflex, blink reflex, stapedial reflex, and the oculomentalis reflex. The latter is a contraction of obicularis oculi and mentalis in relation to loud sound or sudden bright light.

■ Structural Units

Normal motor function of the muscles of facial expression, which is the focus of this discussion, relies on the integrity of the facial nerve. The nucleus of the facial nerve resides in the pons. Seven thousand neuron cell bodies send axons from the pons to the muscles of facial expression. A single neuron can innervate up to 25 muscle fibers.

Each neuron has an axon coated in myelin produced by Schwann cells. Transmission along neurons is by saltatory conduction: depolarization goes from node of Ranvier to node of Ranvier, which are gaps in myelin (**Fig. 2.1a, b**). In the normal physiological state, this saltatory transduction increases the firing rate of the nerve.

Each nerve fiber is surrounded by connective tissue, the endoneurium. The endoneurium is closely adherent to the Schwann cells. Highlighting the structural relevance to normal physiological function, Schwann cells serve as a conduit for regenerating nerve fibers following injury. The perineurium is a sheath of concentric layers of polygonal cells surrounding groups of endoneurium-covered neurons. The perineurium provides tensile strength and intrafunicular pressure. At the outermost layer, the epineurium, loose areolar tissue, holds and separates nerve fasicles. The epineurium contains the vasa nervorum and lymphatic vessels, which provide nutrition to the nerve fibers.

Axons

Axons are the basic structural unit, and axon function relies on:

(1) An ion concentration–mediated negative resting potential. Activation of the cell membrane reverses this potential, generating the action potential. The propagation of the action potential by reversal of the ion gradient is referred to as depolarization.

(2) Each neuron is segmentally insulated by myelin. Where myelin is absent, transmission occurs by a saltatory conduction to the node of Ranvier, propagated along the unmyelinated axon where there is increased cell membrane permeability. Myelination of the nerve allows depolarization to jump from one node of Ranvier to the next, thereby increasing the speed of conduction.

(3) A sufficient stimulus is needed to generate an action potential. Following the action potential, there are refractory and absolute refractory periods during which only large or no stimuli can elicit an action potential.

The action potential is transmitted to the muscle. Each nerve fiber invaginates into the muscle fiber with terminating branches known as sole feet. The space between the sole feet and the muscle fiber membrane is known as the synaptic cleft. Transmission through the synaptic cleft is mediated by acetylcholine. The acetylcholine increases the permeability to sodium ions, changing the resting potential leading to the generation of the action potential.[1]

■ Injuries of the Facial Nerve

Anatomic injury of the facial nerve negatively affects normal function. In general, the purview of the clinician treating facial nerve disorders centers on pathology that negatively affect the structural integrity of the nerve and therefore its normal physiological function. Sunderland has described patterns of facial nerve injury based on histological findings (**Fig. 2.2a–f**).[2] First-degree nerve injury is a neuropraxia: an intraneural compression that prevents conduction of the impulse. First-degree injuries present with sensory-motor problems distal to the site of injury. The endoneurium, perineurium, and epineurium are all intact, and there is no wallerian degeneration. Conduction is intact in the proximal and distal segment of the nerve, but no conduction occurs across the area of injury. If only some fibers are involved, the nerve is still intact and able to transmit signals, but its ability to function normally is reduced. This is typically seen with partial facial nerve paralysis. This type of injury usually does not require surgical intervention, and the nerve will return to normal function

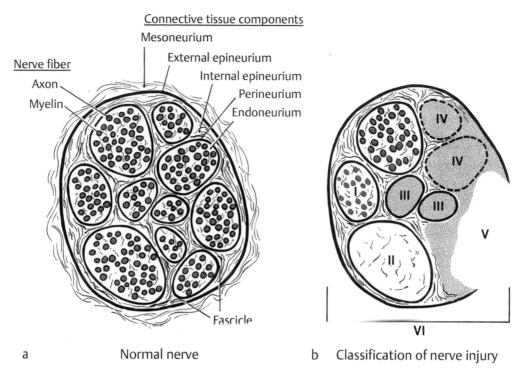

Connective tissue components

Mesoneurium
External epineurium
Internal epineurium
Perineurium
Endoneurium

Nerve fiber
Axon
Myelin

Fascicle

a   Normal nerve   b   Classification of nerve injury

Fig. 2.1a, b (a) Diagrammatic representation of the cross-section of a normal peripheral nerve demonstrating the connective tissue and nerve tissue components. (b) The cross-section of the peripheral nerve demonstrates a mixed, or sixth-degree, injury pattern. This fascicle (bundle of nerve fibers) at 11 o'clock is normal. Moving counterclockwise, the adjacent fascicle demonstrates a first-degree injury (neurapraxia) with segmental demyelination (loss of the myelin that covers many nerve fibers). The next fascicle demonstrates a second-degree injury (axonotmesis). This injury involves both the axon and the myelin. The endoneurial tissue (delicate connective tissue network that holds together the individual fibers of a nerve trunk) is not damaged. The central two fascicles demonstrate a third-degree injury, with injury to the axon, myelin, and endoneurium. The perineurium (sheath of connective tissue that surrounds a bundle of nerve fibers) is intact and normal. The fascicles at 12 and 1 o'clock demonstrate a fourth-degree injury with marked scarring across the nerve, with only the epineurium being intact. In a fifth-degree injury pattern, the nerve is not in continuity but is transected. The surgeon will separate the fourth- and fifth-degree injury patterns, which will require reconstruction from the normal fascicles and the fascicles demonstrating first-, second-, and third-degree injury patterns. These latter patterns of injury require, at most, neurolysis (destruction of nervous tissue). (Used with permission from Mackinnon SE, Dellon AL. Surgery of the Peripheral Nerve. New York, NY: Thieme; 1988: 36.)

within hours to weeks. It is the mildest type of peripheral nerve injury.

Second-degree injury is a compression that results in loss of axons also known as axonotmesis. The axon degenerates distal to the point of injury in a process known as wallerian degeneration. In second-degree injury, the surrounding Schwann cells maintain their integrity. The expectation is complete recovery without synkinesis as the endoneural tubes, and Schwann cells are presumed intact and help guide regenerating nerve fibers. Electromyography demonstrates fibrillation potentials and positive sharp waves (2 to 3 weeks postinjury). Axonal regeneration occurs, and recovery usually returns to normal without surgical intervention. Occasionally, scar tissue may form and is thought to be responsible for incomplete recovery.

Third-degree injury is a neurotmesis. Endoneural tubules are disrupted secondary to neural compression. As the endoneurium can no longer guide axons, regeneration is incomplete. Axon regeneration will be appropriate and inappropriate. Axons that regenerate and make contact

with fibers other than their original endpoint result in synkinetic patterns of facial movement.

First-, second-, and third-degree injuries are mediated by compression. Fourth-degree injury is a disruption of the perineurium, and fifth-degree injury is complete disruption of the nerve. Without intervention, recovery is not expected with fourth- and fifth-degree injury patterns.

Effects of Injury and Mechanisms of Repair

The repair of facial nerve injuries is mediated by a complex array of molecular changes, many that at present are only understood at the gross cellular level. Immune function, a patient's nutritional status, and the degree of neural disruption all affect the ultimate outcome of recovery. It follows that appropriate return of function will be more variable with a greater degree of injury.

Following injury, there is an increase in cell body volume. This physiologically coincides with chromatolysis, loss of Nissl staining ribosomes and rough endoplasmic

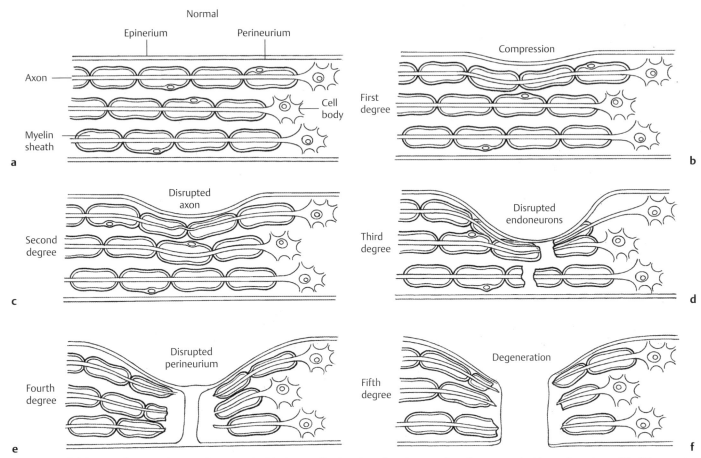

Fig. 2.2a–f (**a**) Normal nerve: the axon is covered with the myelin sheath and each nerve bundle surrounded by perineurium. All of the nerve bundles are covered by the epineurium. (**b**) First-degree injury is neuropraxia: the endoneurium, perineurium, and epineurium are all intact, and there is no wallerian degeneration. (**c**) Second-degree injury also known as axonotmesis: this results when more significant compression causes loss of axons. (**d**) Third-degree injury is a neurotmesis with disruption of endoneural tubules. Regeneration is incomplete, and axon regeneration may be inappropriate resulting in synkinesis. (**e**) Fourth-degree injury is a disruption of the perineurium. (**f**) Fifth-degree injury is complete disruption of the nerve.

reticulum, and increases in ribonucleic acid, enzyme production, and distribution.[3,4] There is an increase in calcitonin-related peptide expression, GAP43, and cytoskeletal proteins such as actin and tubulin.[5] Proximally, the severed axon begins forming a growth cone.[1,3] At 3 days post injury, sprouting begins at the growth cone. Growth occurs at ~1 mm/day; the facial nerve should therefore be able to grow from the cerebellopontine angle to the periphery within 6 months.[6] This activity is usually complete within 3.5 to 4 months.

Favorable and unfavorable factors coincide with this regeneration: axons shrink, allowing new ones to grow around, and microglial cells proliferate, which can interfere with normal synaptic transmission. Sprouting axons maintain a responsiveness to trophic factors. Several neurotrophic factors are known to play a role in regeneration; for a more extensive review, the reader is referred to Tuszynski.[7]

Regenerating axons travel through Bunger bands formed by Schwann cells that have lined the degenerating axons during wallerian degeneration; the Bunger bands serve as

an endoneural tube. The basement membrane of the endoneurium helps to guide regeneration. Regenerating fibers have no known specificity during regeneration; however, the Schwann cell will ultimately myelinate them.[8]

Endoneural tubules are replaced by connective tissue within 3 to 4 months so that the axons that have not found a target will degenerate and axons that are too far apart to form contact may form a neuroma. Nerve repair is therefore advocated as early as the injury occurs. Distal to the site of injury, nerve resorption with Schwann cell proliferation begins quickly and is very advanced by 48 hours. This process is termed axolysis and myelinolysis, and occurs distal to the site of injury.

Denervation at the muscle results in loss of muscle weight with a decrease in muscle fiber diameter. Early changes in the muscle occur at the cellular level within a week of denervation. These cellular changes include increased mitochondria number, deoxyribonucleic acid, satellite cells, and chromatin change. This represents the plastic state of denervated muscle. Over time, fibers disappear and are replaced by fat and connective tissue. The speed of contraction decreases, and spontaneous action potential known as fibrillations can be recorded. The number of motor end plates increase, and inhibitor substances decrease.[9]

Facial muscles can be reinnervated by contralateral axons after injury, especially muscles close to midline structures. Prior to reinnervation, muscle viability is tested by volitional movement which if absent is tested by electromyography. If electromyography shows no response, a muscle biopsy can be performed.

The time at which muscle is no longer available to accept reinnervation is not well established. The literature includes case reports of reinnervation occurring after several years, but a "sooner the better" philosophy is advocated by the time course of the described degenerative and regenerative changes observed.

■ Measuring Physiological Injury and Repair

Electrophysiological testing of the facial nerve in clinical practice is measured by assessing the muscle response. Muscle response can be elicited with voluntary contraction or it can be evoked with electrical signal. Electrophysiological testing provides both quantitative and qualitative measures of physiological degeneration and recovery following facial nerve injury. These tests can be used to predict the degree of injury, the likelihood of recovery, and assist the surgeon in clinical decision making. A detailed discussion on the most commonly used tests is presented in Chapter 4. These tests include the following.

Maximal Stimulation Test

A maximal stimulation test uses electrical stimulation to compare muscle response between sides. Increasing current is used to rate facial movement in the (1) forehead and eyebrow; (2) periorbital area; (3) cheek, upper lip, and nasal ala; (4) lower lip; and (5) cervical and platysma area. Testing is initiated 3 days after injury to account for wallerian degeneration.

Electronystagmography

Electronystagmography or evoked electromyography is an electrically evoked electromyelogram. Electric current is applied to the facial nerve, and the latency and amplitude of the muscle response is recorded and compared with the contralateral normal side.

Electromyography

Electromyography measures voluntary muscle response. The motor unit response morphology provides further information. In addition to the amplitude and latency of the muscle responses, denervation patterns such as positive sharp waves or fibrillation can be recorded. Reinnervation can be documented with polyphasic potentials.

Approximate correlations of degree of injury, using the Sunderland classification, to evoked electromyographic response as a percentage of normal have been described[10]:

First degree: 100% response on evoked electromyography
Second degree: 25% response on evoked electromyography
Third degree: zero to 10% response on evoked electromyography

■ Physiology of Nerve Repair

Although mixed patterns of injury occur, the clinical examination in conjunction with electrophysiological testing helps to determine the overall expected degree of injury. The clinician can correlate this to known cellular responses to injury and expected recovery in the medical and surgical decision-making process.

Nerve injuries that are grades I, II, and III are not amenable to nerve repair or graft. Treatment is aimed at minimizing compression and intraneural pressure. Steroids and surgical decompression are routinely used, with the latter most often reserved for grade III injuries. Nimodipine, a calcium channel blocker, has been shown to accelerate facial nerve recovery in animal models.[11] Continued translational studies will likely increase the number of pharmacological agents available to promote recovery.

Grade IV and V injuries result in partial or complete transection. Treatment is aimed at promoting neurotropism, the factors in nerve regeneration that influence the direction of regeneration, in addition to neurotrophic factors. Surgical repair with direct anastomosis or autologous neural interposition is the gold standard. Neural conduits with neurotrophic factors have been employed and continue to be investigated with the goal of establishing a milieu similar to that seen in injury patterns where the endoneurium is preserved and facial motor outcomes are superior.

■ Synkinesis

Following injury, involuntary facial muscle contraction can occur with voluntary contraction of another facial muscle group. This process is known as synkinesis. The physiology of synkinesis is not completely understood. Aberrant axonal regeneration, nuclear hyperexcitability, and ephaptic transmission have been proposed as mechanisms of synkinesis formation. The nerve does not maintain a topographic distribution from the facial nucleus to the peripheral muscle. Therefore, disruption of individual fibers can result in regeneration patterns where axons innervate the incorrect peripheral muscle group. Recent experimental evidence has shown that this process may occur beyond the site of lesion. In the case of nuclear hyperexcitability, during recovery postsynaptic cells may become more receptive to neurotransmitters from other peripheral muscle axons or with incomplete myelination allow for aberrant contact–mediated cross talk as seen in ephaptic transmission.[12–14]

References

1. Kellman RM. Facial nerve manual. Chapter 3. Physiology and pathophysiology. Am J Otol 1989;10(1):62–67
2. Sunderland S. Nerve and Nerve Injuries, 2nd ed. London, Churchill Livingstone; 1978
3. Nissl F. Uber die Veranderugen am Facialskern des Kaninchen nach Ausreissung der Nerven. Allg Z Psychiatr 1892;48:197–198
4. Kreutzberg GW. Degeneration and regeneration. In: Miehlk A, ed. Surgery of the Facial Nerve. Philadelphia: W.B. Saunders; 1973: 22–35
5. Choi D, Dunn LT. Facial nerve repair and regeneration: an overview of basic principles for neurosurgeons. Acta Neurochir (Wien) 2001;143(2):107–114
6. Schaumburg HH, Berger AR, Thomas PK. Disorders of Peripheral Nerves. Philadelphia: FA Davis; 1992
7. Tuszynski MH. Neurotrophic factors. In: Tuszynski MH, Kordower J, eds. CNS Regeneration. San Diego: Academic Press; 1999: 109–158
8. Fu SY, Gordon T. The cellular and molecular basis of peripheral nerve regeneration. Mol Neurobiol 1997;14(1-2):67–116
9. Diamond J, Cooper E, Turner C, Macintyre L. Trophic regulation of nerve sprouting. Science 1976;193(4251):371–377
10. May M. The Facial Nerve, 2nd ed. New York: Thieme; 2000
11. Lindsay RW, Heaton JT, Edwards C, Smitson C, Hadlock TA. Nimodipine and acceleration of functional recovery of the facial nerve after crush injury. Arch Facial Plast Surg 2010;12(1):49–52
12. Moran CJ, Neely JG. Patterns of facial nerve synkinesis. Laryngoscope 1996;106(12 Pt 1):1491–1496
13. Sadjadpour K. Postfacial palsy phenomena: faulty nerve regeneration or ephaptic transmission? Brain Res 1975;95(2-3): 403–406
14. Choi D, Raisman G. After facial nerve damage, regenerating axons become aberrant throughout the length of the nerve and not only at the site of the lesion: an experimental study. Br J Neurosurg 2004;18(1):45–48

3 Histopathology of Facial Nerve Disorders

Jose N. Fayad and Fred H. Linthicum Jr.

The normal histology of the facial nerve needs defining before discussing the histopathology. The facial nerve is composed of ~10,000 neurons, 7,000 of which are myelinated and innervate the nerves of facial expression. Three thousand of the nerve fibers are somatosensory and secretomotor and make up the nervus intermedius. The nerve fibers, containing microfilaments and microtubules, are surrounded by a multilayered myelin sheath. The fibers are in turn surrounded by endoneurium that encompasses each fiber but also surrounds groups of fibers to form fascicles. In the temporal bone, a tough perineurium surrounds the entire nerve and is cushioned from surrounding tissues and structures by the epineurium (**Fig. 3.1a, b**).

Sitting atop the nerve at the external genu where the nerve makes a sharp turn posteriorly, at the junction of the meatal and tympanic segments, is the geniculate ganglion that carries autonomic fibers from the greater superficial petrosal nerve.

The chorda tympani nerve, which carries taste and glandular secretory fibers, is an integral part of the facial nerve extending from the geniculate ganglion area to the descending mastoid segment, where it leaves the facial nerve to cross the middle ear. The fibers are not recognizable within the nerve unless it has been divided proximal to the geniculate ganglion. In this case, they can be seen as a discrete bundle of fibers near their exit from the tympanic segment (**Fig. 3.2**).

A congenital dehiscence of the tympanic segment of the fallopian canal containing the nerve may occur in 30% of ears, per Shea as quoted by Kaplan (**Fig. 3.3**).[1] The dehiscence may be large enough to allow a prolapse of the nerve so that it appears to be a middle ear tumor.

■ Histopathology

A variety of exogenous circumstances can affect the facial nerve. These can generally be classified as idiopathic, inflammatory, and neoplastic. We describe the various pathologies in each of these categories and provide histopathological examples.

Idiopathic

Bell palsy or idiopathic facial paralysis is a unilateral, sometimes recurrent facial nerve paralysis that usually spontaneously recovers. In a few cases, it may become permanent or result in partial impairment or synkinesis. Although referred to as "idiopathic," there is some suggestion that the etiology may be viral. Inflammatory cells have been seen early in the course of the paralysis, and there

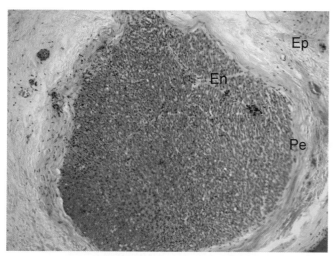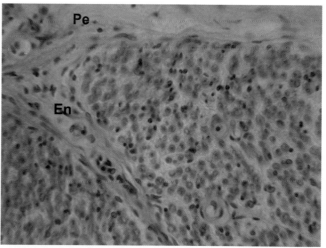

Fig. 3.1a, b (**a**) Normal facial nerve showing endoneurium (*En*) surrounding each fiber and dividing fibers into groups, perineurium (*Pe*) enveloping and containing the nerve, and epineurium (*Ep*) cushioning the nerve from surrounding tissue. Hematoxylin and eosin ×100. (**b**) Higher power (400×) of facial nerve.

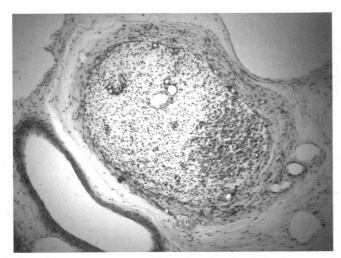

Fig. 3.2 Degenerated nerve, except for a bundle of chorda tympani fibers, following the translabyrinthine removal of a vestibular nerve schwannoma (hematoxylin and eosin ×100).

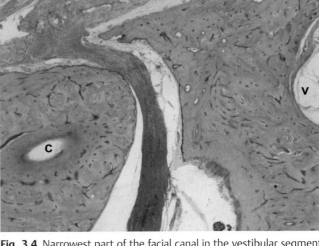

Fig. 3.4 Narrowest part of the facial canal in the vestibular segment between the cochlea (*c*) and the vestibule (*v*). The nerve is artifactually shrunken due to the dehydration process of the temporal bone preparation (hematoxylin and eosin ×20).

is clinical evidence that the paralysis is due to a herpes simplex infection.[2] When the nerve is surgically decompressed at the time of paralysis, there is often evidence of an inflammatory swelling of the nerve. The narrowest area of the facial nerve canal is the labyrinthine segment, and this is believed by many to be the primary site of nerve compression by inflammatory edema (**Fig. 3.4**).

No residual histologic abnormalities are found in the nerves of patients who have been left without residual paralysis. However, in those cases with incomplete recovery, there are varying amounts of residual degenerative changes manifested by areas of the nerve that stain poorly with hematoxylin and eosin, and may exhibit some edema and residual round cell accumulations (**Fig. 3.5**).

Inflammation

Viral

Herpes zoster refers to a reactivation of the latent chicken pox virus. When the process affects the temporal bone, it causes facial nerve paralysis as well as inner ear disturbances (Ramsay Hunt syndrome). The acute phase is manifested by an infiltration of the geniculate ganglion, atop the facial nerve, by lymphocytes and plasma cells.[3] Recovery of the nerve and function is variable. The number of adjacent fibers that are poorly stained depends on the degree of residual function. **Fig. 3.6a, b** shows the partially degenerated nerve of an 83-year-old woman who suffered

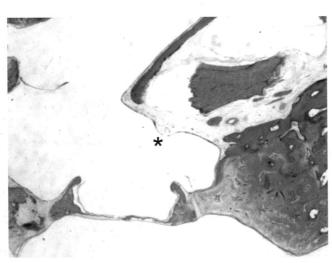

Fig. 3.3 Congenital dehiscence (*asterisk*) of the fallopian canal above the oval window (hematoxylin and eosin ×20).

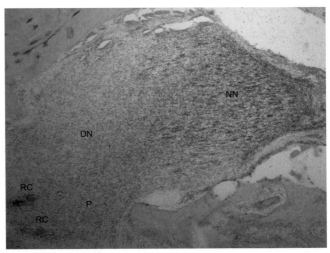

Fig. 3.5 Degenerating facial nerve several weeks after decompression for Bell palsy. DN, degenerating nerve; NN, normal nerve; P, prolapse of nerve through fallopian canal dehiscence; RC, round cells (hematoxylin and eosin ×40).

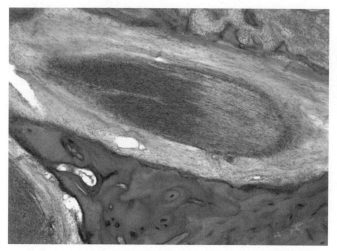
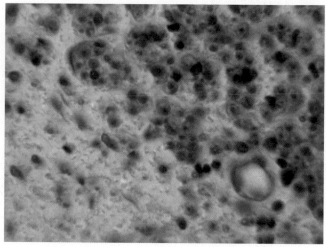

a   b

Fig. 3.6a, b (**a**) Partially degenerated tympanic segment of the facial nerve 7 years after an episode of Ramsey Hunt syndrome (hematoxylin and eosin ×40). (**b**) High-power (100×) image of descending segment of facial nerve with segmental degeneration of a portion of the nerve (*lower left side*).

a total facial paralysis, concha rash, vertigo, and hearing loss 7 years prior to death. Recovery of facial function was to House-Brackmann facial nerve grade II. The vertigo subsided, but a 35 dB hearing deficit remained.

Bacterial

Necrotizing otitis externa (malignant otitis externa) may present as a facial paralysis in what appears to be a mild external otitis usually found in an elderly patient with diabetes. An insidious spread of the pseudomonas organism throughout the temporal bone can first become manifest as a facial paralysis. The suppurative process consisting of dense accumulations of polymorphological leukocytes, macrophages, lymphocytes, and plasma cells destroys the fallopian canal wall and invades and lyses the nerve (**Fig. 3.7**).

Tuberculosis may affect the facial nerve in cases of active or arrested pulmonary disease. Tuberculous microgummas, consisting of a caseous central area surrounded by round cells and multinucleated giant cells, form within the nerve and destroy it (**Fig. 3.8**). Although now relatively unusual in the United States of America, it is still common in developing countries (and in patients with acquired immunodeficiency syndrome in the United States and other developed countries).

Neoplasms

Schwannoma

Facial nerve schwannomas (neuromas) can vary from occult to multilocular. They can occur anywhere in the

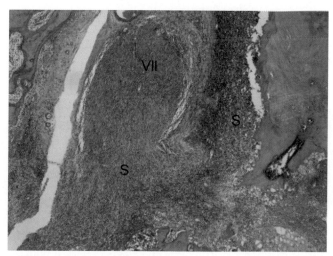

Fig. 3.7 Facial nerve being destroyed by suppuration in the mastoid segment by the spread of suppuration from necrotizing otitis externa. VII, facial nerve; S, suppuration (hematoxylin and eosin ×40).

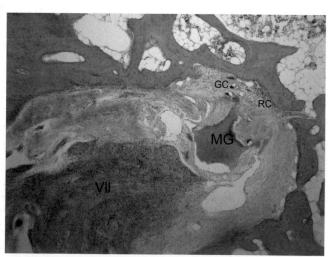

Fig. 3.8 Tuberculous microgumma (*MG*) destroying the tympanic segment of the facial nerve (*VII*) just posterior to the genu. GC, giant cells; RC, round cells (hematoxylin and eosin ×40).

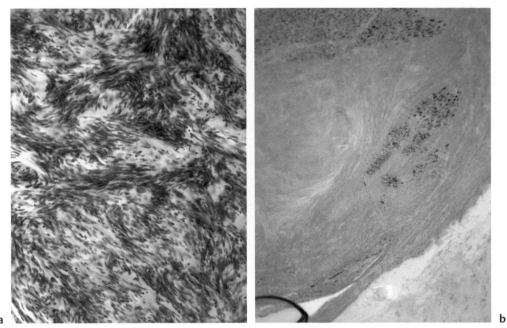

Fig. 3.9a, b (a) Facial nerve schwannoma (hematoxylin and eosin × 200). (b) Nerve fiber bundles within tumor (neurofilament antibody with fast red ×200).

course of the nerve and are common in the area of the geniculate ganglion. Microscopically, they are composed of cells with elongated nuclei arranged in whorls or arbitrarily (**Fig. 3.9a**). They differ from vestibular nerve schwannomas in that they contain nerve fibers within the substance of the tumor, similar to neurofibromatosis type 2 tumors (**Fig. 3.9b**).[4] The location of nerve fibers within the tumor is variable so that removal of even small tumors or biopsy can result in impaired facial function.

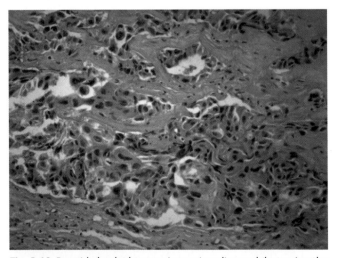

Fig. 3.10 Parotid gland adenocarcinoma invading and destroying the facial nerve (hematoxylin and eosin × 200).

Adenocarcinoma

Adenocarcinomas of the parotid gland have a propensity to travel in nerve sheaths and can travel up into the fallopian canal. **Fig. 3.10** shows the facial nerve from a patient who underwent decompression for what was thought to be Bell palsy. The nerve is largely replaced by adenocarcinoma consisting of groups of poorly differentiated cells with large nuclei. It was subsequently learned that the patient had had a parotid tumor removed years previous to the nerve decompression.

Facial Nerve Hemangioma

Facial nerve hemangiomas frequently occur at the geniculate ganglion and lead to paralysis unless surgically removed.[5] The tumors consist of blood-filled spaces surrounded by fibrous tissue and frequently harbor spicules of new bone (**Fig. 3.11**).

Other Neoplasms

Other neoplasms that may affect the facial nerve, usually by extension from a lesion in the temporal bone, are glomus jugulare or tympanicum, squamous cell carcinoma, leiomyosarcoma, malignant terratoma, and melanoma (**Fig. 3.12a–e**).

Glomus tumors (nonchromaffin, paraganglioma, chemodactoma) arise from epithelioid-like cells found on the surface of the jugular bulb or on Jacobson nerve on the middle ear promontory. Characteristically, they are

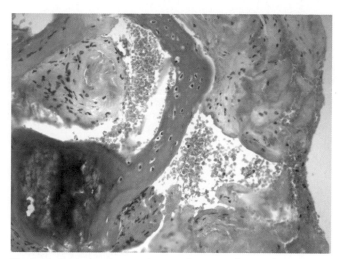

Fig. 3.11 Geniculate hemangioma with neo ossification (hematoxylin and eosin × 200).

Leiomyosarcoma are neoplasms of smooth muscle and, therefore, can be primary anywhere that smooth muscle, including blood vessel walls, is found. **Fig. 3.12c** shows tissue from a female patient who presented with a facial paralysis and was found to have a conductive hearing loss. The middle ear and mastoid were filled with tumor that had destroyed the facial canal and invaded the nerve.

Malignant teratomas are tumors consisting of one or more of the three embryological germ layers that appear on areas that normally do not harbor this type of cell. They may be cystic or solid, such as the case shown in **Fig. 3.12d**.

Melanoma may metastasize to anywhere in the temporal bone, such as the facial nerve in the case shown in **Fig. 3.12e**. The cells are pleomorphic and may or may not be pigmented.

composed of small groups of cells surrounded by a loose stroma. They may compromise facial function by pressure on the nerve or by invasion and destruction of the nerve, as seen in **Fig. 3.12a**.

Squamous cell carcinoma may arise in the external auditory canal or in the epithelium lining radical or modified radical mastoidectomies. They readily spread by direct extension and destroy any structure they encounter (**Fig. 3.12b**).

Trauma

Traumatic damage to the facial nerve may be due to fractures or surgery and can occur anywhere in its course from the internal auditory canal to the parotid. Histologically, there is a loss of normal architecture. The degenerated nerve shown in **Fig. 3.2** is from a patient who underwent a translabyrinthine removal of a vestibular nerve schwannoma. Because the interruption of the nerve was medial to the geniculate ganglion, the afferent fibers from the chorda tympani nerve are

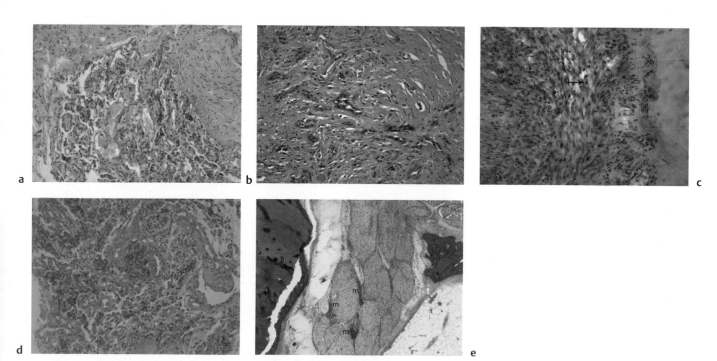

Fig. 3.12a–e Collage showing neoplasms that may affect the facial nerve. (**a**) Glomus tumor (hematoxylin and eosin [H&E] ×200). (**b**) Squamous cell carcinoma (H&E ×200). (**c**) Lyomyosarcoma (arrow) (H&E ×200). (**d**) Malignant terratoma (H&E ×200). (**e**) Melanoma (m) (H&E ×40).

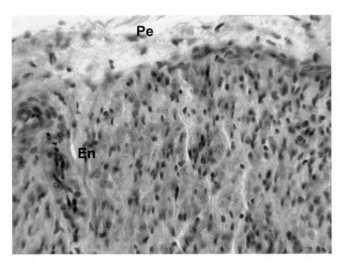

Fig. 3.13 Higher power of a degenerated nerve 5 years after sectioning. Note total loss of nerve fiber morphology as normally seen (see also Fig. 3.1b). En, endoneurium; Pe, perineurium (hematoxylin and eosin ×400).

still viable and appear as a bundle of fibers within the degenerated nerve. **Fig. 3.13** is a high-power (400×) picture of a segmentally degenerated nerve 5 years after transection during removal of a vestibular nerve schwannoma.

References

1. Kaplan J. Congenital dehiscence of the fallopian canal in middle ear surgery. Arch Otolaryngol 1960;72:197–200
2. Adour KK, Byl FM, Hilsinger RL Jr, Kahn ZM, Sheldon MI. The true nature of Bell's palsy: analysis of 1,000 consecutive patients. Laryngoscope 1978;88(5):787–801
3. Devriese PP. Facial paralysis in cephalic herpes zoster. Ann Otol Rhinol Laryngol 1968;77(6):1101–1119
4. Linthicum FH Jr. Unusual audiometric and histologic findings in bilateral acoustic neurinomas. Ann Otol Rhinol Laryngol 1972;81(3):433–437
5. Semaan MT, Slattery WH, Brackmann DE. Geniculate ganglion hemangiomas: clinical results and long-term follow-up. Otol Neurotol 2010;31(4):665–670

4 Facial Nerve Paralysis Examination

Babak Azizzadeh, Jonathan S. Kulbersh, and Brendan P. O'Connell

The facial nerve provides motor, sensory, and parasympathetic innervation to the head and neck. The functional and aesthetic consequences of facial nerve paralysis can potentially be physically and psychologically devastating. Facial palsy is almost invariably accompanied by severe emotional distress. A complete history and thorough examination should be the primary focus of the treating physician. The goal of this chapter is to simplify the clinical evaluation of patients with facial nerve pathology. There are distinct aspects of the history, evaluation, and treatment strategy that differ between patients with acute and chronic paralysis. We separate patients with chronic facial paralysis into the following four categories: facial paresis without synkinesis, facial paresis with mild synkinesis, facial paresis with moderate to severe synkinesis, and complete, flaccid facial paralysis.

■ History

The history for patients presenting with facial palsy serves to narrow the differential diagnosis (**Table 4.1**). In the evaluation of an acute event, the onset and grade of the facial palsy are key determining factors for the etiology, prognosis, and additional laboratory and diagnostic testing. The priority during the evaluation of new onset facial paralysis without a clear cause (e.g., acoustic neuroma surgery, parotidectomy, trauma, etc.) centers on identifying the etiology of the paralysis and preventing ocular complications. All patients presenting with facial nerve paralysis should have the following documented:

(1) Duration of paralysis
(2) Onset: immediate versus progressive
(3) Inciting factors: pregnancy, stress, etc.
(4) History of previous facial nerve paralysis
(5) Family history of facial nerve paralysis
(6) Systemic medical conditions (autoimmune diseases, diabetes)
(7) Skin changes or rashes around ear, face, neck, chest, or back
(8) Prodromal symptoms such as nasal congestion, sore throat, fever, or arthralgias
(9) History of perioral herpes simplex virus infection
(10) Travel history
(11) Otologic symptoms including ear drainage, hearing loss, vertigo, otalgia, or aural fullness

Table 4.1 Common etiologies of facial nerve paralysis

Congenital	Neoplastic	Traumatic	Infectious	Neurologic	Idiopathic	Systemic	Metabolic
Mobius syndrome	Temporal bone tumor	Birth trauma	Lyme disease	Guillain-Barré	Bell palsy	Sarcoidosis	Diabetes mellitus
Congenital unilateral lower lip paralysis	Meningioma	Temporal bone fracture	Herpes simplex virus	Myotonic dystrophy	Recurrent facial palsy		Osteopetrosis
Hemifacial microsomia	Facial neuroma	Facial laceration	Varicella zoster virus	Stroke			
Melkersson-Rosenthal syndrome	Acoustic neuroma	Penetrating trauma	Cytomegalovirus	Multiple sclerosis			
Goldenhar syndrome	Parotid tumor Cholesteatoma Metastatic disease	Iatrogenic	Hepatitis B Hepatitis C Epstein-Barr virus Mumps Rubella Tuberculosis Acute/chronic otitis media Mastoiditis Human immunodeficiency virus Syphilis Petrositis				

(12) Recent tick bite or camping

(13) Full oncologic history including cutaneous neoplasms of the face

(14) Recent trauma

(15) Past surgeries including surgeries to the ear and central nervous system

(16) Neurological symptoms including cranial neuropathies, weakness, or tingling

In patients with long-standing facial nerve paralysis, it is equally important to obtain the history of initial paralysis as detailed previously. In addition, the functional and aesthetic concerns associated with chronic facial nerve paralysis need to be addressed. As aesthetic concerns are common in this population, it is important to document such information in the patient's own words. The possible sequelae of chronic facial nerve paralysis include:

(1) Nasal airway obstruction

(2) Oral incompetence

(3) Aberrant facial nerve regeneration leading to involuntary or uncoordinated facial movements (synkinesis)

(4) Buccal mucosa irritation

(5) Visual changes, ocular irritation, lagopthalmous, dry eye syndrome, epiphora, corneal ulceration, or blindness

(6) Facial asymmetry due to flaccid atrophic muscles, loss of tone, synkinesis, or volumetric loss

(7) Loss of dynamic furrows

(8) Brow ptosis and asymmetry

(9) Effacement or deepening of the nasolabial folds

(10) Drooping or elevation of the oral commissure

(11) Dimpling of the chin (peau d'orange)

It is imperative that an underlying neoplasm is ruled out in all patients with facial nerve pathology, both acute and chronic. The clinical features that raise our suspicion for a neoplastic entity include:

(1) Slowly progressive facial paralysis

(2) Additional cranial neuropathies

(3) History or presence of suspicious skin lesion or cutaneous malignancy

(4) Parotid mass

(5) Facial twitching

(6) Absence of facial nerve recovery 4 months after onset of symptoms

(7) Concurrent sensorineural hearing loss, aural fullness, or tinnitus

(8) Concurrent vestibular symptoms

(9) Ipsilateral recurrence of facial paralysis

(10) History of neoplasm

Any patient with these features requires additional radiological imaging (magnetic resonance imaging, computed tomography) to rule out underlying malignancy.

■ Physical Examination

Head and Neck Examination

In patients presenting with facial nerve paralysis, a complete head and neck physical examination is warranted. Particular focus is placed on the ear, mastoid, parotid gland, facial skin, and cranial nerves.

The external ear is examined for evidence of an erythematous or vesicular rash suggestive of Ramsay-Hunt syndrome, a condition caused by varicella zoster virus. The skin and scalp should also be inspected for scars that could indicate previous cutaneous neoplasm or traumatic injury.

The temporal bone and ear contents should be examined in a comprehensive fashion. The mastoid is palpated for tenderness that can be associated with fractures of the temporal bone or mastoiditis. Ecchymosis over the mastoid process following a traumatic event (Battle sign) is suggestive of a basilar skull fracture. Multiple middle ear processes such as acute or chronic otitis media, middle ear effusion, hemotympanum, tympanic membrane perforation, neoplasm, and cholesteatoma can cause facial nerve paralysis. In patients suspected of having middle ear pathology, it is imperative to perform a complete microscopic examination of the region or refer the patient to a neuro-otologist. If any abnormalities of the middle ear are appreciated or the patient subjectively complains of hearing loss, an audiogram is obtained.

The parotid gland should be palpated for masses or lesions that may impinge on the facial nerve. Sparing of individual branches of the facial nerve increases suspicion for a parotid neoplasm; however, this finding may also be observed with iatrogenic injury. The neck is palpated for masses such as metastatic nodes or parapharyngeal tumors.

A complete neurological examination including vestibular and cranial nerve testing is essential. Additional neuropathies raise suspicion for tumors of the temporal bone, skull base, nasopharynx, or central nervous system.[1] Concurrent vestibulopathy in the setting of facial nerve paralysis is a poor prognostic sign. If clinical suspicion for a nasopharyngeal mass arises, fiberoptic examination of the nasopharynx is undertaken.

Facial Nerve Examination

The majority of patients with a peripheral facial nerve paralysis will demonstrate ipsilateral weakness of all muscles of facial expression, with only 2% of patients having bilateral involvement.[1] Central etiologies of facial paralysis spare the frontalis muscle and are relatively rare.

During the facial nerve examination, all patients are asked to perform a variety of movements including forehead elevation, eye closure, nasal wrinkling, whistling, pursing of lips, soft smile, full smile, and showing of all dentition (**Fig. 4.1**). The muscles of the forehead including

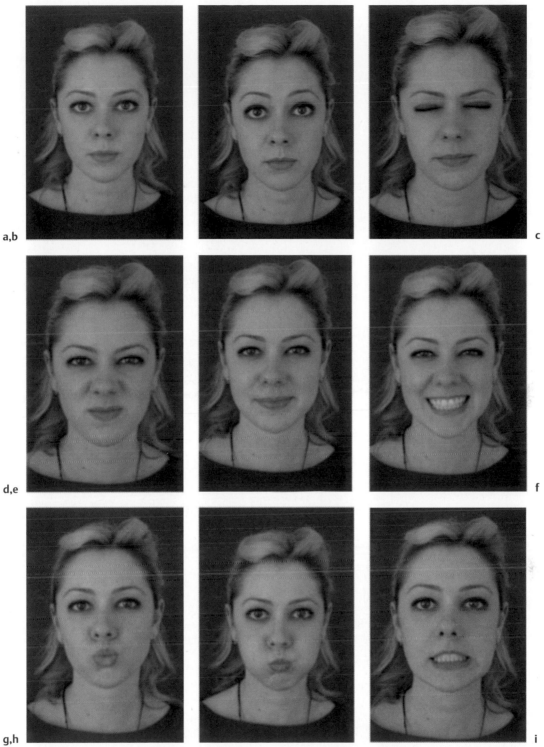

a,b

c

d,e

f

g,h

i

Fig. 4.1a–i Patient with normal facial nerve function demonstrating normal facial movement. (**a**) At rest, the face is symmetric without discrepancy in the position of the oral commissure or lower lid position. (**b**) During raising of the brows, the brows raise to similar heights and dynamic furrows from the frontalis can be appreciated. (**c**) Eye closure is complete. (**d**) During contraction of the nose, the buccal and zygomatic branches are evaluated. (**e, f**) The patient is asked to make a soft and full smile. (**g, h**) The competency of the oral cavity is tested by having the patient make "fish lips" and puff out her cheeks. (**i**) The marginal mandibular branch is best tested by asking the patient to pull down her lower lip.

frontalis, procerus, corrugator supercilli, and depressor supercilli are assessed. The frontalis, a brow elevator, is innervated by the frontal branch of the facial nerve, while the brow depressors such as the procerus, corrugator supercilli, and depressor supercilli have dual innervation from the frontal and zygomatic branches. Position of the eyebrows should be assessed for symmetry as well as location in relation to the supraorbital rim.

Periocular examination emphasizes the shape and function of the eye. Bell phenomenon, or upward rotation of the eye on attempted eye closure, should be confirmed in all patients. Patients with facial paralysis that demonstrate poor Bell phenomenon are at an exceedingly high risk of developing corneal ulceration and blindness if proper eye protection measures are not instituted (**Fig. 4.2**). The height of the lateral canthus should be 2 mm superior to the medial canthal angle. The orbicularis oculi and the levator palpebrae are responsible for eyelid opening, closure, shape, support, and tear pumping. The orbicularis oculi receives dual innervation from the frontal and zygomatic branches. The levator palpebrae, an upper eyelid elevator, is innervated by the oculomotor cranial nerve and therefore not affected by facial nerve palsy. Normal palpebral fissure and ocular width is ~12 mm and 29 mm, respectively. Patients with total facial paralysis have poor eye closure leading to lagophthalmos. On the other hand, patients with synkinesis often have narrowing of their palpebral fissure leading to asymmetric eyes.

The lower lid lash line should be positioned at the lower border of the lower limbus (**Fig. 4.3**). If it is inferiorly

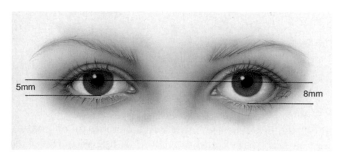

Fig. 4.3 The marginal reflex distance-2 (MRD_2) is used in the evaluation of lower lid retraction. Lower lid malposition is present if the MRD2 is greater than 5.5 cm. (Used with permission from Azizzadeh B, Murphy MR, Johnson CM Jr., eds. Master Techniques in Facial Rejuvenation. Philadelphia, PA: Saunders; 2007:8.)

displaced, then the patient has lower lid malposition. Marginal reflex distance−2 (MRD_2) is the distance measured between the light reflex and central portion of the lower lid when a patient's eye is in the neutral position. Lower lid malposition is present if the MRD_2 is significantly > 5.5 mm. Lower eyelid tone and support should be verified by the snap and lid retraction test (**Fig. 4.4**). If the lid does not snap back into its anatomical position within 1 second, the puncta displaces > 3 mm, or the lid distracts > 7 mm, lid laxity is diagnosed.

The midface region has significant arborization of the buccal and zygomaticus branches of the facial nerve and as a result, all muscles in this region likely have dual innervation. The buccal nerve is the dominant branch to the buccinators and supplies part of the dual innervation to the orbicularis oris and the depressor angulii oris. The zygomatic nerve is the dominant branch to the orbicularis oris, zygomaticus major, zygomaticus minor, levator angulii oris, levator labii superiorus, and levator labii superiorus alaeque nasi (all lip elevators). The mentalis, depressor angulii oris, depressor labii inferioris, and platysma are innervated by the marginal mandibular branch. The cervical branch of the facial nerve innervates the platysma muscle (**Table 4.2**; **Fig. 4.5**). The marginal mandibular nerve is a terminal branch and as a result is less likely to recover from injury.

There are three types of smiles that can be appreciated: zygomatic, canine, and full denture (**Fig. 4.6**). Zygomatic smile is dominated by the zygomaticus major and is present in 67% or the population. The canine teeth and lower teeth are typically not visible. Canine smile usually involves the activation of zygomaticus muscles as well as levator labii alequae nasi and is present in 31% of the population. Two percent of the population has a full denture smile where all upper and lower teeth are appreciated due to the activation of both elevators and depressors.[2] Knowing the characteristics of the smile will allow the physician to better understand what procedures are necessary to create a natural appearing smile.

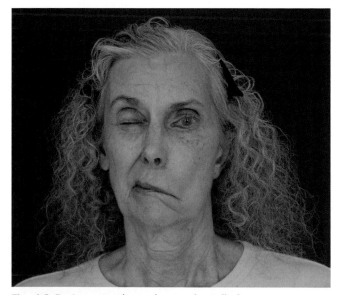

Fig. 4.2 During normal eye closure, the Bell phenomenon stimulates the eye to rotate superiorly to protect the cornea. In patients with abnormal Bell phenomenon, as here, the eye does not rotate superiorly during attempted eye closure, leaving the cornea exposed and at risk for injury.

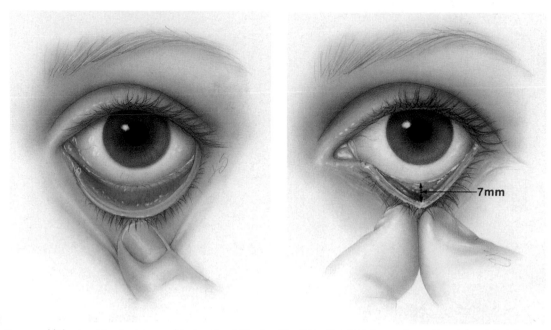

a   b

Fig. 4.4a, b Snap and lid retraction test is used to test for lid laxity. The lid is distracted away from the globe. (**a**) If the puncta displaces > 3 mm from the medial canthal tendon or does not snap back into place in < 1 second, then lid laxity is present. (**b**) The lid is lax if it can be distracted > 7 to 10 mm from the globe. (Used with permission from Azizzadeh B, Murphy MR, Johnson CM Jr., eds. Master Techniques in Facial Rejuvenation. Philadelphia, PA: Saunders; 2007:9.)

Table 4.2 Innervation of the muscles of facial expression

Facial Nerve Branch	Muscle Innervated	Muscle Origin	Muscle Insertion
Temporal	Frontalis	Galea aponeurotica	Skin above the eyebrows
	Procerus	Fascia of the nasal bone and upper nasal cartilage	Skin in center of the forehead between eyebrows
	Corrugator supercilli	Orbital rim near the medial canthus	Deep surface of the frontalis muscle
	Orbicularis oculi	Medial palpebral ligament, lacrimal crest, or from bone on the medial orbital wall	Circumferentially around the orbit
Zygomatic	*Procerus*	*As above*	
	Corrugator supercilli	*As above*	
	Orbicularis oculi	*As above*	
	Zygomaticus major	Zygomatic bone	Orbicularis oris near angle of the mouth
Buccal	*Zygomaticus major*	*As above*	
	Zygomaticus minor	Zygomatic bone	Orbicularis oris near angle of the mouth
	Levator labii superioris	Maxilla just above the infraorbital foramen	Upper lip
	Levator labii superioris alaeque nasi	Frontal process of the maxilla	Ala of the nose and upper lip
	Risorious	Fascia of masseter below zygomatic arch	Corner of the mouth
	Levator anguli oris	Maxilla inferior to the infraorbital foramen	Corner of the mouth
	Nasalis	1. Transverse portion: upper jaw near the canine tooth	1. Transverse portion: nasal cartilage on the bridge of the nose
		2. Alar portion: upper jaw and nasal cartilage	2. Alar portion: skin of nostril
	Depressor anguli oris	Mandible near the attachment of the platysma	Corner of the mouth
	Depressor labii inferioris	Mandible	Skin and muscles of the lower lip
	Orbicularis oris	Maxilla and mandible	Skin around the lips
	Buccinator	Pterygomandibular ligament and lateral surfaces of mandible and maxilla	Orbicularis oris
Marginal mandibular	*Depressor anguli oris*	*As above*	
	Depressor labii inferioris	*As above*	
	Mentalis	Mandible	Skin of the chin near midline
Cervical	Platysma	Inferior margin of the body of the mandible	Skin over the upper portion of the breast area

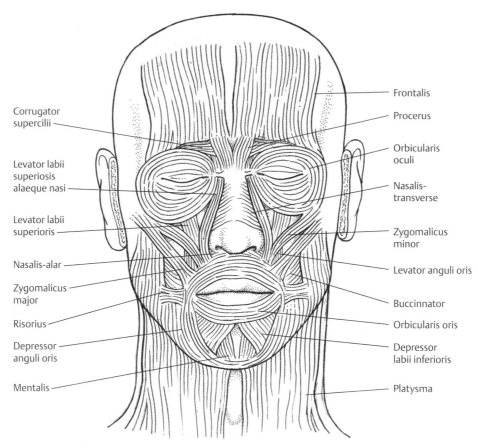

Fig. 4.5 Facial musculature.

Assessment of Muscles for Facial Expression

The naïve examiner may look at the face and simply notice the presence of the facial paralysis. The more experienced examiner will look at the face and examine each muscle group individually. Each muscle group is tested twice; the first time the movement is examined is to determine how well the individual the muscle group functions. The second time the muscle group is tested is to determine if any other muscle group has abnormal muscle movement. Additional abnormal movement may indicate the presence of synkinesis or hyperkinesis.

An overall assessment of the muscle function is determined and then individual groups are tested starting superior to inferior. When examining the patient with a facial paralysis, the examiner should first observe the patient's facial movements when he or she is speaking. Next, the examiner will start with top of the face and notice how the patient moves the forehead. The patient is asked to raise his or her eyebrows to assess the action of the frontalis muscle. The eyebrows should elevate similarly and equally on both sides. There should be symmetric furrowing of the forehead. Abnormal movement of the obicularis oculi muscle is next tested by asking the patient to close his or her eyes. The patient is asked to close the eyes as tightly as possible. The patient is then asked

to close the eye gently, allowing the examiner to notice how well the eye closes under less tension. The purpose of eye closure testing is twofold: assessment of orbicularis oculi function and to determine how well the cornea is protected. When poor function of eye closure is present, the examiner should observe for a Bell phenomenon, described as protective movement of the globe superior and lateral to protect the cornea under the upper lid when the lid cannot close. The amount of corneal exposure should be noted.

Next, the zygomaticus major muscle is tested by asking the patient to smile. A broad open mouth smile is first followed by a gentle closed mouth smile. This demonstrates if the patient has significant movement and can also assess for abnormal muscle movements such as synkinesis. The patient is asked to move or wiggle his or her nose, testing nasalis muscle movement. This can also assess the effect the paralysis is having on the nasal valve area. Loss of this function can cause the patient to complain of nasal obstruction. Testing of the mouth area can assess any difficulty the patient may have with eating and articulation. The patient is asked to pucker and press the lips firmly together (pressing the lips together is an excellent test of syskinetic muscle movement). Chronic facial paralysis patients that develop syskinesis

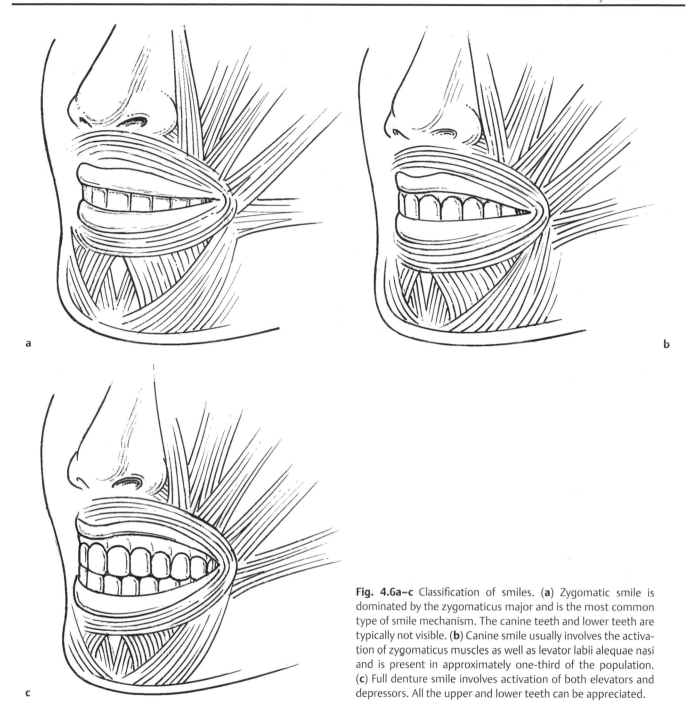

Fig. 4.6a–c Classification of smiles. (**a**) Zygomatic smile is dominated by the zygomaticus major and is the most common type of smile mechanism. The canine teeth and lower teeth are typically not visible. (**b**) Canine smile usually involves the activation of zygomaticus muscles as well as levator labii alequae nasi and is present in approximately one-third of the population. (**c**) Full denture smile involves activation of both elevators and depressors. All the upper and lower teeth can be appreciated.

will complain of abnormal movement; pressing of the lips together is the best test of oral-ocular syskinesis. The eye will close or narrow with lip tightening when syskinesis is present. The patient is asked to press the jaw forward and tighten the neck muscles. This assesses the platysma's movement. This can be important when longstanding facial paralysis is present as abnormal bands of platysma tightening may be seen. After complete assessment of the facial nerve function, a facial nerve grade may be given to the patient; see Chapter 5 for grading scales (**Figs. 4.7, 4.8, 4.9, and 4.10**).[3,4]

Occasionally, it is helpful to have the patient videotape his or her facial nerve function for documentation purposes. This may be helpful if the patient lives a distance from the treating physician. A videotaping procedure is included in the Appendix at the end of this chapter.

Isolated Facial Nerve Paralysis

Patients may present with isolated paralysis of one or more branches of the facial nerve. This is most commonly secondary due to trauma or iatrogenic injury. Patients with

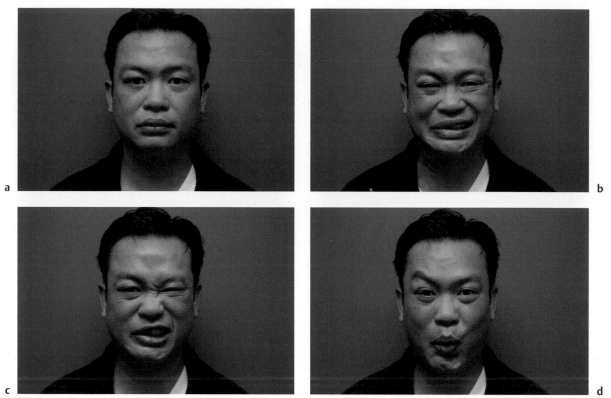

Fig. 4.7a–d Patient with mild facial paralysis (House-Brackmann grade II). (**a**) At rest, there is general symmetry and similar volumes of each side of the face. (**b–d**) During animation, the face becomes asymmetric while the paretic side displays minimal movement.

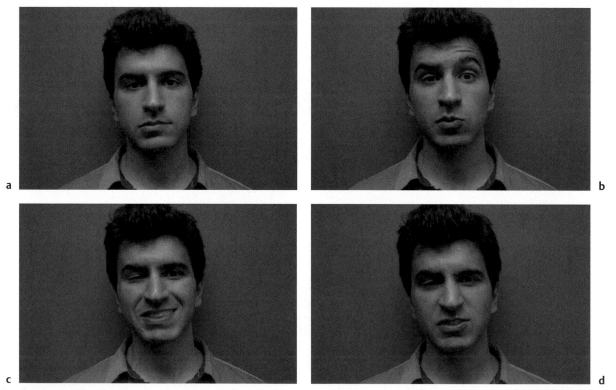

Fig. 4.8a–d Patient with moderate facial paralysis (House-Brackmann grade III). (**a**) At rest, minor asymmetries can be noticed including depression of the oral commisure and elevation of the brow. (**b**) During brow elevation, minimal movement of the paretic face is observed. (**c**) During smile, there is moderate synkinesis with dimpling of the chin and moderate narrowing of the palpebral fissure. (**d**) Showing lower teeth produces minimal movement of the paretic side.

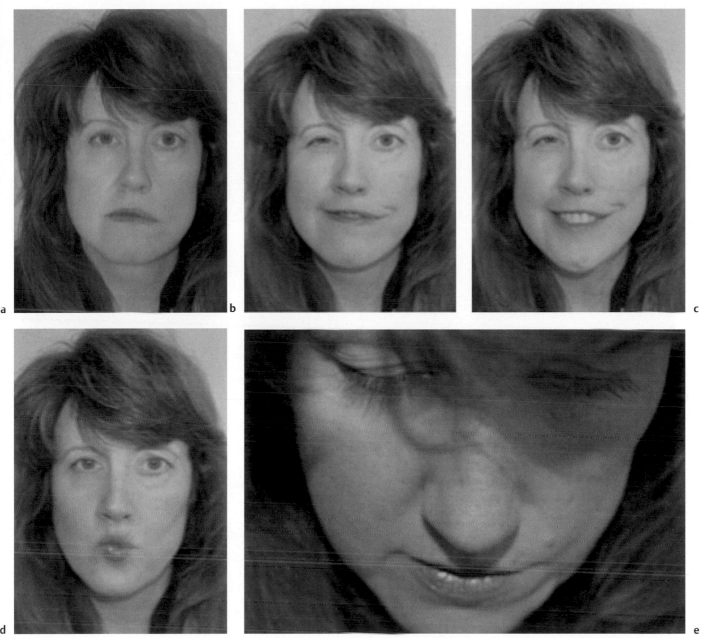

Fig. 4.9a–e Patient with moderate facial paralysis (House-Brackmann grade IV). (**a**) Patient with right-sided partial facial paralysis without synkinesis. Asymmetry at rest including lower lid malposition and drooping of the corner of the mouth. (**b**) On gentle smile, the pulling of the risorus can be appreciated. (**c**) On full smile, the asymmetry of the eyes is exaggerated and the smile appears "pulled" on the right paretic side. (**d**) Patient has good movement of the marginal mandibular nerve and little synkinesis. (**e**) Volume loss is appreciated on the paretic side.

a frontal nerve paralysis will present with brow ptosis, loss of dynamic rhytids of the forehead, and crow's feet. Lagophthalmos is rarely seen with an isolated frontal branch palsy. With loss of the zygomatic branch, patients may have difficulty closing the eye, effacement of the nasolabial angle, and decreased elevation of the lip with animation. Buccal branch injuries are subtle in nature. Patients will have a diminished ability to depress the lower lip and may complain of biting their buccal mucosa, owing to denervation to the buccinator. In marginal mandibular nerve injury, patients have reduced capability to depress the lip during smile.

Congenital unilateral lower lip paralysis is secondary to agenesis of the depressor anguli oris, so it is not a true disorder of the facial nerve.[5,6] Its clinical picture is similar to a marginal mandibular nerve injury (**Fig. 4.11**).

Isolated paralysis of the cervical branch has little sequelae and patients rarely complain of functional deficits.

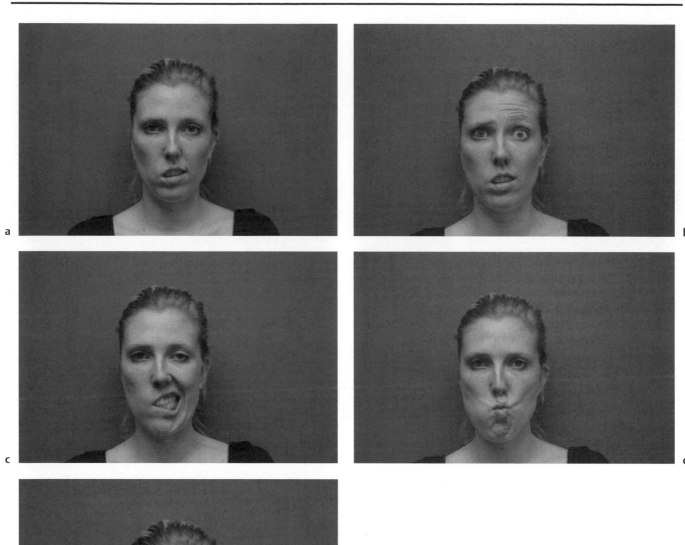

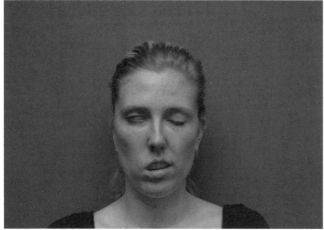

Fig. 4.10a–e Patient with severe facial paralysis (House-Brackmann grade V). (**a**) At rest, a complete right flaccid facial paralysis produces volumetric loss, effacement of the nasolabial fold, descent of oral commissure, and severe asymmetry. (**b**) Patient raising the brows. (**c**) Substantial asymmetry and absence elevation of the oral commissure during smile. (**d**) Difficulty pursing the lips. (**e**) Right orbit displaying lagophthalmus, lower lid laxity, lower lid malposition, and ocular irritation.

Bilateral Paralysis

A subset of patients may have bilateral paralysis and either side may be categorized into the previously discussed functional categories. These patients most commonly have Mobius syndrome or bilateral Bell palsy. Patients with complete bilateral paralysis have significant functional deficits including oral incompetence and speech impediments. The adverse psychological effects secondary to the inability to demonstrate facial expression are also significant. Frequently, patients feel isolated and struggle to effectively communicate.

■ Differential Diagnosis

Facial paralysis is uncommon, with an estimated 30 cases per 100,000 people each year. There is a wide ranging differential diagnosis for facial paralysis; the common

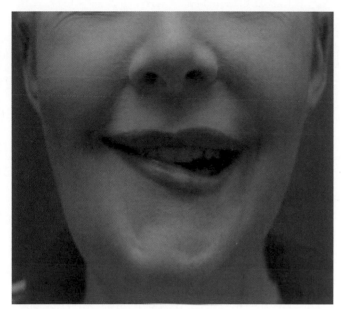

Fig. 4.11 Congenital unilateral lower lip palsy.

etiologies are outlined in **Table 4.1**. Bell palsy (idiopathic facial nerve paralysis) is the most common diagnosis, accounting for up to 70% of cases of unilateral facial paralysis.[7] Bell palsy is a diagnosis of exclusion, and all other potential etiologies should be ruled out prior to making this diagnosis.

Trauma is the second leading cause of facial nerve paralysis, followed by Ramsay Hunt syndrome and neoplasm.[8] Facial paralysis in a patient with history of a previous cancer, particularly skin cancer, should be attributed to metastatic disease until proven otherwise.

Congenital etiologies include syndromes and teratogens, both of which are commonly associated with a wide variety of other congenital anomalies in addition to facial palsy. Orobello believes congenital facial nerve paralysis is an error in embryogenesis, not fetogenesis, and should be appropriately termed developmental facial nerve paralysis.[9]

Möbius syndrome, a rare congenital disorder of unclear etiology, is predominately characterized by unilateral or bilateral facial nerve paralysis and abducens nerve palsy; however, involvement of other cranial nerves has also been reported. This disorder is associated with a variety of limb, orofacial, and chest-wall abnormalities.[10]

Roughly 30% of patients with ipsilateral recurrence of facial palsy were found to have tumors of the facial nerve or parotid gland; therefore, recurrent facial paralysis warrants diagnostic tests and imaging.[11] In cases of adult onset bilateral facial nerve palsy, entities such as brainstem tumors, intracranial infection, Guillain-Barré syndrome, and Lyme disease are most common.[1]

■ Special Testing

Audiometry

Pure tone and speech audiometry should be considered in patients with facial nerve paralysis. This allows for documentation of hearing and identifies patients that may have simultaneous involvement of the eighth cranial nerve. Further, it establishes baseline hearing in cases requiring surgical or nonsurgical intervention.

Topognostic Testing

Topognostic testing has historically been used in an effort to identify the exact site of a lesion. Theoretically, facial nerve branches proximal to the lesion should respond normally. Topognostic testing in localizing facial nerve lesions remains unreliable due to the variable anatomy of the facial nerve and its branches, the fact that lesions often fail to localize to one site of the nerve, and the variable recovery rates of differing neural segments.[8] The tear, salivary flow, and taste tests are not reliable predictors of outcome in cases of Bell palsy.[12,13] Because of difficulty in obtaining accurate results, lack of prognostic applications, and the emergence of improved imaging techniques, topognostic testing is only useful to supplement other diagnostic information and has a restricted role in current practice.

Shirmer Test

Shirmer test evaluates the function of the greater superficial petrosal nerve, which supplies secretory fibers to the lacrimal gland. The greater superficial petrosal nerve branches from the facial nerve at the geniculate ganglion. This test involves placing sterile paper strips in the conjunctival fornix to stimulate tear production. Tear production after 5 minutes is measured, and this value is compared between the eyes. A 25% decrease in tearing or < 25 mm of lacrimation on the pathological side is an abnormal test. An abnormal test would suggest a lesion proximal to the geniculate ganglion.

The Stapedial Reflex

The stapedial reflex tests the integrity of the stapedial nerve, a branch arising from the mastoid segment of facial nerve innervating the stapedial muscle. This bilateral reflex is elicited by either ipsilateral or contralateral acoustic stimulation. Responses are measured through alterations in acoustic immitance. A 50% decrease in the amplitude of the reflex is considered abnormal, signifying a lesion proximal to the stapedial nerve. The prognostic value of stapedial testing in acute facial paralysis has been studied. In a small series, all patients who had a normal stapedial reflex within 2 weeks of facial paralysis completely recovered in 12 weeks.[14] Conversely, an abnormal reflex is common in the first 2 weeks after facial paralysis limiting its prognostic role in predicting poor outcomes.[8]

Taste Tasting

The chorda tympani arises just proximal to the point at which the facial nerve exits the skull base through the stylomastoid foramen. The chorda tympani passes through the middle ear and petrotympanic fissure to join the lingual nerve. It carries taste fibers to the anterior two-thirds of the tongue and secretory fibers of the submandibular and sublingual glands. Taste testing involves application of stimuli to different sites on the tongue and qualitatively compares responses. Taste testing results were abnormal in almost all patients who were tested in the acute phase of Bell palsy. Further, the results of the taste testing could not identify patients with a poor prognosis, thus it has little prognostic value.[15]

Salivary Flow Test

The salivary flow test measures the secretion rates of the submandibular and sublingual glands. This technique requires cannulation of Wharton ducts. Collected saliva is compared between sides. Reduced flow suggests a lesion proximal to chorda tympani branching. Salivary flow testing can be both uncomfortable for the patient and time consuming. Further, it has little prognostic value and is rarely used.[8]

■ Electrical Testing of the Face

Nerve Excitability Test

The use of the nerve excitability test (NET) in the evaluation of facial nerve paralysis was first described in 1962.[16,17] This technique became popularized when Hilger introduced a nerve stimulator that was compact, inexpensive, and easy to use in 1963.[18] NET requires placement of a stimulating electrode over the facial nerve trunk or a peripheral branch. During a minimal excitability test, a low energy pulsed current is steadily increased to the normal facial nerve until facial muscle twitching is observed. The threshold of excitation is defined as the lowest current producing a visible twitch. This process is then repeated on the paralyzed side, and the threshold difference is calculated.

NET is particularly useful in differentiating physiologic blockage, or neuropraxia, from axonal degeneration.[16] With neuropraxia, electrical stimulation distal to the site of conduction block will produce a propagated action potential and subsequent muscle twitch. In these cases, NET will not demonstrate differences in threshold potential between healthy and paralyzed sides at any time point after symptom onset. Conversely, in patients with more severe injuries ranging from partial axonal degeneration to complete axonal transection, NET can provide valuable information. Nerve excitability will remain normal until distal axonal degeneration occurs. However, this can take

up to 3 to 4 days even after complete transection. Thus the usefulness of a NET in the first days after pathological insult is limited.[19,20]

Variability exists amongst authors as to a significant threshold difference between paretic and normal facial nerves.[21-23] Laumens et al proposed that a threshold difference > 3.5 mA is a reliable sign of nerve degeneration and accurate predictor of poor prognosis.[17] Devi et al followed patients with facial palsy for 6 months with serial minimal excitability tests. Patients with a NET of > 5 mA had poor recovery unless the difference significantly improved within 1 week of symptom onset.[24]

The differences in the stimulation thresholds obtained in a NET may assist in predicting severity of injury and probability of recovery. The test relies, however, on subjective scoring, and the standard value of significant threshold difference may fluctuate between institutions, making generalized guidelines difficult to describe. Due to the development of newer, objective electrophysiological testing methods, the applicability of NET is restricted in current practice but useful in select clinical scenarios.

Maximal Stimulation Test

The maximal stimulation test (MST) is a modification of the NET that employs similar neurostimulators, electrodes, and electrode placement. While the NET measures the minimum current necessary to elicit a facial twitch, MST uses a level of current (maximal stimulus) at which the greatest amplitude of facial movement is observed. The maximal stimulus provides sufficient electricity to depolarize all axons. Current levels greater than maximal stimulus, or supramaximal stimulus, can be used as well. The movements of the facial muscles on the paralyzed side are subjectively described in comparison to the healthy side as follows: equal, slightly decreased, markedly decreased, or absent when compared with the healthy side.[25] In a study evaluating the prognostic application of MST in patients with idiopathic complete facial paralysis, patients demonstrating equal MST in the affected and paretic sides had a 92% chance of complete recovery.[6] An additional study supported this finding and found that complete recovery occurred in 3 to 6 weeks.[18] Conversely, in patients with markedly decreased or absent responses on the affected side, there was an 86% chance of incomplete recovery of facial function.[26]

The MST can be a useful test in the evaluation of a facial paralysis patient but it has similar limitations to the NET. It is a qualitative method relying on subjective observations, and testing can be limited by pain experienced by the patient. As with NET, MST will be normal until the onset of wallerian degeneration, which can take up to 4 days. MST has been shown to become abnormal earlier than NET, suggesting it may be a superior test.[25]

Electroneuronography

Electroneuronography (EnoG), or evoked electromyography, measures muscle action potentials elicited by supramaximal stimulation of the facial nerve. First described by Esslen and Fisch, this method involves placement of a bipolar stimulating electrode at the stylomastoid foramen and a second recording electrode in the nasolabial groove.[27,28] The exact placement of the second electrode has been challenged in recent studies; however, the most appropriate muscle is likely the nasalis.[29] Supramaximal electrical stimulation is applied and the amplitude and latency of the elicited compound muscle action potential (CMAP) is recorded. The amplitude of the maximum response is compared between the affected and normal facial nerve. Expressed as a percentage, this value theoretically reflects the extent of facial musculature denervation and correlates to the number of degenerated motor nerve fibers. This information can be used to objectively assess the amount of neural degeneration.[30] Therefore, if the amplitude of the response on the paralyzed side is 30% of the response elicited on the healthy side, ~70% of the motor axons on the injured side have degenerated.

The role for EnoG in cases of partial paralysis is limited because a full, spontaneous recovery can generally be expected in these patients. However, its use as a prognostic tool in complete facial nerve paralysis has been well studied and advocated by many experts.[15,26,28,31–33] Given that neural wallerian degeneration does not occur until 3 to 4 days after the pathological event, EnoG testing before this time will demonstrate normal muscle responses, and therefore not be of any practical value.[32,34] Most proponents of EnoG support daily or every other day serial examinations until reductions in amplitude on the paralyzed side cease. Once this steady state is reached, the maximum amount of nerve degeneration is determined. EnoG has limited clinical value after this point because clinical improvement will almost always manifest prior to electrical changes seen on an EnoG.

Most data predicts complete recovery when the paralyzed side shows less than a 30% reduction in amplitude of CMAP. For reductions in CMAP amplitude between 70 and 90%, full recovery can take from 2 to 8 months and mild to moderate residual deficits can be expected.[31] Many authors have shown that CMAP amplitude reduction, or nerve degeneration, > 90% correlates with a poor recovery (**Fig. 4.12**).[26,31,32] Residual function will be moderately to severely limited, and maximum recovery will be delayed between 6 and 12 months.[31] Conversely, a prospective multicenter trial demonstrated that patients who did not reach 90% nerve degeneration on EnoG within 14 days of symptom onset returned to House-Brackmann grade I or II by 7 months.[33]

The reliability of EnoG in identifying candidates who will benefit from surgical intervention has been studied.[28,33]

Right Facial Nerve ENoG- Nasalis

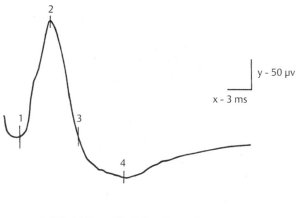

Left Facial Nerve ENoG- Nasalis

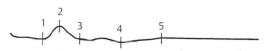

Fig. 4.12 Electroneuronography (ENoG) demonstrating > 90% reduction in compound muscle action potential in the paralyzed left facial nerve when compared with the contralateral side.

Fisch established criteria for surgical decompression after neural degeneration of > 90% observed within 3 weeks of symptom onset. Using these guidelines, patients who underwent decompression had more satisfactory return of facial function than patients in the nonsurgical group.[28] Gantz et al studied the value of surgery in patients with Bell palsy that had > 90% reduction in CMAP amplitudes and no voluntary motor unit potentials on electromyography (EMG). Decompression within 2 weeks of symptom onset was associated with a 91% chance of returning to House-Brackmann grade I or II by 7 months. Patients who were treated with steroids only had a 42% chance of achieving a similar functional outcome. No benefit to surgical decompression after 2 weeks of symptom onset was demonstrated.[33]

May et al studied the value of surgical decompression in patients with Bell palsy demonstrating > 75% reduction in Shirmer test, salivary flow test, MST, and EnoG. Patients meeting these criteria underwent decompression of the facial nerve. Contrary to prior results published by Fisch and Gantz et al, no benefit of surgical decompression was demonstrated.[35] It is important to note that different types of surgical decompression were performed in the various studies. Fisch and Gantz et al decompressed the meatal foramen, labyrinthine segment, geniculate ganglion, and tympanic segment of the facial nerve while May et al did not decompress the meatal foramen.

While the role of surgery in Bell palsy remains controversial, critics of EnoG cite poor test accuracy in predicting unfavorable outcomes. In a series of 23 patients meeting the surgical criteria originally proposed by Fisch, 80% were shown to have moderate to complete return of facial function.[36] EnoG is also susceptible to test-retest variability evidenced by amplitude ratios that are not constant with repeat measurements on the same subject.[37] However, there are reports of test-retest variability as low as 6.2%.[38] Taking an average of multiple tests performed during a single examination and stimulating the nerve 10 to 20 times before recording amplitude has been shown to improve the accuracy of measurements.[39]

EnoG is currently the best available electrodiagnostic technique available for evaluation of acute facial nerve palsy in the immediate postoperative setting.[13,22,26,40-43] In cases of acute onset complete paralysis, it provides physicians with vital information concerning the degree and rate of nerve damage. Most agree that valuable prognostic information can be extracted from EnoG data; however, no consensus concerning the use of EnoG in selecting patients for surgical decompression exists.

Electromyography

Facial nerve EMG involves placement of bipolar needle electrodes in the facial musculature that record electrical action potentials generated by spontaneous and voluntary muscle contraction. In contrast to other neurophysiologic tests, this test does not require active stimulation of the facial nerve and is the only test that can document reinnervation of the facial nerve.

During an injury to the facial nerve, there will be a decrease in the number of voluntary motor units that are innervated. EMG measures the voluntary firing of motor units of the facial musculature. In the acute phase of facial nerve paralysis, the continued presence of voluntary motor units 72 hours after symptom onset suggests that some motor axons remain intact, although the degree

of injury cannot be assessed. Lack of voluntary motor units at this time confers a poor prognosis to complete recovery.[26] Motor units that fail to become reinnervated develop unstable resting membrane potentials and will begin to spontaneous depolarize in positive sharp waves and fibrillation potentials (**Fig. 4.13**). These may develop between 10 and 21 days after the injury.[44-46] Two studies evaluated patients that displayed fibrillation potentials at 10 to 14 days after facial paresis and reported 80.8% and 86% positive predictive values of incomplete recovery.[44,46]

EMG is a vital tool in attempting to prognosticate outcomes for patients with complete nerve palsy and > 90% degeneration with EnoG. In some cases, > 90% degeneration recording on EnoG may be due to dyssynchronous discharges of the neurapraxic fibers. This haphazard firing prevents adequate summation of the myogenic action potential, resulting in a significantly reduced or absent CMAP suggesting severe nerve degeneration.[33] In this scenario, the value of EMG in conjunction with the EnoG cannot be underestimated as it is imperative to identify false-positive EnoG. It has been demonstrated that despite markedly decreased EnoG (> 90%), the prognosis for recovery is excellent if voluntary motor potentials are present on EMG.[15,32] Fisch has termed this the "early de-blocking" phenomenon. He attributes the presence or return of voluntary motor units to early reversal of the physiological conduction block responsible for the neuropraxia.[32] These patients would not need surgical decompression.

In patients with acute facial nerve palsy and no clinical resolution of symptoms 2 to 3 weeks after onset of paralysis, EMG is particularly useful. At this time point, many neurophysiological tests are no longer useful as the facial nerve may have lost excitability. The appearance of small, rapid, polyphasic potentials on EMG is an indicator of nerve regeneration and suggests that further functional

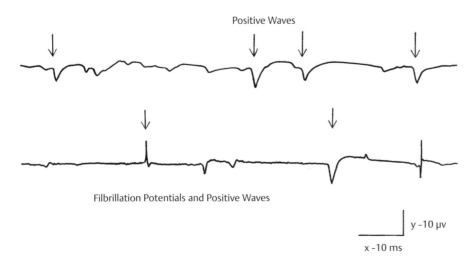

Positive Waves

Filbrillation Potentials and Positive Waves

y -10 μv

x -10 ms

Fig. 4.13 Positive waves and fibrillation potentials are signs of deinnervation.

Polyphasic Motor Unit Potential

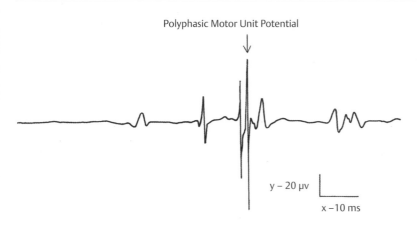

y – 20 μv

x –10 ms

Fig. 4.14 Polyphasic motor unit potential is an indication of active reinnervation.

recovery is still to come (**Fig. 4.14**).[21,27] The return of voluntary motor unit firing often precedes clinical recovery of the facial nerve. Serial EMG is the only test that can follow the degree and pace of facial nerve recovery and reinnervation.

EMG is complementary to other neurophysiological tests in patients with facial paralysis. It is the only test to document and follow recovery of the facial nerve. It is invaluable in situations where > 90% degeneration occurs on EnoG to identify patients that have a good prognosis for recovery.

Blink Reflex

The afferent and efferent limbs of the blink reflex are mediated by the trigeminal nerve and facial nerve, respectively. The reflex can be routinely elicited in healthy patients by either mechanical or electrical stimulation of the supraorbital nerve.[47] Resultant orbicularis oculi muscle consists of an oligosynaptic early response ipsilaterally (R1) and polysynaptic late responses bilaterally (R2, R2').[48,49] Abnormal blink reflex responses are characterized by differences in amplitude or latency of R1, R2, or R2' responses between affected and unaffected sides. In contrast to direct facial nerve testing, blink reflex testing provides information on the neurophysiological status of the trigeminal nerve, pons, and the proximal intracranial segments of the facial nerve. The previously mentioned direct electrophysiological facial nerve stimulation techniques cannot evaluate these neural pathways.[21,50]

Patients with facial nerve paralysis are expected to have amplitude reductions, increased latencies, or absence of ipsilateral R1 and R2 responses on the paretic side.[48,50] No significant difference in median value of amplitude or latency of the contralateral R2' component has been demonstrated when comparing a paralyzed facial nerve to controls.[50] In a study of 32 patients with Bell palsy, increased R1 latency was the most common change occurring in 34.4% of patients.[51] Few studies have examined the utility of blink reflex as a prognostic measurement in peripheral facial nerve injuries. Kimura et al suggested

that a return of the R1 reflex after 1 week is a good prognostic sign.[52]

Blink reflex abnormalities in patients with acoustic neuroma has also been described. This technique was first used as an adjunct in the diagnosis of cerebellopontine tumors; however, it has been largely replaced by more sensitive and specific radiographic studies.[53]

The blink reflex provides valuable information concerning neurophysiological status of trigemino-facial connections and function of the intracranial facial nerve.

■ Electrophysiological Features of Residual Nerve Deficits

Synkinesis is common after a facial nerve insult. Clinically, synkinesis presents as involuntary contraction of one facial muscle upon voluntary contraction of a separate muscle. Various mechanisms have been proposed to explain the development of clinical synkinesis including peripheral ephaptic transmission, aberrant regeneration of facial nerve fibers, and hyperexcitability of the facial nucleus.[54] While aberrant nerve regeneration is the most widely accepted theory, no consensus has yet been reached.

Synkinetic Spread

Synkinetic spread can be quantitatively evaluated with blink reflex testing. Stimulation of the supraorbital nerve normally elicits a response only in the orbicularis oculi. Abnormal wave responses are recorded simultaneously from both the ipsilateral orbicularis oculi and orbicularis oris muscles in patients with clinical evidence of synkinesis. In a heterogeneous study population of 29 patients, Kimura et al described increased latency and decreased amplitude for R1 and R2 in both muscle groups. Comparison of reflex responses between the two muscle groups did not reveal any significant differences.[52]

Lateral Spread

Lateral spread, or ephaptic spread, can be evaluated electrophysiologically. It is characterized by stimulation of one facial nerve branch resulting in a late response of a facial muscle not normally innervated by that branch.[55,56] Formation of an artificial synapse at the site of injury and crossing over of impulses from one nerve fiber to another is the proposed mechanism.

Though synkinetic and lateral spread can be demonstrated electrophysiologically as described previously, these responses appear after the development of clinical synkinesis in almost all cases. Therefore, they are not used to predict the development of synkinesis.[57] However, objective measurements can be helpful in distinguishing volitional movement from synkinetic movement, especially in cases of subclinical synkinesis.

■ Blood Testing

In patients with facial nerve palsy, no single laboratory study exists that definitively confirms the diagnosis. Many studies have examined the prevalence of antibodies to herpes simplex virus and varicella zoster virus.[7,58–64] Studies have demonstrated that patients with Bell palsy had significantly higher levels of immunoglobulin M antibodies to vesicular stomatitis virus and immunoglobulin M and immunoglobulin G antibodies to herpes simplex virus than controls.[58,60,64] Additional serologic studies may be considered to suggest or rule out other potential causes. These should be dictated by the clinical history and setting. Though nonspecific, erythrocyte sedimentation rate and white blood cell count can help differentiate between infectious and noninfectious processes. When history involves tick bites or travel to endemic areas of Lyme disease, Lyme titers are indicated. Testing for human immunodeficiency virus is indicated if signs of immunocompromise are noted or if the patient has a history of intravenous drug use. Serum angiotensin levels may also be considered if sarcoidosis is suspected.

■ Conclusion

Facial neuropathy has wide ranging effects both in form and function of the head and neck. A comprehensive and detailed history and examination is fundamental in the evaluation and treatment of patients with facial neuropathy. Recent advances in electrophysiological technology have greatly improved our ability to accurately prognosticate outcomes and guide further treatment. Interpreting electrophysiological results in the context of history, physical examination, laboratory values, and radiographic findings will continue to improve patient care and ultimately clinical outcomes.

■ Appendix: Facial Protocol for Video Picture Assessment: Instructions for Videotaping

Camera Setup

(1) An appropriate light source will be placed ~4 to 5 feet from the video camera.
(2) The camera will be ~4 feet from the stool where the patient will be sitting.
(3) The camera, lighting, and patient's eyes should be in the same horizontal plane.
(4) During videotaping, the patient should fixate at all times at the light source located at the back of the camera.
(5) A new tape should be used for each patient evaluation.

Patient Instructions

(1) The patient's upper body will be videotaped briefly to record the patient at rest.
(2) Full face: The full face of the patient should be videotaped for approximately 1 minute. During this period, the patient will be asked to:
  (A) Smile forcefully for 5 seconds and relax for 5 seconds
  (B) Pucker lips for 5 seconds and relax for 5 seconds
  (C) Chew for 5 seconds and relax for 5 seconds
(3) Upper face: The upper face should be recorded on the videotape with the camera positioned so that the nostrils are in the lower portion of the videoframe and the mid forehead is in the upper aspect. During this period, the patient will be asked to:
  (A) Smile forcibly for 5 seconds and relax for 5 seconds, repeating this facial maneuver five times
  (B) Pucker lips for 5 seconds and relax for 5 seconds, repeating this facial maneuver five times
  (C) Chew for 5 seconds and relax for 5 seconds, repeating this facial maneuver five times
(4) Return to full face: The following actions should be performed for 5 seconds. Each action will be repeated for the 5-second period. Allow 5 seconds between each action. The patient will be asked to complete the following with the full face exposed:
  (A) Raise the eyebrows
  (B) Gently close the eyes
  (C) Gently close the eyes starting with the lower eye lids
  (D) Close the eyes tightly
  (E) Flare or open the nose more
  (F) Smile evenly with the mouth closed
  (G) A big wide smile with the mouth open
  (H) Raise the upper lip while wrinkling the nose

(I) Raise the left or right upper lip while wrinkling the nose (do each side, start with the noninvolved side)

(J) Move the right or left corner of the mouth back toward the ear (do each side, start with the noninvolved side)

(K) Pucker the lips

(L) Press the lips together

(M) Pull the lips back and in, over the teeth

(N) Push the lips out as far as they will go

(O) Roll the lower lip out and down

(P) Move/turn the corners of the mouth downward

(Q) Tighten the chin

(R) Tighten the neck

(S) Stick out the tongue

Miscellaneous

It is helpful if one individual is running the camera while the patient is seated on the stool. The individual running the camera can read the requested action aloud and have the patient/subject perform the exercise.

References

1. Keane JR. Bilateral seventh nerve palsy: analysis of 43 cases and review of the literature. Neurology 1994;44(7):1198–1202

2. Cheney ML. Facial surgery: plastic and reconstructive, 1st ed. Baltimore: Williams & Wilkins: 20

3. House JW, Brackmann DE. Facial nerve grading system. Otolaryngol Head Neck Surg 1985;93(2):146–147

4. Ross BG, Fradet G, Nedzelski JM. Development of a sensitive clinical facial grading system. Otolaryngol Head Neck Surg 1996; 114(3):380–386

5. Udagawa A, Arikawa K, Shimizu S, et al. A simple reconstruction for congenital unilateral lower lip palsy. Plast Reconstr Surg 2007;120(1):238–244

6. Kobayashi T. Congenital unilateral lower lip palsy. Acta Otolaryngol 1979;88(3–4):303–309

7. Adour KK, Byl FM, Hilsinger RL Jr, Kahn ZM, Sheldon MI. The true nature of Bell's palsy: analysis of 1,000 consecutive patients. Laryngoscope 1978;88(5):787–801

8. May M, Schaitkin BM. The facial nerve, May's 2nd ed. New York: Thieme: 27

9. Orobello P. Congenital and acquired facial nerve paralysis in children. Otolaryngol Clin North Am 1991;24(3):647–652

10. Bianchi B, Copelli C, Ferrari S, Ferri A, Sesenna E. Facial animation in children with Moebius and Moebius-like syndromes. J Pediatr Surg 2009;44(11):2236–2242

11. May M, Hardin WB. Facial palsy: interpretation of neurologic findings. Laryngoscope 1978;88(8 Pt 1):1352–1362

12. Kerbavaz RJ, Hilsinger RL Jr, Adour KK. The facial paralysis prognostic index. Otolaryngol Head Neck Surg 1983;91(3):284–289

13. Hughes GB. Practical management of Bell's palsy. Otolaryngol Head Neck Surg 1990;102(6):658–663

14. Ide M, Morimitsu T, Ushisako Y, Makino K, Fukiyama M, Hayashi A. The significance of stapedial reflex test in facial nerve paralysis. Acta Otolaryngol Suppl 1988;446(Suppl):57–63

15. Sillman JS, Niparko JK, Lee SS, Kileny PR. Prognostic value of evoked and standard electromyography in acute facial paralysis. Otolaryngol Head Neck Surg 1992;107(3):377–381

16. Campbell ED, Hickey RP, Nixon KH, Richardson AT. Value of nerve-excitability measurements in prognosis of facial palsy. BMJ 1962;2(5296):7–10

17. Laumans EP, Jongkees LB. On the Prognosis of Peripheral Facial Paralysis of Endotemporal Origin. Ann Otol Rhinol Laryngol 1963; 72:621–636

18. Lewis BI, Adour KK, Kahn JM, Lewis AJ. Hilger facial nerve stimulator: a 25-year update. Laryngoscope 1991;101(1 Pt 1):71–74

19. Gilliatt RW, Taylor JC. Electrical changes following section of the facial nerve. Proc R Soc Med 1959;52:1080–1083

20. Groves J, Gibson WP. Bell's (idiopathic facial) palsy: The nerve excitability test in selection of cases for early treatment. J Laryngol Otol 1974;88(9):851–854

21. Gilchrist JM. Seventh cranial neuropathy. Semin Neurol 2009; 29(1):5–13

22. Dumitru D, Walsh NE, Porter LD. Electrophysiologic evaluation of the facial nerve in Bell's palsy. A review. Am J Phys Med Rehabil 1988;67(4):137–144

23. Kasse CA, Cruz OL, Leonhardt FD, Testa JR, Ferri RG, Viertler EY. The value of prognostic clinical data in Bell's palsy. Braz J Otorhinolaryngol 2005;71(4):454–458

24. Devi S, Challenor Y, Duarte N, Lovelace RE. Prognostic value of minimal excitability of facial nerve in Bell's palsy. J Neurol Neurosurg Psychiatry 1978;41(7):649–652

25. May M, Harvey JE, Marovitz WF, Stroud M. The prognostic accuracy of the maximal stimulation test compared with that of the nerve excitability test in Bell's palsy. Laryngoscope 1971;81(6): 931–938

26. May M, Blumenthal F, Klein SR. Acute Bell's palsy: prognostic value of evoked electromyography, maximal stimulation, and other electrical tests. Am J Otol 1983;5(1):1–7

27. Esslen E. The acute facial palsies: investigations on the localization and pathogenesis of meato-labyrinthine facial palsies. Schriftenr Neurol 1977;18:1–164

28. Fisch U. Surgery for Bell's palsy. Arch Otolaryngol 1981;107(1):1–11

29. Glocker FX, Magistris MR, Rösler KM, Hess CW. Magnetic transcranial and electrical stylomastoidal stimulation of the facial motor pathways in Bell's palsy: time course and relevance of electrophysiological parameters. Electroencephalogr Clin Neurophysiol 1994;93(2):113–120

30. Gutnick HN, Kelleher MJ, Prass RL. A model of waveform reliability in facial nerve electroneurography. Otolaryngol Head Neck Surg 1990;103(3):344–350

31. Olsen PZ. Prediction of recovery in Bell's palsy. Acta Neurol Scand Suppl 1975;61:1–121

32. Fisch U. Prognostic value of electrical tests in acute facial paralysis. Am J Otol 1984;5(6):494–498

33. Gantz BJ, Rubinstein JT, Gidley P, Woodworth GG. Surgical management of Bell's palsy. Laryngoscope 1999;109(8):1177–1188

34. Thomander L, Stålberg E. Electroneurography in the prognostication of Bell's palsy. Acta Otolaryngol 1981;92(3–4):221–237

35. May M, Klein SR. Differential diagnosis of facial nerve palsy. Otolaryngol Clin North Am 1991;24(3):613–645

36. Sinha PK, Keith RW, Pensak ML. Predictability of recovery from Bell's palsy using evoked electromyography. Am J Otol 1994; 15(6):769–771

37. Sittel C, Guntinas-Lichius O, Streppel M, Stennert E. Variability of repeated facial nerve electroneurography in healthy subjects. Laryngoscope 1998;108(8 Pt 1):1177–1180

38. Hughes GB, Nodar RH, Williams GW. Analysis of test-retest variability in facial electroneurography. Otolaryngol Head Neck Surg 1983;91(3):290–293

39. Hughes GB, Josey AF, Glasscock ME, Jackson CG, Ray WA, Sismanis A. Clinical electroneurography: statistical analysis of controlled measures in twenty-two normal subjects. Laryngoscope 1981;91(11):1834–1846

40. Coker NJ. Facial electroneurography: analysis of techniques and correlation with degenerating motoneurons. Laryngoscope 1992;102(7):747–759

41. Coker NJ, Fordice JO, Moore S. Correlation of the nerve excitability test and electroneurography in acute facial paralysis. Am J Otol 1992;13(2):127–133

42. Engström M, Jonsson L, Grindlund M, Stålberg E. Electroneurographic facial muscle pattern in Bell's palsy. Otolaryngol Head Neck Surg 2000;122(2):290–297

43. Kennelly KD. Electrophysiological evaluation of cranial neuropathies. Neurologist 2006;12(4):188–203

44. Sittel C, Stennert E. Prognostic value of electromyography in acute peripheral facial nerve palsy. Otol Neurotol 2001;22(1):100–104

45. Grosheva M, Guntinas-Lichius O. Significance of electromyography to predict and evaluate facial function outcome after acute peripheral facial palsy. Eur Arch Otorhinolaryngol 2007;264(12):1491–1495

46. Grosheva M, Wittekindt C, Guntinas-Lichius O. Prognostic value of electroneurography and electromyography in facial palsy. Laryngoscope 2008;118(3):394–397

47. Bischoff C, Meyer BU, Fauth C, Liscic R, Machetanz J, Conrad B. Blink reflex investigation using magnetic stimulation. Eur Arch Otorhinolaryngol 1994;S267–S268

48. Valls-Solé J. Electrodiagnostic studies of the facial nerve in peripheral facial palsy and hemifacial spasm. Muscle Nerve 2007;36(1):14–20

49. Ongerboer de Visser BW, Kuypers HG. Late blink reflex changes in lateral medullary lesions. An electrophysiological and neuroanatomical study of Wallenberg's Syndrome. Brain 1978;101(2):285–294

50. Mikula I, Miskov S, Negovetić R, Demarin V. Blink reflex in the prediction of outcome of idiopathic peripheral partial facioparesis: follow-up study. Croat Med J 2002;43(3):319–323

51. Hill MD, Midroni G, Goldstein WC, Deeks SL, Low DE, Morris AM. The spectrum of electrophysiological abnormalities in Bell's palsy. Can J Neurol Sci 2001;28(2):130–133

52. Kimura J, Giron LT, Young SM. Electrophysiological study of Bell palsy: electrically elicited blink reflex in assessment of prognosis. Arch Otolaryngol 1976;102(3):140–143

53. Darrouzet V, Hilton M, Pinder D, Wang JL, Guerin J, Bebear JP. Prognostic value of the blink reflex in acoustic neuroma surgery. Otolaryngol Head Neck Surg 2002;127(3):153–157

54. Meier JD, Wenig BL, Manders EC, Nenonene EK. Continuous intraoperative facial nerve monitoring in predicting postoperative injury during parotidectomy. Laryngoscope 2006;116(9):1569–1572

55. Nielsen VK. Pathophysiology of hemifacial spasm: II. Lateral spread of the supraorbital nerve reflex. Neurology 1984;34(4):427–431

56. Nielsen VK. Pathophysiology of hemifacial spasm: I. Ephaptic transmission and ectopic excitation. Neurology 1984;34(4):418–426

57. Celik M, Forta H, Vural C. The development of synkinesis after facial nerve paralysis. Eur Neurol 2000;43(3):147–151

58. Adour KK, Bell DN, Hilsinger RL Jr. Herpes simplex virus in idiopathic facial paralysis (Bell palsy). JAMA 1975;233(6):527–530

59. Makeieff M, Venail F, Cartier C, Garrel R, Crampette L, Guerrier B. Continuous facial nerve monitoring during pleomorphic adenoma recurrence surgery. Laryngoscope 2005;115(7):1310–1314

60. Morgan M, Moffat M, Ritchie L, Collacott I, Brown T. Is Bell's palsy a reactivation of varicella zoster virus? J Infect 1995;30(1):29–36

61. Morrow MJ. Bell's Palsy and Herpes Zoster Oticus. Curr Treat Options Neurol 2000;2(5):407–416

62. Musani MA, Farooqui AN, Usman A, et al. Association of herpes simplex virus infection and Bell's palsy. J Pak Med Assoc 2009;59(12):823–825

63. Sweeney CJ, Gilden DH. Ramsay Hunt syndrome. J Neurol Neurosurg Psychiatry 2001;71(2):149–154

64. Vahlne A, Edström S, Arstila P, et al. Bell's palsy and herpes simplex virus. Arch Otolaryngol 1981;107(2):79–81

5 Measurement of Facial Nerve Function

John W. House and Mark Brandt Lorenz

The House-Brackmann (HB) facial nerve grading scale was adopted as the official metric of the International Facial Nerve Study Group in Bordeaux in 1984 and the American Academy of Otolaryngology-Head and Neck Surgery in 1985. The HB remains the most widely accepted scale in otolaryngology literature since its introduction.[1] Its simplicity, quickness, and general descriptive power are its strengths, but the scale does not discriminate regional facial weakness or secondary deficits such as synkinesis, gustatory tearing, or hemifacial spasm. These secondary deficits are generally associated with the degree of facial weakness, however. It remains a fast and highly reliable assessment of clinical facial nerve function and has been proven predictive of multiple clinical outcomes. It does not require special equipment, can be performed anywhere, and has provided a common language for literature concerning facial nerve function.

The utility of a common standard for clinical tracking and reporting of facial nerve function has long been recognized in facial nerve surgery. As recently as 1980, the otolaryngology literature supported multiple facial nerve systems based on subjective or measured assessment of gross motor or regional motor function.[2-7] Many scientific articles discussing facial nerve function would begin with a lengthy explanation of their specific metric, prior to discussion of results. This lack of standardization led to significant heterogeneity in the literature and made meta-analysis impossible. Several facial nerve scales suggested high levels of accuracy by assignment of a percentile from 0–100%, but poor interrater reliability and complexity rendered them impractical for widespread clinical usage. To aid with prediction of functional impairment, other scales allocated additional numerical weight to specific regions of the face. These scales were likewise challenging to administer, time-consuming, and had poor agreement among clinicians. In general, as systems attempted to improve descriptive accuracy, they became vulnerable to increased subjective interpretation. Of all the early facial nerve grading systems, few remain in use, except the Yanagihara scale, which still remains in widespread usage in Japan.[8] It was developed in 1976 and is a regional system that measures 10 separate aspects of function on a scale of 0 to 4. It is easy to administer but does not address synkinesis or secondary deficits (**Table 5.1**).

While developing the HB scale, the authors acknowledged that a system that assessed gross motor function would reduce variability in scoring at the expense of fine motor detail. The scale was then designed incorporating these clinical observations (**Table 5.2**). Completely normal facial nerve function is HB grade I and complete absence of facial motion is HB grade VI. Minimal weakness and dynamic asymmetry is HB grade II, whereas minimal function and tone is considered HB grade V. Patients in these four grades are rarely afflicted by synkinesis or hemifacial spasm to a degree requiring therapy. The ability to activate musculature of the forehead is the dividing line between moderate (HB grade III) and moderately severe (HB grade IV) paralysis. Forehead function, although considered the least important functionally and cosmetically, suggests that the facial nerve has not degenerated, and portends excellent facial nerve recovery.[9] Along this line, eye closure has significant clinical implications and was seen as a useful dividing line for patients with moderately severe paralysis. In this way, certain regional deficits are used to distinguish moderate to moderately severe forms of facial weakness.

In its original format, patients with synkinesis and hemifacial spasm severe enough to interfere with function were considered to have moderately severe dysfunction regardless of motor activity. The stipulations regarding synkinesis were subsequently removed prior to its acceptance by the American Academy of Otolaryngology-Head and Neck Surgery, and a modified HB scale is most commonly accepted in the literature. Although the scale was initially designed to record long-term facial nerve function, subsequent studies found that these minor modifications made it applicable for immediate postoperative facial nerve function.[10]

Table 5.1 The Yanagihara facial nerve scale

At rest	0	1	2	3	4
Wrinkle forehead	0	1	2	3	4
Blink	0	1	2	3	4
Slight closure of eye	0	1	2	3	4
Tight closure of eye	0	1	2	3	4
Closure of eye on the involved side only	0	1	2	3	4
Wrinkle nose	0	1	2	3	4
Whistle	0	1	2	3	4
Grin	0	1	2	3	4
Depress lower lip	0	1	2	3	4

Note: This is a scale of normal, slight paralysis, moderate paralysis, severe paralysis, and total paralysis for which points of 4, 3, 2, 1, and 0, respectively, are awarded.
Used with permission from Yanagihara N. Grading of facial palsy. In: Fisch U, ed. Facial nerve surgery. Proceedings: Third International Symposium on Facial Nerve Surgery, Zurich, 1976. Kugler Medical Publications, Amstelveen, Netherlands; and Aesculapius Publishing Co., Birmingham, AL; 1977:533–535.

Table 5.2   The House-Brackmann facial nerve grading system

Grade	At Rest	Dynamic	Regional Findings	Secondary Deficits
(I) Normal	Normal symmetry and tone	Normal facial function in all areas	Normal facial function in all areas	
(II) Mild dysfunction	Normal symmetry and tone	Slight weakness noticeable only on close inspection	Some to normal movement of forehead Ability to close eye with minimal effort and slight asymmetry Ability to move corners of mouth with maximal effort and slight asymmetry	*No synkinesis, contracture, or hemifacial spasm*
(III) dysfunction	Normal symmetry and tone	Obvious but not disfiguring difference between two sides, no functional impairment	Ability to close eye with maximal effort and obvious asymmetry	*Patients with obvious but not disfiguring synkinesis, contracture, and/or hemifacial spasm are grade III, regardless of degree of motor activity*
(IV) Moderately severe dysfunction	Normal symmetry and tone	Obvious weakness and/or disfiguring asymmetry	No movement of forehead, inability to close eye completely with maximal effort, asymmetrical movement of corners of mouth with maximal effort	*Patients with synkinesis, mass action, and/or hemifacial spasm severe enough to interfere with function are grade IV regardless of degree of motor activity*
(V) Severe dysfunction	Possible asymmetry with droop of corner of mouth and decreased or absent nasolabial fold	Only barely perceptible motion	No movement of forehead, incomplete closure of eye and only slight movement of lid with maximal effort, slight movement of corner of mouth	*Synkinesis, contracture, and hemifacial spasm usually absent*
(VI) Total paralysis	Loss of tone, asymmetry	No motion		*No synkinesis, contracture, or hemifacial spasm*

Note: This is the scale in its initial format, and the column labeled "secondary deficits" was omitted prior to its adoption by the American Academy of Otolaryngology-Head and Neck Surgery. Used with permission from House JW, Brackmann DE. Facial nerve grading system. Otolaryngol Head Neck Surg 1985;93(2):146–147.

Table 5.3   The facial nerve grading questionnaire

1) Are you able to raise your eyebrow on the surgery side?

 Yes/No

2) Are you able to move the corner of your mouth, as in a smile on the surgery side?

 Yes/No

3) Please estimate the percentage of facial motion on the surgery side of your face compared with the normal side.

 0% (no motion)

 20%

 40%

 60%

 80%

 100% (normal or same)

4) When you smile, does the eye on the surgery side close?

 Yes/No

5) Which of the following treatments do you use for your eye?

 Ointment

 Drops

 Patch

 Other

6) Have you had surgery on your eye? If yes, type of surgery: _____

7) Have you had other surgery for your facial nerve function?

 Nerve transfer

 Muscle transfer

 Cosmetic

 Other: _____

8) How many months passed before the beginning of the return of facial movement on the surgery side?

 1

 2–3

 4–9

 More than 9

 No movement has returned

Used with permission from Cullen RD, House JW, Brackmann DE, Luxford WM, Fisher LM. Evaluation of facial function with a questionnaire: reliability and validity. Otol Neurotol 2007;28(5):719–722.

There is a degree of subjectiveness involved in the modified HB scale, which is most apparent for patients with moderate to moderately severe facial paralysis.[11] For example, a patient with no brow movement who can completely close his/her eye with effort may be graded HB III or HB IV depending on the observer. Modifications recommended by the authors to improve scoring accuracy in moderately severe paralysis with objective measurement of brow elevation and commissure excursion have been largely overlooked, and the HB scale is most commonly used in the format excluding these measurements.[1]

A self-assessment facial nerve function questionnaire, based on the HB scale, has been validated for patients after acoustic neuroma treatment (**Table 5.3**).[12] High interrater reliability coefficients were found between clinicians and patients at 1 year after therapy. The HB scale has been found to have important implications for facial nerve recovery after acoustic neuroma surgery. Tumor size, intraoperative facial nerve stimulation, and severity of immediate postoperative paralysis can be used with the HB scale to make predictions regarding facial nerve recovery.[13–15]

■ Additional Scoring Metrics

Since its introduction, the modified HB Facial Nerve Grading Scale was found to be more efficient and reliable than the existing grading systems of that time.[16] Multiple grading systems have developed in the past 25 years that have been suggested as refinements or replacement systems to further describe patients with moderate to moderately severe paralysis and their secondary deficits.

Attempting to reduce subjective influence on scoring, the Burres-Fisch system was developed in 1986, in which the observer compares a subject's facial expressions against seven standard facial expressions. Although it demonstrated excellent correlation with the modified HB scale, this scale takes over 20 minutes to administer and does not account for secondary defects.

The Nottingham system was later proposed as a replacement system to address the subjectivity of the modified HB scale.[17] At rest and at maximal effort, measurements are obtained from above the brow and below the orbit, as well as from the lateral canthus to the lateral oral commissure. These values are then averaged and compared between the two sides. Synkinesis and hemifacial spasm are considered modifiers, as are dry eyes, dysgeusia, and gustatory tears (**Fig. 5.1**). The scale cannot be used in patients with bilateral weakness and requires more time than the HB scale, although it can still be administered in less than 5 minutes.

The Sunnybrook scale was introduced as an alternative to the HB scale in 1996 (**Table 5.4**). An observer subjectively scores regional symmetry at rest on a scale of 0 to 2. Next, the observer rates facial movement in five different expressions from 1 to 5. Synkinesis is judged on a four-point scale in five basic facial expressions. These values are combined on weighted scales to become a single numerical value. The scale is relatively easy to administer and is sensitive to fine changes in facial nerve function. However, there is a significant time commitment to administering it, and it retains a subjective component, which limits its precision. Measurements for this scale can be obtained in approximately 5 minutes.

The Facial Nerve Grading Scale 2.0 is a recently proposed substitute for the modified HB scale.[18] This adaptation has been developed to describe regional weakness, synkinesis, and other secondary deficits (**Table 5.5**). In a series of facial movements, the examiner grades the function of the brow, eye, nasolabial fold, and oral commisure on a scale of 1 to 6. Synkinesis is given a score of 0 to 3. The cumulative score, from 4 to 24, is then ranked on a scale of I to VI. Using this scale, interobserver reliability in cases of moderately severe facial paralysis made modest improvements over the modified HB scale, from 57.5% to 64%.[16] Additional work may demonstrate that this is a viable alternative to the modified HB scale that is quick, conveys a significant amount of information, and is easy to administer.

Computer-assisted grading has been suggested to be a rapid, reliable scoring method for the paralyzed face. Several programs have been developed that use image subtraction, luminescence, or moiré topography to generate a composite score evaluating dynamic facial function.[19–21] While promising, computer-assisted techniques will always be limited by the requirements of specialized, proprietary software, and additional personnel training required to operate the equipment.

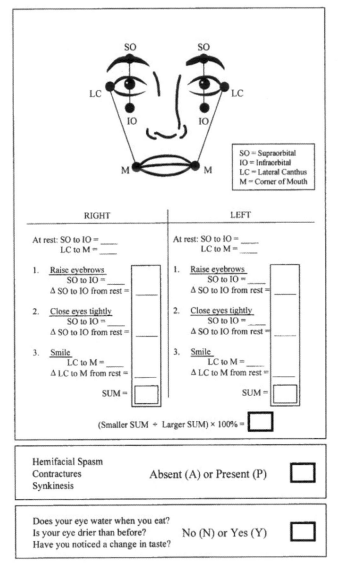

Fig. 5.1 The Nottingham facial nerve grading system. (Used with permission from Kang TS, Vrabec JT, Giddings N, Terris DJ. Facial Nerve Grading Systems (1985-2002): Beyond the House-Brackmann Scale. Otology & Neurology. 2002; 23:767-771.)

■ Conclusion

Studies have shown that scales such as the Sunnybrook, HB, and Yanagihara scales demonstrate similar levels of agreement for the clinician evaluating the paralyzed face.[22] Still, decades of research that have utilized the modified HB scale would need to be re-interpreted if a new scale is implemented. Currently, the HB scale remains the most widely accepted scale for facial nerve measurement because of its ease, quickness, and predictive value.

Table 5.4 The Sunnybrook facial nerve grading scale

Resting Symmetry		Symmetry of Voluntary Movement						Synkinesis			
			No movement	Slight movement	Mild excursion	Movement almost complete	Movement complete		None	Mild	Moderate	Severe
Eye	Normal	0	Forehead wrinkle	1	2	3	4	5		1	2	3	4
	Narrow	1											
	Wide	1											
	Eyelid surgery	1											
Cheek (nasolabial fold)	Normal	0	Gentle eye closure	1	2	3	4	5		1	2	3	4
	Absent	2											
	Less pronounced	1											
	More pronounced	1	Open mouth smile	1	2	3	4	5		1	2	3	4
Mouth	Normal	0											
	Corner drooped	1	Snarl	1	2	3	4	5		1	2	3	4
	Corner pulled Up/out	1	Lip pucker	1	2	3	4	5		1	2	3	4
Resting symmetry score			**Voluntary movement score**						**Synkinesis score**				

Note: This regional weighted system is based on evaluation of different facial regions including resting symmetry, symmetry of voluntary movement, and synkinesis to form a composite score of 0 to 100. Voluntary movement score × 4 − resting symmetry score × 5 − synkinesis score × 1 = composite score
Used with permission from Ross BG, Fradet G, Nedzelski JM. Development of a sensitive clinical facial grading system. Otolaryngol Head Neck Surg 1996; 114:380–6.

Table 5.5 The facial nerve grading scale 2.0 by region

Score	Brow	Eye	Nasolabial Fold	Oral
1	Normal	Normal	Normal	Normal
2	Slight weakness > 75% of normal	Slight weakness > 75% of normal Complete closure with mild effort	Slight weakness > 75% of normal	Slight weakness > 75% of normal
3	Obvious weakness > 50% of normal Resting symmetry	Obvious weakness > 50% of normal Complete closure with maximal effort	Obvious weakness > 50% of normal Resting symmetry	Obvious weakness > 50% of normal Resting symmetry
4	Asymmetry at rest < 50% of normal	Asymmetry at rest < 50% of normal Cannot close completely	Asymmetry at rest < 50% of normal	Asymmetry at rest < 50% of normal
5	Trace movement	Trace movement	Trace movement	Trace movement
6	No movement	No movement	No movement	No movement

Grade	Total score
I	4
II	5–9
III	10–14
IV	15–19
V	20–23
VI	24

Score	Degree of movement
0	None
1	Slight synkinesis; minimal contracture
2	Obvious synkinesis; mild to moderate contracture
3	Disfiguring synkinesis; severe contracture

Used with permission from Vrabec JT, Backous DD, Djalilian HR, et al; Facial Nerve Disorders Committee. Facial Nerve Grading System 2.0. Otolaryngol Head Neck Surg 2009 Apr;140(4):445-50.

References

1. House JW, Brackmann DE. Facial nerve grading system. Otolaryngol Head Neck Surg 1985;93(2):146–147
2. Botman JW, Jongkees LB. The result of intratemporal treatment of facial palsy. Pract Otorhinolaryngol (Basel) 1955;17(2):80–100
3. May M. Facial paralysis, peripheral type: a proposed method of reporting. (Emphasis on diagnosis and prognosis, as well as electrical and chorda tympani nerve testing). Laryngoscope 1970;80(3):331–390
4. Peiterson E. Natural history of Bell's palsy. In: Graham MD, House WF, eds. Disorders of the Facial Nerve: Anatomy, Diagnosis and Management. New York: Raven Press; 1982:307–312
5. Adour KK, Swanson PJ Jr. Facial paralysis in 403 consecutive patients: emphasis on treatment response in patients with Bell's palsy. Trans Am Acad Ophthalmol Otolaryngol 1971;75(6):1284–1301
6. Yanagihara N. Grading of facial palsy. In: Fisch U, ed. Facial nerve surgery. Proceedings: Third International Symposium on Facial Nerve Surgery, Zurich, 1976. Kugler Medical Publications, Amstelveen, Netherlands; and Aesculapius Publishing Co., Birmingham, AL; 1977:533–535
7. Stennerl E. Facial nerve paralysis scoring system. In: Fisch U, ed. Facial nerve surgery. Proceedings: Third International Symposium on Facial Nerve Surgery, Zurich, 1976. Kugler Medical Publications, Amstelveen, Netherlands; and Aesculapius Publishing Co., Birmingham, AL; 1977:543–547
8. Yanagihara N. Grading system for evaluation of facial palsy. In: Portmann M, ed. Proceedings of the Fifth International Symposium on the Facial Nerve. New York, NY: Masson, Inc; 1985: 41–42.
9. House JW, Brackmann DE. Facial nerve grading system. Otolaryngol Head Neck Surg 1985;93(2):146–147
10. Friedman RA, House JW. Use of the House-Brackmann facial nerve grading scale with acute and subacute facial palsy. In: Yanagihara N, ed. New Horizons in Facial Nerve Research and Facial Expression. The Hague, The Netherlands: Kugler Publications; 1998:529–532
11. King TT, Sparrow OC, Arias JM, O'Connor AF. Repair of facial nerve after removal of cerebellopontine angle tumors: a comparative study. J Neurosurg 1993;78(5):720–725
12. Cullen RD, House JW, Brackmann DE, Luxford WM, Fisher LM. Evaluation of facial function with a questionnaire: reliability and validity. Otol Neurotol 2007;28(5):719–722
13. Fenton JE, Chin RY, Fagan PA, Sterkers O, Sterkers JM. Predictive factors of long-term facial nerve function after vestibular schwannoma surgery. Otol Neurotol 2002;23(3):388–392
14. Isaacson B, Telian SA, El-Kashlan HK. Facial nerve outcomes in middle cranial fossa vs translabyrinthine approaches. Otolaryngol Head Neck Surg 2005;133(6):906–910
15. Wiet RJ, Mamikoglu B, Odom L, Hoistad DL. Long-term results of the first 500 cases of acoustic neuroma surgery. Otolaryngol Head Neck Surg 2001;124(6):645–651
16. Croxson G, May M, Mester SJ. Grading facial nerve function: House-Brackmann versus Burres-Fisch methods. Am J Otol 1990;11(4):240–246

17. Kang TS, Vrabec JT, Giddings N, Terris DJ. Facial nerve grading systems (1985–2002): beyond the House-Brackmann scale. Otol Neurotol 2002;23(5):767–771
18. Vrabec JT, Backous DD, Djalilian HR, et al; Facial Nerve Disorders Committee. Facial Nerve Grading System 2.0. Otolaryngol Head Neck Surg 2009;140(4):445–450
19. Neely JG, Cheung JY, Wood M, Byers J, Rogerson A. Computerized quantitative dynamic analysis of facial motion in the paralyzed and synkinetic face. Am J Otol 1992;13(2):97–107
20. Yuen K, Inokuchi I, Maeta M, Kawakami SI, Masuda Y. Evaluation of facial palsy by moiré topography index. Otolaryngol Head Neck Surg 1997;117(5):567–572
21. Sargent EW, Fadhli OA, Cohen RS. Measurement of facial movement with computer software. Arch Otolaryngol Head Neck Surg 1998;124(3):313–318
22. Berg T, Jonsson L, Engström M. Agreement between the Sunnybrook, House-Brackmann, and Yanagihara facial nerve grading systems in Bell's palsy. Otol Neurotol 2004;25(6):1020–1026

6 Imaging of the Facial Nerve

Ajay Gupta and C. Douglas Phillips

With the advent of high-resolution multidetector computed tomography (CT; using 16- and 64-detector arrays) and increasing field strength (3 teslas and greater) for magnetic resonance imaging (MRI) scanners, CT and MRI images have continued to improve. It is apparent that CT and MRI play complementary roles in imaging of the facial nerve in the normal and pathologic state. In this chapter, we briefly summarize some of the imaging techniques involved in evaluating the facial nerve and then turn our attention to the imaging findings of several specific forms of facial nerve pathology.

■ Imaging Techniques

Computed Tomography Imaging of the Facial Nerve

Though imaging protocols vary, in most cases, intravenous contrast is not necessary for CT evaluation of the facial nerve. In general, 0.625 mm or thinner helically acquired axial images with reconstructions in the coronal plane form the basis of most CT protocols. Despite its inability to directly image the facial nerve itself, CT can play an important role in the appropriate clinical settings. Given its high resolution of bony structures (including of the facial nerve canal in all segments), CT is particularly well suited for evaluation of facial nerve injury related to temporal bone fracture, destructive osseous facial nerve lesions, or calcification that can be seen with hemangioma of the facial nerve.[1] In addition, CT can play a critical role in assessing the intratympanic facial nerve and its relation to bony structures such as the footplate of the stapes or the lateral semicircular canal. More distally in its course, the relationship of the canal of the mastoid segment of the facial nerve and the jugular foramen is also well evaluated on CT. Besides the inability to directly visualize the facial nerve, another disadvantage of CT is its use of ionizing radiation, a particularly important consideration in pediatric populations. Nonetheless, when correctly utilized, CT demonstrates bony detail not possible with MRI and can serve as an important component of the imaging of facial nerve pathology.

Magnetic Resonance Imaging of the Facial Nerve

Generally, high-resolution multiplanar T1- and T2-weighted images along with gadolinium-enhanced, fat-suppressed T1-weighted images should be included in most standard imaging protocols of the facial nerve. Unlike CT, MRI allows direct visualization of the facial nerve, especially in the cisternal, intracanalicular, mastoid, and extracranial segments. In addition, if clinical findings suggest a lesion from the origin of the pontine nuclei of the facial nerve (or even from the cortex in a supranuclear facial palsy), MRI can offer far greater anatomic detail and contrast resolution of the brain. Heavily T2-weighted three-dimensional images are particularly useful in evaluating neural and vascular structures adjacent to the bright cerebrospinal fluid (allowing, for example, separation of the facial nerve from the components of the vestibulocochlear nerve in the internal auditory canal). In addition, MRI is valuable in demonstrating abnormal enhancement of the facial nerve in its cisternal, intracanalicular, and intratemporal segments, which can be seen in infectious, inflammatory, and neoplastic pathologies. In this regard, it is important to keep in mind that mild, symmetric perineural venous enhancement can normally be seen within the geniculate ganglion and the tympanic and mastoid segments.[2] Finally, in the evaluation of suspected vascular lesions causing facial nerve symptoms (such as hemifacial spasm), magnetic resonance angiography can play a valuable role in assessing the relationship between anomalous/tortuous central vascular structures and the adjacent facial nerve.[1]

The authors' simplified approach to choice of modality for imaging of facial nerve lesions is seen in **Fig. 6.1**. Should physical exam and clinical findings localize a facial nerve deficit anywhere from cortical motor inputs to the cisternal segment of the internal auditory canal (IAC), precontrast and contrast-enhanced MRI should be the initial examination of choice. From the level of the IAC distally to the exit of the facial nerve through the stylomastoid foramen, both CT and MRI play complementary roles, and the first exam of choice depends on multiple factors as discussed and detailed as follows. Finally, distal to the stylomastoid foramen (e.g., for the evaluation of a suspected intraparotid lesion causing a facial nerve deficit) with its ability to resolve and characterize soft tissue lesions, MRI is the imaging exam of choice.

■ Imaging of Specific Pathology of the Facial Nerve

Bell Palsy

Patients with the typical symptoms of acute onset peripheral facial nerve palsy are frequently referred for imaging evaluation. Contrast-enhanced MRI is the mainstay for

The Facial Nerve: In Schematic

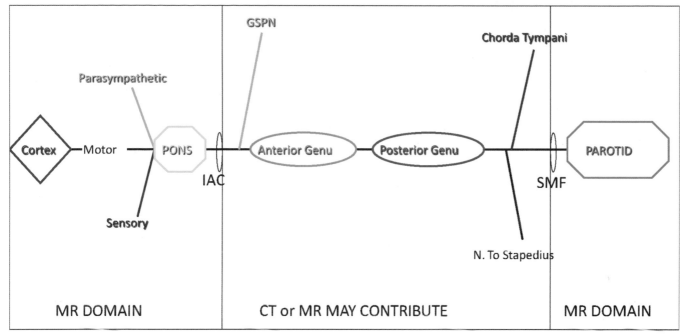

Fig. 6.1 Imaging of the facial nerve can require computed tomography (*CT*) and/or magnetic resonance (*MR*) imaging. The schematic illustrates that the preference of imaging study is dependent on the anatomical location. GSPN, greater superficial petrosal nerve; IAC, internal auditory canal; SMF, stylomastoid foramen.

imaging of this clinical presentation, and the typical imaging is abnormal uniform enhancement of the facial nerve, which is usually normal in size or only slightly enlarged (**Fig. 6.2a, b**).[3] Focal linear enhancement in the fundus of the IAC is a classic finding, with enhancement also frequently noted along the intratemporal portion of the nerve.[4,5] Enhancement of more distal portions of the facial nerve, such as the mastoid segment, can occur, but is less frequently observed. Persistent enhancement of the nerve can lag clinical symptomatic improvement and can be seen for up to about 1 year in some cases. The mechanism of facial nerve enhancement in Bell palsy is not entirely clear but may be a function of the hyperemia of the perineural structures from inflammation or may be secondary to frank breakdown of the blood–nerve barrier. Nonetheless, depending on the timing of imaging, not all cases of Bell palsy demonstrate pathologic facial nerve enhancement with reported rates varying from 57–100%.[1]

Given its generally benign and self-limited clinical course, when a classic clinical presentation for Bell palsy is noted, imaging findings add little to patient management. However, in atypical presentations (slow insidious onset, progressive worsening of symptoms, failure of normal resolution within 4 months, etc.), MRI can provide valuable insight into other possible causes for facial nerve dysfunction along the entire course of the visualized nerve.[6] In such cases, focal facial nerve enlargement or nodular, nonlinear enhancement should suggest an alternate diagnosis, and the possibility of a neoplastic entity should be entertained in the correct context. Slow insidious onset of facial paralysis or weakness requires imaging of the complete facial nerve including the entire parotid, temporal bone, and the central (brainstem) course.

Ramsay Hunt Syndrome

Thought to result from a similar reactivation of varicella zoster infection from the geniculate ganglion, the acute onset of symptoms including clinically apparent, sometimes hemorrhagic vesicles on the pinna and external auditory canal often result in the request for an imaging examination. Contrast-enhanced MRI is the imaging exam of choice, with variable findings, often indistinguishable from Bell palsy, including enhancement of the tympanic, geniculate, and mastoid segments of the facial nerve; it should be noted, however, that up to 50% of patients may not demonstrate abnormal enhancement of any component of the facial nerve.[1] Though the physical exam findings should make the presence of lesions along the pinna and external auditory canal clear, MRI can confirm findings in cases with florid subcutaneous vesicular disease by demonstrating abnormal soft tissue enhancement (**Fig. 6.3a, b**).

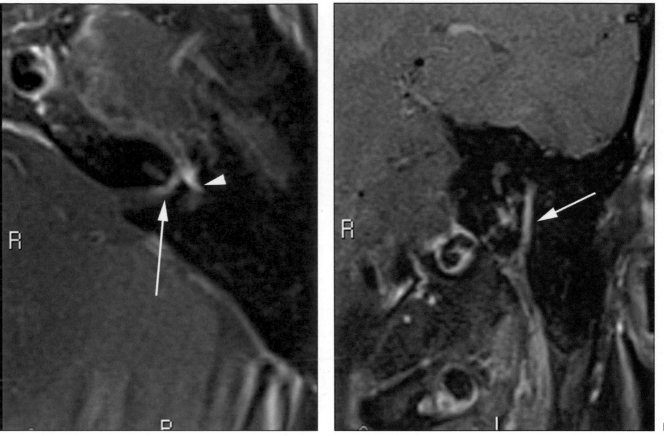

Fig. 6.2a, b Bell palsy. (**a**) Axial T1-weighted postcontrast image shows enhancement extending from the fundus (*white arrow*) of the internal auditory canal into the proximal tympanic segment (*arrowhead*) including the geniculate ganglion. (**b**) Coronal T1-weighted postcontrast image shows abnormal enhancement of the mastoid segment of the facial nerve (*arrow*) through the stylomastoid foramen.

Hemifacial Spasm

The anatomic basis for the clinical syndrome of hemifacial spasm is, in > 90% of cases, a redundant or tortuous vascular loop that causes compression of proximal cisternal segment of the facial nerve.[1] The anterior inferior cerebellar, posterior inferior cerebellar, and vertebral arteries are most commonly responsible for this syndrome.[7] MRI (typically combined with magnetic resonance angiography) can display, often in exquisite anatomic detail, the cisternal segment of the facial nerve and the culprit compressing vascular structure (**Fig. 6.4a, b**). The vessel causing compression usually exerts mass effect near the root exit zone of the facial nerve near the brainstem. Here, normally the medially positioned motor fibers are compressed by the anterolaterally positioned offending vessel.

Though a vascular loop can often be identified, absence of this finding on high-resolution MRI may occur because focal nerve compression may be secondary to a vessel that is below the spatial resolution threshold of MRI; therefore, a negative MRI study should not discourage surgical decompression in clinically appropriate cases.[8] Conversely, an enlarged or prominent vessel in the cerebellopontine angle (CPA) cistern can be seen in up to a third of asymptomatic patients, many of whom display vertebrobasilar

dolichoectasia secondary to long-standing hypertension. As such, imaging work-up for this syndrome should be considered an adjunct to clinical history and physical exam findings.[8]

Primary Tumors of the Facial Nerve

Schwannoma

Both CT and MRI play important roles in the preoperative imaging of suspected facial nerve schwannomas. The imaging findings for this entity vary based on the location of the lesion, which can occur anywhere along the course of the facial nerve. Frequently, these lesions can present with findings similar to the more common vestibular schwannoma, with an enhancing, possibly fusiform mass on MRI seen within the CPA and/or IAC (**Fig. 6.5a, b**).

Extension of the CPA/IAC mass into the labyrinthine segment with associated expansion of the labyrinthine canal on CT should raise facial nerve schwannoma to the top of the imaging differential. Lesions involving the geniculate ganglion cannot only demonstrate marked expansion of the bony canal of the ganglion, but may occasionally demonstrate extension into the adjacent middle cranial fossa,

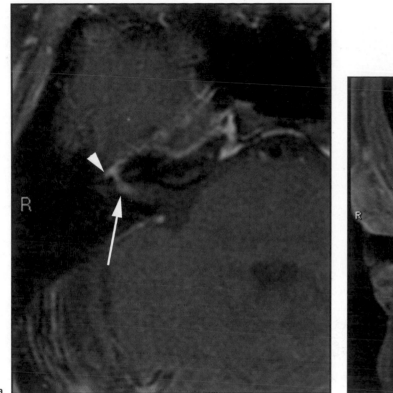

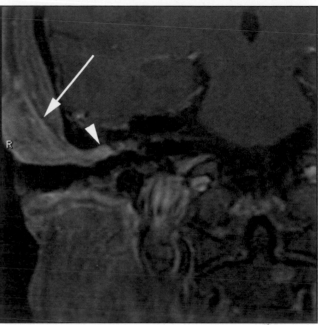

Fig. 6.3a, b Ramsay Hunt syndrome. (**a**) Axial T1-weighted postcontrast image demonstrates abnormal enhancement from the fundus of the internal auditory canal (*arrow*) into the geniculate ganglion and to the proximal tympanic segment (*arrowhead*) of the facial nerve in a patient with facial nerve paralysis and clinically apparent Ramsay Hunt syndrome. (**b**) Coronal T1-weighted postcontrast image demonstrates marked abnormal enhancement along the soft tissues surrounding the subcutaneous tissues of the external auditory canal (*arrow*) extending to the level of the tympanic membrane (*arrowhead*) in a patient with hemorrhagic vesicular rash visible on physical exam.

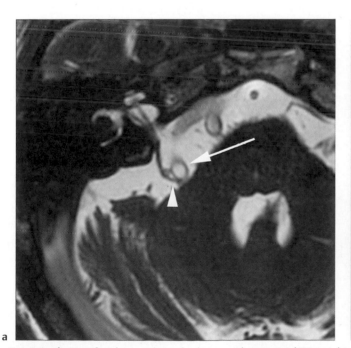

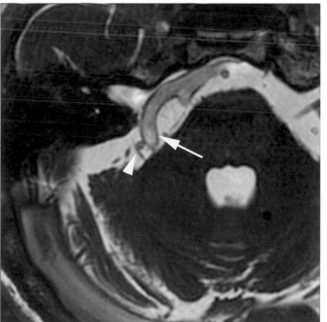

Fig. 6.4a, b Hemifacial spasm/vascular loop syndrome. Axial T2-weighted images (**a, b**) show marked vertebrobasilar dolichoectasia (*arrows*) causing posterolateral displacement and mass effect on the cisternal segment of the right facial and vestibulocochlear nerve complex (*arrowheads*). The patient also had right-sided sensorineural hearing loss.

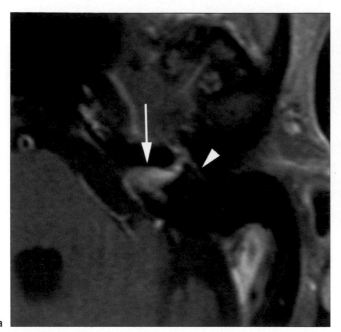 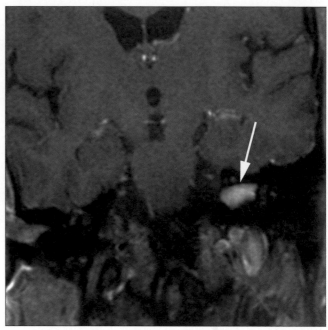

a

b

Fig. 6.5a, b Facial nerve schwannoma. (**a**) Axial T1-weighted postcontrast image demonstrates an enhancing left cerebellopontine angle mass extending into the left internal auditory canal (*arrow*). Note the enhancement extending into the labyrinthine segment (*arrowhead*) via the geniculate ganglion, differentiating the lesion from vestibular schwannoma. (**b**) Coronal T1-weighted postcontrast image demonstrates enhancing mass filling left internal auditory canal (*arrow*) in a patient with facial nerve schwannoma.

possibly mimicking an extra-axial meningioma.[6] Involvement of the labyrinthine bony canal or the geniculate fossa are two important imaging findings that may allow appropriate preoperative distinction of this lesion from the more common vestibular schwannoma, and distinction that has important prognostic significance. Examining intratemporal facial nerve schwannomas with CT is helpful not only to evaluate for possible bony canal expansion, but also to examine lesion relationship to the adjacent otic capsule, ossicles, and semicircular canals.

Though the normal intraparotid facial nerve cannot be consistently seen on any imaging modality, MRI is useful to demonstrate an intraparotid mass and possible continuity with the more proximal facial nerve in patients with a suspected intraparotid schwannoma. In these patients, a fusiform or tubular enhancing lesion along the expected course of the intraparotid facial nerve should raise suspicion for an intraparotid schwannoma.

Hemangioma

Though relatively rare lesions, both CT and MRI can help suggest an image-specific diagnosis. Facial nerve hemangiomas are generally intratemporal bone lesions and are most commonly seen in the region of the geniculate ganglion. CT can be valuable to evaluate the temporal bone for changes suggestive of facial nerve hemangioma, which include multiseptated expansile osseous change (sometimes referred to as a "honeycomb" appearance) and small calcifications within the hemangioma itself (**Fig. 6.6a**).[1,9] Although this honeycomb bone appearance

is seen in about half of all hemangiomas, MRI can further characterize this lesion. Given the vascular nature of this tumor, facial nerve hemangiomas are T2 hyperintense and can demonstrate avid homogenous contrast enhancement on postcontrast T1-weighted imaging (**Fig. 6.6b**).[10]

Metastasis to the Facial Nerve

Perineural Spread of Tumor

Because perineural spread of tumor along the facial nerve can be clinically silent and its presence can dramatically alter therapeutic options for patients with malignancy, imaging can play a vital role in diagnosis. In patients with head and neck malignancies known to have perineural spread such as adenoid cystic or squamous cell carcinoma, involvement of the facial nerve typically occurs through retrograde spread along motor facial branches at the level of the parotid gland.[11]

Alternatively, spread of tumor can occur along the greater superficial petrosal nerve via adjacent tumor-involved nerves in the pterygopalatine fossa, or via the auriculotemporal nerve, or other potential neural connections between other cranial nerves and the facial nerve. In either case, MRI with T1-weighted precontrast and postcontrast imaging are the mainstays of imaging diagnosis (**Fig. 6.7a, b**).[12]

On precontrast T1 images, obliteration of the normal bright fat signal in the pterygopalatine fossa or any of the bony canals containing the facial nerve should be viewed with suspicion. On postcontrast images, a typical

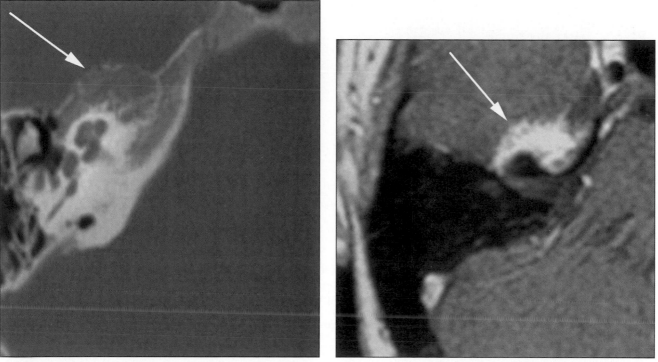

Fig. 6.6a, b Facial nerve hemangioma. (**a**) Axial computed tomography image shows expansile lesion with classic multiseptated honeycomb appearance involving the region of geniculate ganglion (*arrow*) in a patient with pathologically proven facial nerve hemangioma. (**b**) Axial T1-weighted postcontrast magnetic resonance image at the same level shows avid enhancement of the lesion (*arrow*).

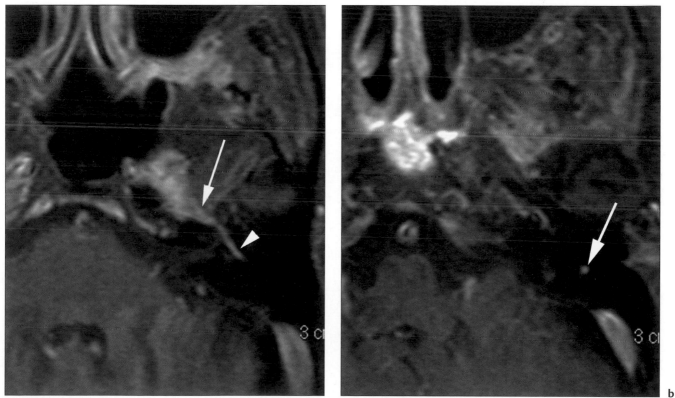

Fig. 6.7a, b Perineural tumor spread, extension from trigeminal nerve branches to the facial nerve. (**a**) Axial postcontrast T1-weighted image shows abnormal enhancement along Meckel cave (*arrow*) from the trigeminal nerve with abnormal enhancement extending posteriorly into the tympanic segment of the facial nerve (*arrowhead*) via the greater superficial petrosal nerve in a patient with squamous cell carcinoma involving left masticator space (not shown). (**b**) Axial postcontrast T1-weighted image shows abnormal enhancement along the mastoid segment of the facial nerve (*arrow*) illustrating more inferior extent of perineural tumor.

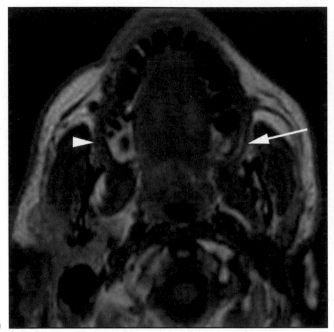
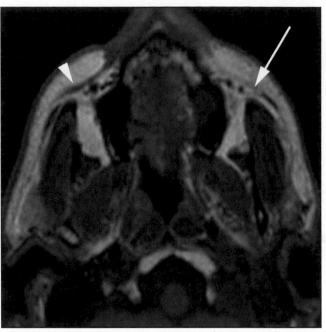

a   b

Fig. 6.8a, b Denervation atrophy. (**a**) Axial T1-weighted image shows atrophy and partial fatty degeneration of left buccinator musculature (*arrow*), compared with normal contralateral side (*arrowhead*). The patient underwent prior parotid resection for neoplasm. (**b**) More cephalad axial T1-weighted image at the inferior aspect of the maxillary sinuses demonstrates similar, asymmetric left levator labii atrophy (arrow), compared with normal contralateral side (arrowhead).

appearance is an enhancing, invasive parotid mass extending along through the stylomastoid foramen into the mastoid segment of the facial nerve. In these patients, denervation of muscles supplied by the facial nerve can occasionally be seen on MRI by evidence of asymmetric muscle atrophy and possible associated high intramuscular signal from edema/fatty change (**Fig. 6.8a, b**).[6]

Leptomeningeal Metastasis

In patients with tumors that have a propensity for leptomeningeal metastases such as lung, breast, melanoma, lymphoma, or leukemia, contrast-enhanced MRI can be valuable in identifying lesions involving the cisternal and intracanalicular segments of the facial nerve. On postcontrast images, abnormal enhancement of the nerves within the CPA-IAC can be seen unilaterally or bilaterally (**Fig. 6.9**). Enhancement is generally smooth and linear though nodular, mass-like enhancement can sometimes occur.[13] Findings can be unilateral or bilateral. Though nonspecific, the imaging diagnosis can be suggested in the correct patient population. Additional imaging clues include evidence of parenchymal brain metastases or enhancing meningeal disease elsewhere in the brain.

Congenital Abnormalities of the Facial Nerve

Congenital abnormalities of the facial nerve that can be identified on imaging studies can range from asymptomatic lesions to those that cause profound facial nerve

dysfunction or paralysis.[6] The most common structural abnormality seen on imaging is bony dehiscence of the tympanic segment of the facial nerve, an abnormality that can be seen in up to 50% of the general population and is most commonly noted at the level of the oval window.[1] This finding is almost always asymptomatic, though rarely can be a cause of conductive hearing loss when the stapes anomalously abuts the dehiscent nerve. Because the normal bony canal is extremely thin, dehiscence can only

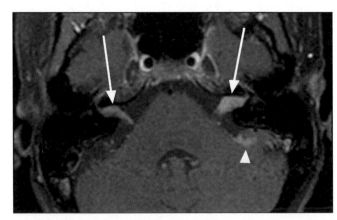

Fig. 6.9 Leptomeningeal metastases to bilateral facial nerve. Axial T1-weighed postcontrast image in a patient with breast cancer demonstrates marked, smooth bilateral enhancement of the internal auditory canals, consistent with leptomeningeal metastases along facial and vestibulocochlear nerve complexes (*arrows*). Note the enhancing left cerebellopontine nodular leptomeningeal metastases (*arrowhead*).

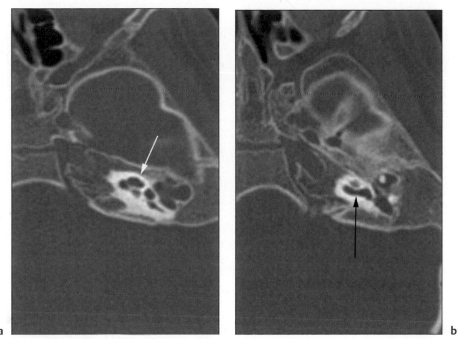

Fig. 6.10a, b Complete facial nerve aplasia. (**a**) Computed tomography image of the left inner ear structure demonstrates relatively normal bony structure of cochlea (*arrow*) with no internal auditory canal visible in this infant with right hemifacial paralysis. (**b**) Caudal computed tomography image shows relatively normal bony architecture of inner ear structures including basal turn of cochlea (*arrow*) with no internal auditory canal or expected bony canal of facial nerve.

reliably be diagnosed on CT in those cases where nerve protrusion is noted and can be best demonstrated on coronal images showing a smooth soft tissue density at the level of the oval window with an inferior rounded convexity at the undersurface of the lateral semicircular canal.[14]

Other congenital abnormalities of the facial nerve include hypoplasia or aplasia of the facial nerve as may be seen in rare sporadic abnormalities (**Fig. 6.10a, b**) or as a part of congenital syndromic abnormalities such as Möbius (**Fig. 6.11a, b**), CHARGE (coloboma of the

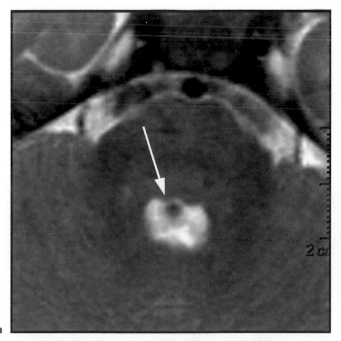

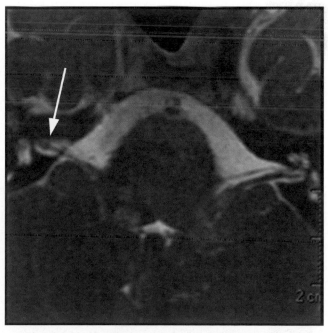

Fig. 6.11a, b Möbius syndrome. (**a**) Axial T2-weighted image in a newborn with right-sided facial nerve paralysis and abducens nerve dysfunction. Note the subtle hypoplasia of right facial colliculus (*arrow*), a feature that has been described with this rare congenital syndrome of sixth and seventh nerve palsies. (**b**) Axial T2-weighted image more inferiorly demonstrates mild hypoplasia of right internal auditory canal (*arrow*) and absence of cisternal segment of facial nerve.

eye, *h*eart defects, *a*tresia of the choanae, *r*etardation of growth and/or development, *g*enital and/or urinary abnormalities, and *e*ar abnormalities and deafness), Goldenhar, DiGeorge, or Poland syndromes.[6] In these cases, MRI can help establish a diagnosis and obviate the need for additional testing. In addition, in those entities with an anomalous facial nerve course, MRI can provide valuable information that may help avoid inadvertent iatrogenic injury at surgery.

■ Conclusion

With careful attention and with good technique, MRI and CT evaluation of the facial nerve can provide valuable clinical information that can aid in the management of a wide variety of pathology. With the ability of CT to display the fine bony details of the temporal bone and skull along with direct visualization of the facial nerve made possible by high-resolution MRI, these modalities should be considered complementary tools in the evaluation of suspected facial nerve disease.

References

1. Phillips CD, Hashisaki G, Veillon F. Anatomy and Development of the Facial Nerve. In: Swartz, JD and Loevner LA, eds. Imaging of the Temporal Bone. 4th ed. New York: Thieme Medical Publishers; 2009:444–479
2. Saremi F, Helmy M, Farzin S, Zee CS, Go JL. MRI of cranial nerve enhancement. AJR Am J Roentgenol 2005;185(6):1487–1497
3. Tien R, Dillon WP, Jackler RK. Contrast-enhanced MR imaging of the facial nerve in 11 patients with Bell's palsy. AJNR Am J Neuroradiol 1990;11(4):735–741
4. Engström M, Thuomas KA, Naeser P, Stålberg E, Jonsson L. Facial nerve enhancement in Bell's palsy demonstrated by different gadolinium-enhanced magnetic resonance imaging techniques. Arch Otolaryngol Head Neck Surg 1993;119(2):221–225
5. Sartoretti-Schefer S, Wichmann W, Valavanis A. Idiopathic, herpetic, and HIV-associated facial nerve palsies: abnormal MR enhancement patterns. AJNR Am J Neuroradiol 1994;15(3):479–485
6. Raghavan P, Mukherjee S, Phillips CD. Imaging of the facial nerve. Neuroimaging Clin N Am 2009;19(3):407–425
7. Sobel D, Norman D, Yorke CH, Newton TH. Radiography of trigeminal neuralgia and hemifacial spasm. AJR Am J Roentgenol 1980;135(1):93–95
8. Digre K, Corbett JJ. Hemifacial spasm: differential diagnosis, mechanism, and treatment. Adv Neurol 1988;49:151–176
9. Curtin HD, Jensen JE, Barnes L Jr, May M. "Ossifying" hemangiomas of the temporal bone: evaluation with CT. Radiology 1987;164(3):831–835
10. Shelton C, Brackmann DE, Lo WW, Carberry JN. Intratemporal facial nerve hemangiomas. Otolaryngol Head Neck Surg 1991;104(1):116–121
11. Parker GD, Harnsberger HR. Clinical-radiologic issues in perineural tumor spread of malignant diseases of the extracranial head and neck. Radiographics 1991;11(3):383–399
12. Rumboldt Z, Gordon L, Gordon L, Bonsall R, Ackermann S. Imaging in head and neck cancer. Curr Treat Options Oncol 2006;7(1):23–34
13. Lakshmi M, Glastonbury CM. Imaging of the cerebellopontine angle. Neuroimaging Clin N Am 2009;19(3):393–406
14. Swartz JD. The facial nerve canal: CT analysis of the protruding tympanic segment. Radiology 1984;153(2):443–447

7 Differential Diagnosis of Acute Facial Paralysis

Maurizio Barbara

Facial paralysis (FP) consists of weakness of the face musculature. The timing of this weakness usually is immediate, taking place within a few hours (**Table 7.1**), although some etiologies of facial weakness cause paralysis over weeks to months. The most common type of FP occurs overnight so that patients wake up and notice the paralysis when they look in the mirror. Acute FP (AFP) is generally unilateral, being bilateral in rare cases. While Bell palsy represents the most common type of unilateral FP (50–66%), the bilateral forms may appear during the clinical course or onset of several systemic, sometimes life-threatening diseases or events that need to be recognized to arrange an appropriate treatment of the affected patient.

When examining patients with AFP, a thorough history taking is of utmost importance, especially focusing on some of the factors that may be helpful to the clinician: age, geographic localization, race of the patient, season of the year, preexisting at-risk syndromes or diseases, and concomitant signs or symptoms.

Table 7.1 Differential diagnosis of facial paralysis

Congenital	Botulism	Metastatic carcinoma (breast, kidney, lung, stomach, larynx, prostate, thyroid)
Forceps delivery and cranial molding	Mucormycosis	
Myotonic dystrophy	Lyme disease	**Toxicity**
Möbius syndrome	Leptospirosis	Thalidomide
	Genetic and metabolic	Tetanus
Traumatic	Diabetes	Diphtheria
Cortical injury	Hyperthyroidism	Carbon monoxide
Skull base fractures	Pregnancy	Lead intoxication
Brainstem injury	Hypertension	Anticancer drugs
Direct middle ear injury	Alcoholic neuropathy	
Barotrauma	Bulbopontine paralysis	**Iatrogenic**
	Oculopharyngeal muscular dystrophy	Mandibular block anesthesia
Neurologic		Antitetanus serum
Facial motor area lesion	**Vascular**	Rabies vaccination
Millar-Gubler syndrome	Anomalous sigmoid sinus	Otologic, neurotologic, skull base, and parotid surgery
	Benign intracranial hypertension	
Infectious	Intratemporal internal auditory canal aneurysm	Embolization
Malignant external otitis		
Acute or chronic otitis media	External carotid artery embolization for epistaxis	**Idiopathic**
Congenital or acquired cholesteatoma		Familial Bell palsy
Mastoiditis	**Neoplastic**	Melkersson-Rosenthal syndrome
Parotitis	Schwannoma	Hereditary hypertrophic neuropathy (Charcot-Marie-Tooth syndrome, Dejerine-Sottas syndrome)
Chickenpox	Paraganglioma	
Herpes zoster oticus	Leukemia	
Encephalitis	Meningioma	Periarterite nodosa
Type 1 poliomyelitis	Hemangioblastoma	Thrombotic thrombocytopenic purpura
Mumps	Pontine glioma	Guillain-Barré syndrome
Epstein-Barr	Sarcoma	Multiple sclerosis
Leprosy	Hydroadenoma	Myasthenia gravis
Human immunodeficiency virus	Facial nerve schwannoma	Sarcoidosis
Influenza	Teratoma	Wegener granulomatosis
Coxsackie	Fibrous dysplasia	Eosinophilic granuloma
Malaria	Neurofibromatosis type 2	Amyloidosis
Syphilis	Carcinomatous encephalitis	Hyperostoses (Paget disease, osteopetrosis)
Scleroma	Cholesterol granuloma	Kawasaki disease
Tubercolosis		

When considering age, the earliest AFP is the one occurring during or just after birth, with an incidence of 0.2% of live infants.[1] While congenital FP is rare, it may cause significant problems for the newborn such as difficulty with nursing and eye protection. This problem, if unresolved, may affect the child's speech, facial expression, emotional expression, and cause difficulty with eating. Possible etiologies include intrauterine posture, perinatal trauma, intrapartum compression, and familial and congenital aplasia of the nucleus, the latter being most frequently reported for bilateral cases, Möbius syndrome.[2] A complete examination is required to identify other associated congenital anomalies that may be associated with the FP (hemifacial microsomia).

■ Pediatric Acute Facial Paralysis

The most common acquired causes of AFP in childhood are represented by Kawasaki disease, Lyme disease, and Melkersson-Rosenthal syndrome.

Kawasaki Disease

This disease, named after the Japanese pediatrician who first described it in 1967, consists of a systemic vasculitis that manifests with coronary vessels aneurysms and is accompanied by high fever, skin rash, and enlarged neck lymph nodes. Other symptoms, such as painful and swollen joints, abdominal pain, diarrhea, irritability, and headaches, can also be observed. Most reports in the literature come from Asian countries and involve children under the age of 5. Facial nerve involvement is possible as a neurological manifestation of Kawasaki disease, presumably due to ischemia resulting from inflammation of the surrounding arteries. In the majority of cases, FP is unilateral, but bilateral involvement has also been reported.[3]

Kawasaki disease is a rare disease in which an infectious or genetic cause can be suspected; however, as yet no specific etiology has been identified. Diagnosis is not helped by any laboratory test and relies mainly on the age group involved (mostly children) and the presence of the heart disease. Aspirin and high-dosage intravenous gamma globulin are usually the treatment of choice that decreases, in the majority of the cases, the morbidity of the disease.

Neuroborreliosis or Lyme Disease

This pathological entity has been named after the report from a city in Connecticut (i.e., Lyme), where it was provoked in a school community by the bite of an insect (genus *Ixodes*, commonly called ticks) that caused multiple neurological involvement.[4] Facial nerve palsy is part of the syndrome along with other typical signs, like redness, fatigue, malaise, and fever. The insect's bite produces a bacterial infection via the spirochete *Borrelia burgdorferi*, mostly carried by white-tailed deer and white-footed mice (**Fig. 7.1**).

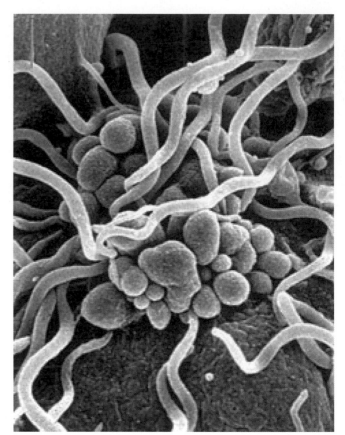

Fig. 7.1 Scanning electron micrograph of *Borrelia burgdoferi*, the agent causing Lyme disease or neuroborreliosis.

Neuroborreliosis (NBD) usually evolves in three stages: the first is characterized by erythema migrans at the site of the bite. This is often described as a "bull's eye" rash: a flat or slightly raised red spot at the site of the tick bite. This can be quite large and expanding in size with a clear arc in the center. In the second phase, days to weeks later, dissemination of the infection takes place and neurological symptoms may be seen; the third phase (months to years later) only develops in untreated subjects and corresponds to the chronic stage of the disease. Ten percent of patients with NBD develop unilateral or bilateral FP during the second or third stage of the disease, which usually resolves completely, although electrophysiological testing may reveal an incomplete facial recovery in a certain number of affected subjects.[5]

NBD must be considered when AFP occurs in the northern hemisphere and during summertime. These cases are often bilateral. A correct diagnostic work-up should include, among suspected cases, serologic testing like single step VIsE (IR6) enzyme-linked immunosorbent assay for detection of immunoglobulin G antibodies to *Borrelia burgdorferi* peptide, and of immunoglobulin G and immunoglobulin M antibodies to sonicate *Borrelia burgdorferi* antigens.[6] This test has been shown to express positivity during all stages of the disease, be less time-consuming, and as reliable as the formerly recommended two-tier test, which may, instead, be negative in the early stages.[7] Treatment consists of 10 to 14 days of antibiotics (ceftriaxone, 2 g/day; doxycycline, 100 mg twice a day; or azithromycin, 500 mg/day) that allow complete remission of the disease when administered in the early, first stage of NBD.

Melkersson-Rosenthal Syndrome

This rare disease of unknown etiology (with supposed genetic predisposition) consists of a triad of symptoms: recurrent orofacial edema (mainly the upper lip), relapsing facial palsy, and fissured (folds and furrows) tongue. Interestingly enough, Melkersson in 1928 described the coexistence of recurrent facial palsy with angioneurotic edema, and Rosenthal (1931) added the fissured tongue to the clinical picture that was eventually named after both of them by Luscher in 1949. The most frequent sign is fissured tongue (granulomatous chcilitis of Miescher), while association with FP occurs in half of the patients and the complete triad is only present in 25% of patients. This condition usually starts in the second decade of life, and the manifestations usually occur sequentially and alternating (rarely simultaneously). Bilateral, sequential FP with relapses generally coincides with the side of facial swelling. Melkersson-Rosenthal syndrome may at times conceal Crohn disease or sarcoidosis. Attacks may occur as frequently as days apart or be separated by years. Swelling may persist and increase after recurrent attacks, eventually becoming permanent. Treatment is symptomatic and may include medication therapies with nonsteroidal anti-inflammatory drugs and corticosteroids to reduce swelling, as well as antibiotics and immune-suppressants. Facial nerve decompression in its entire course has also been proposed to avoid or reduce the number of relapsing episodes.[8]

■ Adult Acute Facial Paralysis

When considering unilateral AFP in adults, the diagnosis of Bell palsy is usually formulated after exclusion of other possible causes, mostly rare systemic diseases that often prompt an immediate treatment.

Amyloidosis

Amyloidosis is a rare disease characterized by deposition of extracellular fibrillar protein in various tissues. Several clinical variants have been described, with two main forms of systemic amyloidosis: primary and secondary. In primary systemic amyloidosis, the heart, tongue, and gastrointestinal tract are usually affected, while in secondary systemic amyloidosis (tuberculosis, osteomyelitis, or rheumatoid arthritis) the disease usually involves the spleen, adrenals, liver, and kidneys. In the localized form of amyloidosis, the amyloid deposits are restricted to specific anatomic regions, such as isolated tongue involvement. In addition, a systemic form of amyloidosis associated with multiple myeloma, where the tissues affected are the same as in primary systemic amyloidosis, has been described. One also has to consider that normal aging encompasses amyloid deposition in joints, the heart, and vasculature, but the disease is usually asymptomatic until a major substitution of the functional tissue by amyloid takes place. Type 2 diabetes and Alzheimer disease, for instance, have also been put in relation to amyloid deposition. Apart from isolated reports on localization of amyloid in the facial nerve, it has to be mentioned that the most common form is hereditary systemic amyloidosis (familial amyloid polyneuropathy). Type IV familial amyloid polyneuropathy was first described as an autosomal dominant disease by the ophthalmologist Jouko Meretoja in the Finnish population.[9] Similar cases were also described in other European countries, like Germany,[10] the United Kingdom,[11] and outside Europe.[12] The clinical expression is characterized by lattice corneal dystrophy, usually found in third decade of life, followed by a slowing progressive cranial neuropathy, including bilateral facial palsy.

Sarcoidosis

Sarcoidosis is a chronic, noncaseating granulomatous disease characterized by hilar or peripheral adenopathy, polyarthralgias, anergy, elevated serum calcium, and hepatic dysfunction. One variant of sarcoidosis, Heerfordt disease (uveoparotid fever), consists of uveitis, mild fever, nonsuppurative parotitis, and cranial nerve paralysis. The facial nerve is the most commonly involved among the cranial nerves, and paralysis usually occurs days to months after parotid inflammation. In these circumstances, paralysis is thought to be caused by direct invasion of the nerve by the granulomatous process.[13] An elevated serum angiotensin-converting enzyme generally confirms the diagnosis, and treatment consists of steroid administration.

Wegener Granulomatosis

Wegener granulomatosis, first described by Friedrich Wegener in 1936, is a systemic disease characterized by granuloma formation and widespread necrotizing vasculitis. An autoimmune origin has been proposed, with a peak age during the fifth to sixth decade, and prevalence in men. It classically appears with involvement of upper/lower respiratory tracts and renal system. Mortality, in the late stages, is usually related to renal insufficiency. FP, as well as other otologic manifestations, has been reported during the course of the disease, although it represents an extremely rare feature. FP is considered to occur in

5% of the cases[14] and is generally unilateral, while only few reports with bilateral involvement have so far been published.[15,16] FP as first sign of Wegener granulomatosis has also been reported.[17] Early diagnosis, by testing of anticytoplasmic antibodies versus neutrophil polymorphonucleate granules, which are positive in 97% of the cases, prompts a timely medical treatment (steroids plus cyclophosphamide), with high rates of remission of an otherwise lethal disease.

■ Bilateral Facial Paralysis

Bilateral FP is defined as deficit of the facial musculature that involves both sides of the face (**Table 7.2**). It is an extremely rare condition occurring in 0.3–2.0% of patients with facial nerve paralysis[18] with an annual incidence of 1 case per 5 million.[19]

According to timing of clinical manifestation, bilateral FP can be either simultaneous, when occurring in both sides within 4 weeks, or sequential, when the second paralyzed side appears at a longer distance of time. Grading of facial nerve deficit can be different between the two affected sides, and the first side is not necessarily more severe than the second. Resolution is also independent from the timing of FP and is usually related to the causative agent or disease.

Simultaneous bilateral FP is much more frequent than the sequential form, for which only a few reports have been published in relation to sarcoidosis[13] and chickenpox.[20]

Table 7.2 Bilateral facial paralysis

Simultaneous	Sequential
Bell palsy	Bell palsy
Lyme disease	Varicella zoster virus
Guillain-Barré syndrome	Melkersson-Rosenthal syndrome
Leukemia	Sarcoidosis
Sarcoidosis	Infections (chickenpox)
Meningitis	Non-Hodgkin lymphoma
Syphilis	
Leprosy	
Amyloidosis	
Möbius syndrome	
Wegener granulomatosis	
Infections (Epstein-Barr, human immunodeficiency virus, chickenpox, leptospirosis)	
Temporal bone fractures	
Mandibular fractures	
Refractory anemia with excess of blasts	
Pontine infarction	
Pregnancy	
Kawasaki disease	
Familial and congenital aplasia of the facial nuclei	

In contrast to idiopathic unilateral FP, for which the cause cannot be rescued on many occasions—often driving the clinician to diagnosis of a new Bell palsy case—bilateral FP is more often related to a systemic disease. Therefore, its diagnosis has to be considered an emergency due to possible life-threatening situations, such as congenital abnormalities (Möbius syndrome, myotonic dystrophy), cranial or mandibular trauma, infections (Lyme disease, Guillain-Barré syndrome, herpes zoster, syphilis, leprosy, infectious mononucleosis, influenza, mumps, chickenpox, malaria, poliomyelitis, human immunodeficiency virus [HIV], leptospirosis, sarcoidosis, bilateral otitis media, encephalomyelitis), metabolic disorders (acute porphyria, diabetes mellitus), neoplasms (leukemia, myeloproliferative syndromes, lymphoma, neurofibromatosis type 2), vasospasm, vascular insufficiency, autoimmune phenomena (rheumatoid arthritis), pregnancy, Wegener granulomatosis, electrical injury, and anticancer drug assumption (vincristine, placlitaxel).

Patients with bilateral FP often look dull and idle due to the incapacity to smile or show emotions. These patients also experience speech difficulty with bilabial incompetence causing flaccid dysarthria, with substitution, distortion, or omission of the bilabial and alveolar phonemes. Among the other functional impairments, eating and drinking problems are also noteworthy.

Bell Palsy

Bell palsy may present, although rarely, with a bilateral deficit and represents around 20% of cases of bilateral FP. Diagnosis should only be made after exclusion of other possible causes. Prognosis does not differ from that of unilateral cases. Sequential bilateral FP is more common as opposed to simultaneous bilateral FP with Bell palsy.

Guillain-Barré Syndrome

Guillain-Barré syndrome is an acute inflammatory polyradiculoneuropathy that may evolve into a paralytic disease, for which an association with *Campylobacter jejuni* infection has been reported.[21] Nowadays, it is recognized as a heterogeneous syndrome, with demyelinating (prevailing in the United States) and axonal forms, and usually manifests as an ascending compromising of the voluntary muscles from the legs to arms, trunk, and face, so that facial nerve involvement generally occurs at a later stage. In a single report, facial weakness has been described prior to involvement of the other muscular groups.[22] Around 50% of Guillain-Barré syndrome displays bilateral FP.[23] Diagnosis is based on raised cerebrospinal fluid proteins content, without increased cell count. Treatment is performed either by plasmapheresis or immunoglobulin infusions. A single report of bilateral simultaneous facial palsy has been reported during plasmapheresis.[24]

Human Immunodeficiency Virus

Simultaneous bilateral FP during human immunodeficiency syndrome has been reported to occur with a variable incidence depending on geographical localization. In fact, against the 4.1–7.2% reported in Europe[25] and the United States,[26] in African endemic areas it has been associated with 77–100% of HIV-infected individuals.[27] FP has been described in the early, preclinical stages, when antibodies are developing,[28,29] as well as in the late stages of the disease.[30] In the first case, FP may represent the most common clinical sign as a single cranial nerve presentation of HIV (1–4% of cases), displaying after the primary HIV infection or seroconversion stages. In the late stages (acquired

immunodeficiency syndrome and advanced HIV infection, occurring years after virus transmission), FP may present in the cohort of multiple neurological involvement. Although bilateral FP is less frequent than unilateral, its occurrence should alert the clinician and prompt him or her to envision this possible cause within the diagnostic work-up.

■ Conclusion

The diagnosis of FP, either unilateral or bilateral, prompts the clinician to consider all possible causes, before formulating diagnosis of a new Bell palsy episode. As previously mentioned, important issues, primarily careful history taking, may facilitate this task (**Table 7.3**). Whenever available, laboratory testing is significant for eventually confirming the clinical diagnosis.

Table 7.3 Diagnosis and treatment of unusual causes of facial paralysis

Suspected Diagnosis	Laboratory Testing Positivity	Other Clinical Findings/Signs	Treatment
Lyme disease	Single step VlsE (IR6) enzyme-linked immunosorbent assay Enzyme-linked immunosorbent assay-Western Blot (two-tier test)	Insect bite Erythema migrans Northern hemisphere summertime	Ceftriaxone, 2 g/day Doxycycline, 100 mg twice a day Azithromycin, 500 mg/day
Kawasaki disease	None	Age (infancy, childhood) coronary vessels aneurysms high fever, skin rash, enlarged neck lymph nodes, painful and swollen joints, abdominal pain, diarrhea, irritability, and headaches	Aspirin (100 mg/kg/day) High-dosage intravenous gamma globulin (2 g/kg)
Melkersson-Rosenthal syndrome	None	Fissured tongue Angioneurotic edema Relapsing facial palsy	Nonsteroidal anti-inflammatory drugs Corticosteroids Antibiotics Immunosuppressants (Total facial nerve decompression)
Amyloidosis	Byoptic material Gelsolin mutation (familial amyloid polyneuropathy)	Familiarity (Meretoja disease or familial amyloid polyneuropathy)	Liver transplantation
Sarcoidosis	Angiotensin-converting enzyme	Parotid inflammation	Steroids
Wegener granulomatosis	Cytoplasmic antineutrophil cytoplasmic antibodies	Upper and lower respiratory tracts disease Kidney disease	Steroids Cyclophosphamide
Guillain-Barré syndrome	High proteins in the cerebrospinal fluid, without increased cell count Electromyography: prolonged distal latencies with a reduction in the amplitude of the compound muscle action potential, decrease in the conduction velocity and abnormalities of the F waves	Ascending muscular weakness Bilateral facial palsy	Plasmapheresis Immunoglobulin
Human immunodeficiency virus Early (seroconversion) stage Late stage	Human immunodeficiency virus test	Bilateral facial palsy Flu-like illness Manifest signs of disease	Famcyclovir, acyclovir

References

1. Falco NA, Eriksson E. Facial nerve palsy in the newborn: incidence and outcome. Plast Reconstr Surg 1990;85(1):1–4

2. Jemec B, Grobbelaar AO, Harrison DH. The abnormal nucleus as a cause of congenital facial palsy. Arch Dis Child 2000;83(3): 256–258

3. Lim TC, Yeo WS, Loke KY, Quek SC. Bilateral facial nerve palsy in Kawasaki disease. Ann Acad Med Singapore 2009;38(8): 737–738

4. Steere AC, Malawista SE, Snydman DR, et al. Lyme arthritis: an epidemic of oligoarticular arthritis in children and adults in three connecticut communities. Arthritis Rheum 1977;20(1):7–17

5. Bagger-Sjöbäck D, Remahl S, Ericsson M. Long-term outcome of facial palsy in neuroborreliosis. Otol Neurotol 2005;26(4): 790–795

6. Peltomaa M, McHugh G, Steere AC. The VlsE (IR6) peptide ELISA in the serodiagnosis of lyme facial paralysis. Otol Neurotol 2004;25(5):838–841

7. Centers for Disease Control and Prevention. Recommendations for test performance and interpretation from the second National Conference on Serologic Diagnosis of Lyme disease. Morbid Mortal Weekly Rep 1995;44:590–591.

8. Dutt SN, Mirza S, Irving RM, Donaldson I. Total decompression of facial nerve for Melkersson-Rosenthal syndrome. J Laryngol Otol 2000;114(11):870–873

9. Meretoja J. Familial systemic paramyloidosis with lattice dystrophy of the cornea, progressive cranial neuropathy, skin changes and various internal symptoms. A previously unrecognized heritable syndrome. Ann Clin Res 1969;1(4):314–324

10. Lüttmann RJ, Teismann I, Husstedt IW, Ringelstein EB, Kuhlenbäumer G. Hereditary amyloidosis of the Finnish type in a German family: clinical and electrophysiological presentation. Muscle Nerve 2010;41(5):679–684

11. Hornigold R, Patel AV, Ward VMM, O'Connor AF. Familial systemic amyloidosis associated with bilateral sensorineural hearing loss and bilateral facial palsies. J Laryngol Otol 2006;120(9): 778–780

12. Starck T, Kenyon KR, Hanninen LA, et al. Clinical and histopathologic studies of two families with lattice corneal dystrophy and familial systemic amyloidosis (Meretoja syndrome). Ophthalmology 1991;98(8):1197–1206

13. Sharma SK, Mohan A. Uncommon manifestations of sarcoidosis. J Assoc Physicians India 2004;52:210–214

14. McCaffrey TV, McDonald TJ, Facer GW, DeRemee RA. Otologic manifestations of Wegener's granulomatosis. Otolaryngol Head Neck Surg (1979) 1980;88(5):586–593

15. Nikolaou AC, Vlachtsis KC, Daniilidis MA, Petridis DG, Daniilidis IC. Wegener's granulomatosis presenting with bilateral facial nerve palsy. Eur Arch Otorhinolaryngol 2001;258(4):198–202

16. Magliulo G, Parrotto D, Alla FR, Gagliardi S. Acute bilateral facial palsy and Wegener's disease. Otolaryngol Head Neck Surg 2008; 139(3):476–477

17. Calonius IH, Christensen CK. Hearing impairment and facial palsy as initial signs of Wegener's granulomatosis. J Laryngol Otol 1980;94(6):649–657

18. Stahl N, Ferit T. Recurrent bilateral peripheral facial palsy. J Laryngol Otol 1989;103(1):117–119

19. Adour KK, Byl FM, Hilsinger RL Jr, Kahn ZM, Sheldon MI. The true nature of Bell's palsy: analysis of 1,000 consecutive patients. Laryngoscope 1978;88(5):787–801

20. van der Flier M, van Koppenhagen C, Disch FJ, Mauser HW, Bistervels JH, van Diemen-Steenvoorde JA. Bilateral sequential facial palsy during chickenpox. Eur J Pediatr 1999;158(10): 807–808

21. Rees JH, Soudain SE, Gregson NA, Hughes RA. Campylobacter jejuni infection and Guillain-Barré syndrome. N Engl J Med 1995;333(21):1374–1379

22. Narayanan RP, James N, Ramachandran K, Jaramillo MJ. Guillain-Barré Syndrome presenting with bilateral facial nerve paralysis: a case report. Cases J 2008;1(1):379

23. May M. The Facial Nerve. New York: Thieme; 1986:181.

24. Stevenson ML, Weimer LH, Bogorad IV. Development of recurrent facial palsy during plasmapheresis in Guillain-Barré syndrome: a case report. J Med Case Reports 2010;4:253

25. Schielke E, Pfister HW, Einhäupl KM. Peripheral facial nerve palsy associated with HIV infection. Lancet 1989;1(8637):553–554

26. Lalwani AK, Sooy CD. Otologic and otoneurologic manifestations in acquired immunodeficiency syndrome. Otolaryngol Clin North Am 1992;25:1183

27. Di Costanzo B, Belec L, Testa J, Georges AJ, Martin PM. [Seroprevalence of HIV infection in a population of neurological patients in the Central African Republic]. Bull Soc Pathol Exot 1990;83(4):425–436

28. Kim MS, Yoon HJ, Kim HJ, et al. Bilateral peripheral facial palsy in a patient with Human Immunodeficiency Virus (HIV) infection. Yonsei Med J 2006;47(5):745–747

29. Yeo JCL, Trotter MI, Wilson F. Bilateral facial nerve palsy associated with HIV seroconversion illness. Postgrad Med J 2008;84(992):328–329

30. Abboud O, Saliba I. Isolated bilateral facial paralysis revealing AIDS: a unique presentation. Laryngoscope 2008;118(4): 580–584

8 Congenital Facial Weakness

Randolph Sherman and Ronald M. Zuker

Each of us enters this world in a profoundly dramatic way. Either by unrelenting naturally propulsive physical forces through vaginal birth or abrupt, overwhelming surgical intervention, we are thrust into a radically different, startlingly harsh environment. Our first reaction, if we've successfully run the gauntlet, is to wave our arms and legs around in protest and shriek unmercifully. Hopefully at the other end there will await a highly skilled attendant, who will not only take care of our initial needs for comfort and warmth, but also catalogue our responses; count fingers and toes; note skin color, heart rate, and breathing; and meet our visible and audible objections with a warm reassuring gaze and loving smile. If all is in order, we will sooner or later smile, or more probably, contract all facial muscles in response, demonstrating normal function of our muscles of facial animation. Rarely, in those precious, very first moments of the outside world, we might not be able to return that simple gesture. Our attendant's smile will then bleed into a look of consternation as the unmistakable presence of a congenital facial palsy will be recognized.

Fortunately, an event such as the one described happens only rarely, as the incidence of facial palsies at birth is between 1 and 2 for every 1,000 live births. A wide range of presentations are included in this finite cohort with only an extremely small fraction of those representing profound, complete facial nerve paralyses. An overwhelming majority of congenital facial palsies reported in the literature are associated with problematic labor or specific birth trauma, presumably associated with the use of forceps and most of those are transient.[1] With the abandonment of this procedure in nearly all modern day obstetrical practices, we can expect that the overall rate of congenital facial nerve injuries has almost certainly decreased in kind. As with acquired forms of this disease, congenital palsies can present as unilateral or bilateral, complete or incomplete, transient or permanent.

■ Work-up

The initial work-up of a patient presenting with any degree of facial paralysis should begin immediately with a thorough cranial nerve examination highlighting careful observation and annotation of the presence or absence of function of all relevant cranial nerve innervated facial muscles. These involve not only muscles controlling facial expression but those responsible for ocular control, sphincter competency, chewing, and deglutition. While still photo documentation is required, video sequencing is critical for more reflective study of the specific deficiency and can be entered into standardizing databases that currently have the capacity to quantify deficiencies and more accurately track changes, thus helping guide long-term therapeutic decision making. Of course, early appreciation of facial palsy, in some cases, may lead to a more precise diagnosis. Important points to be noted should include any history of prolonged or otherwise difficult birth such as cephalopelvic disproportion, arrested descent, or protracted labor. Family history of facial paralysis either alone or with other deformities should raise suspicions of syndromic presentations. Any use of forceps should be documented and should lead the investigator to search for and make particular note of even the smallest signs of bruising, swelling, or deformation in the region of the temporomandibular joint area as well as hemotympanum in the ear canal.

Even in the newborn, identification of uni- or bilaterality as well as degree of completeness should be assessed as soon as possible. Initial component evaluation of upper, mid, and lower facial nerve function helps better define each particular defect.[2] As follow-up evaluations are done, the precision and thoroughness of the initial assessment becomes crucial in measuring progress toward resolution and restoration of function or lack thereof. Of the several quantitative evaluation tools available, the most widely used and longest standing grading system to aid in categorizing severity is the House-Brackmann scale (see **Table 5.2** in Chapter 5).[3] The enduring nature of this device is (1) its simplicity of use, asking the observer to critique the face at rest, then in motion; and (2) its reliable correlate to eventual return of function. The severity of the condition is reflected in a higher score, grade I being normal, through to grade VI describing total facial paralysis. The Sunnybrook scale (see **Table 5.5** in Chapter 5) is in common use as well. Ahrens et al have developed a downloadable program that allows observed data entered to be measured across multiple grading scales.[4]

Unlike in the acquired varieties of facial paralysis, laboratory testing and analysis does not aid in the differential diagnosis in any substantive way with congenital facial paralysis. If there is either a history of similar problems in other family members or associated findings in the affected patient, genetic screening tools might be utilized to help characterize syndromic conditions. In the rare instances where chromosomal abnormalities are diagnosed, timely and appropriate genetic counseling may be appropriate.

Imaging studies, including plain skull series, computed tomography scanning, and/or magnetic resonance imaging, do not have a substantial role in the diagnosis and treatment of congenital facial paralysis. The one exception is in those positively diagnosed cases of birth-related trauma. Radiologic examination of the temporal bone may reveal evidence of fracture, tumor, stenosis, or other malformations in extremely rare cases but will not contribute to a decision to treat any particular functional deficiency. Consequently, these tests should be obtained judiciously, especially in the newborn.

Electrophysiologic examination may offer some insight into the status of the facial nerve in the days and weeks after birth. These tests are done to primarily differentiate between a posttraumatic palsy and developmental paralysis. Accordingly, a high index of suspicious should predate the ordering of neurologic stimulation studies. Electromyography, the most commonly used tool for most peripheral nerve disorders, records motor unit potential response to an electrical stimulus as well as spontaneous activity. This test becomes increasingly insightful many weeks after an injury, precluding its use as an immediate discriminator of injury. Electroneurography will differentiate acute injury from developmental disease by giving normal results in the former process while revealing little to no function in the latter.

■ Causes

Paralysis of the facial nerve identified at birth is either posttraumatic or developmental. Cranial nerve VII palsies stemming from birth-related injuries are almost exclusively unilateral. As mentioned previously, these have been historically linked to the use of obstetrical forceps. Other factors can include arrested descent of labor or positional injury. Initial physical examination will usually reveal some cutaneous manifestation of an adverse perinatal event. When coupled with the appropriate historical findings, a traumatic etiology for the observed paresis must be suspected.

Developmental causes are either isolated or syndromic. These account for an extremely small minority of cases but can present across the clinical spectrum, ranging from unilateral to bilateral, mild to severe, one facial nerve branch or all. Of the many isolated syndromes that can present with facial weakness or paralysis, Möbius syndrome is the most dramatic. Occurring in only 1 out of 50,000 live births, these patients often have bilaterally complete loss of facial nerve function and have no ability to trigger any degree of facial movement. The effect is immediately profound and worsens with time. In this particular syndrome, the abducens nerve (cranial nerve VI) is affected as well and compromises eye movement and coordination. Other possible nerve deficits, however rare, may include cranial nerves V, IX, X, and XII. Patients afflicted with Möbius syndrome, aside from lacking any facial expression, will suffer from the following in various degrees: drooling, deficiency of bilabial speech, sucking, swallowing, dry eyes, strabismus, and dental problems. Associated anomalies include cleft palate, club foot, syndactyly, auditory problems, and, even more rarely, Poland syndrome. Males and females are affected equally. While there seems to be a slight increased risk in the offspring of those

affected, there is no identifiable genetic locus and no specific laboratory marker for disease identification. Intellectual capacity does not seem to be impaired in children afflicted.[6]

Other causes or associated conditions attributed to congenital facial weakness include hemifacial microsomia, velocardiofacial syndrome, DiGeorge syndrome, osteopetrosis (Albers-Schonberg disease), CHARGE syndrome (*c*olobomata, *h*eart disease, *a*tresia of choanae, *r*etarded growth, *g*enital hypoplasia, and *e*ar anomalies), facioscapulohumeral muscular dystrophy, congenital unilateral lower lip paralysis/asymmetric crying facies, and the maternal use of teratogens including thalidomide and misoprostol.[7–11]

■ Therapy

Conservative

Once a diagnosis of congenital facial paralysis is made, therapy in the neonatal period is completely supportive. Ophthalmological concerns involve protection against dry eye, corneal irritation, and outright exposure leading to abrasion. Frequent exams with lacrimal tear support throughout the day are recommended. As these children grow, speech therapy and careful dental hygiene monitoring are essential. Patients with unilateral lower segment palsies can be managed expectantly with administration of Botox periodically given to relax the depressors on the normal side.

Surgical

Urgent Intervention

When a unilateral facial paralysis is positively attributed to birth trauma, iatrogenic or otherwise, surgical intervention might be considered in a very small number of circumstances. Fortunately, 9 of 10 cases will resolve spontaneously. While early surgical decompression has not been proven advantageous over observation, those patients who have suffered from temporal bone fracture documented on computed tomography scan with abnormal electrophysiological testing in the postpartum period and again in the second month of life may be candidates. In those rare circumstances where surgery is being contemplated in the acute phase after diagnosis, simple decompression of the temporal bone at the fracture site is, by far, the most straightforward approach possible. Problems arise in this environment stemming from our inability to differentiate the degree of internal architectural injury to the nerve. Once having decompressed the temporal bone, grossly visible anatomic disruption of the nerve must be addressed by debridement of the affected segment and either reapproximation of the nerve directly or interpositional nerve grafting using autologous donor nerve such as the sural, greater auricular, or either antebrachiocutaneous branch. Nerve reapproximation and neurorrhaphy or interpositional nerve grafting, all in the total absence of tension, is thought to be of paramount importance toward maximizing any chance of axonal regeneration.

In those rare instances where it is determined that proximal injury has precluded any chance of ipsilateral facial nerve regrowth, cross facial nerve grafting (CFNG) should be considered. This can be done as a one- or two-staged procedure. Targeted donor and recipient branches can be matched but rapidly increase the degree of complexity of the reconstructive procedure. Transposition of the ipsilateral hypoglossal to the distal segment of the injured facial nerve while waiting for CFNG regrowth is commonly accepted.[12]

■ Elective Reconstruction: Mid Face

There are several surgical options available to those patients who suffer from permanent congenital facial palsies long after any hope for functional recovery has passed. Timing of intervention may occur early, after the third year of life or sooner, dependent on the predicted size of vessels and the surgeon's anastomotic skill. Issues to be considered are timing of the reconstruction, regional requirements (upper, lower, unilateral, bilateral), and whether static or dynamic transfers best meet the patient's needs. The primary goals to be met by the reconstructive surgeon include maximizing facial symmetry both at rest and in motion, improving oral competency to diminish drooling, aiding in bilabial speech

in patients with Möbius syndrome, limiting synkinesis, and assisting with eye closure. Repositioning of the forehead in older patients with acquired palsies can be helpful as a static procedure but is almost never used in the pediatric patient with congenital palsies. Similarly, static slings with tensor fascia lata strips or alloplastic materials are mostly reserved for old patients with acquired deficiencies.

Facial reanimation using functional muscle transplantation remains the standard of care for this population. Local muscle transposition using the temporalis transfer was first described a generation ago and served its purpose well prior to the advent of free tissue transplantation. This procedure still has its place in the elderly population and in those that may not be suitable for prolonged surgical procedures. Free tissue transfer techniques were introduced by Harii with the description of the gracilis muscle transplant after CFNG.[13] Others have reported the use of the pectoralis minor, the serratus, and the rectus abdominis. Most recently, Harii has introduced the segmental latissimus dorsi as a one-stage procedure. Despite the variety of transplant options available, the gracilis transfer stands alone as the most advantageous, adaptable, and effective donor and has yielded excellent results in reports of large series from several authors.

The gracilis muscle is ideally suited for facial reanimation because of its configuration, vascular pedicle orientation, innervation, flexibility for subdivision, ease of harvest, and minimal donor site morbidity (**Figs. 8.1** and **8.2**). The obturator

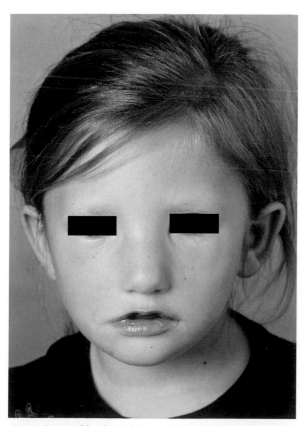

Fig. 8.1 A 5-year-old girl with bilateral Möbius syndrome.

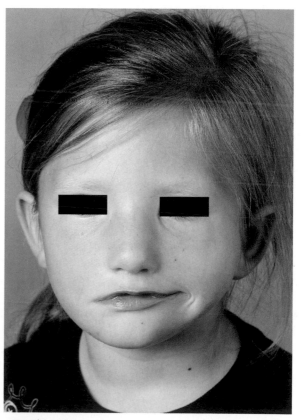

Fig. 8.2 The same 5-year-old girl after left-sided innervated free gracilis transfer.

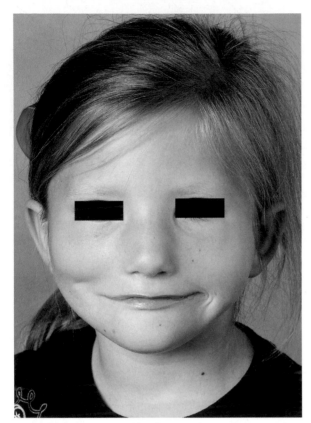

Fig. 8.3 The same 5-year-old girl 1 year later, after second-stage, right-sided innervated free gracilis transfer.

subsequently approached for a separate intraoral neurorraphy or brought across to the opposite preauricular side with the second stage neurorrhaphy being done in the same operative field as the facial to medial circumflex femoral pedicle anastamoses.

In cases of bilateral paralysis as presents with Möbius syndrome, the absence of a normal contralateral facial nerve donor as described previously demands an alternative donor power unit (**Fig. 8.4**). Historically, cranial nerve XII, the hypoglossal, and much less often, cranial nerve XI, the accessory, were considered and sometimes used via nerve transposition as either a direct donor to the inactivated ipsilateral facial nerve or as a motor input to a muscle transplant. The XII-VII transfer earned the name "babysitter" and was described as an interim maneuver to maintain tone and bulk (referred to previously) in the ipsilateral facial musculature once it was determined that direct reconstruction of the involved facial nerve was not an option.[18] More recently, in the hands of many surgeons, cranial nerve V, the motor branch to the masseter muscle, has become the donor of choice when cranial nerve VII is not available, either from the proximal segment, or the nerve grafted contralateral side. Used primarily to motor a one-stage, innervated muscle transfer, the motor branch to masseter has the advantages of being almost always available, conveniently located, powerful, and, once harvested, sparing any real or measurable loss of masseteric function

nerve supplying innervation to the gracilis is ideally suited as a neural donor as are the medial circumflex femoral vessels in regard to length and circumference. The muscle can be tailored to the exact length and width needed in the recipient bed without compromising functional restoration after revascularization and reinnervation (**Fig. 8.3**). This is not so with the other donor muscles described. Additionally, given the degree of excursion achieved in most transfers, the muscle bulk needed is surprisingly minimal. Interestingly enough, one of the most important nuances in gracilis muscle harvest is the appropriate calculation of muscle volume to be transferred so as to avoid overcorrection.

Dynamic muscle transfers are most often done following a previously placed CFNG. In the case of bilateral facial paralysis as in Möbius syndrome where no such option is available, a one-stage procedure is performed using the ipsilateral motor branch to the masseter (cranial nerve V). CFNGs are most often harvested from the sural nerve in the lower leg, leaving small cutaneous scars and resulting in a limited area of hypesthesia in the dorsolateral aspect of the involved foot. Intraoperative mapping of the contralateral zygomaticobuccal branches of the normal facial nerve is crucial to maximize the potential for dynamic symmetry and spontaneity once the gracilis transfer is subsequently reinnervated. The CFNG may either be banked in the superior labial sulcus and

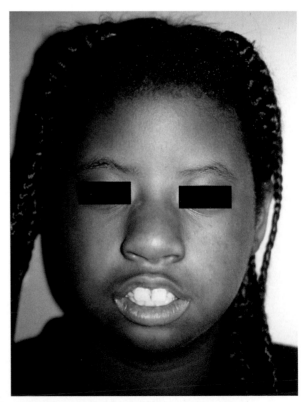

Fig. 8.4 An 8-year-old girl with Möbius syndrome at rest.

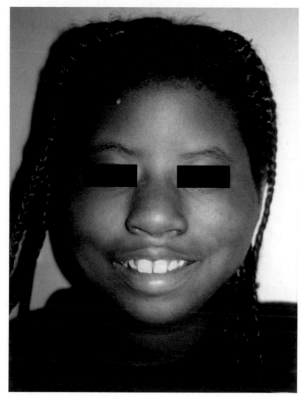

Fig. 8.5 The same 8-year-old girl 1 year later, after bilateral sequential innervated free gracilis transfers.

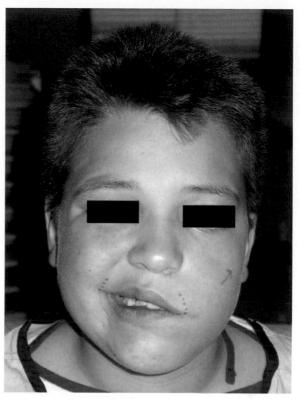

Fig. 8.7 Preoperative vector analysis and marking for directional placement of gracilis muscle transfer.

(because of remaining intact motor branches) (**Figs. 8.5 and 8.6**).[19]

Whether it is used with cranial nerve VII, via CFNG, or cranial nerve V, through direct neurorrhaphy, the gracilis transplant should be preceded by careful smile analysis of the recipient's particular needs. Vector analysis in the awake patient comparing the length and angle of excursion of the normal corner of the mouth with transposition

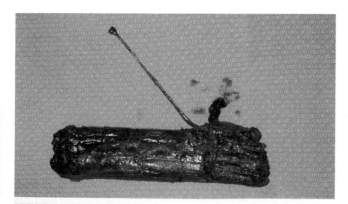

Fig. 8.6 Segmental gracilis muscle harvested demonstrating vascular pedicle and obturator nerve.

of those measurements to the paralyzed side is critical (**Fig. 8.7**).

Replication of the nasolabial crease on the reconstructed side is instrumental in restoring balance and symmetry. The recipient site is prepared by creating an appropriate pocket through an extended rhytidectomy incision, isolating and skeletonizing the facial vessels, then freshening the CFNG or exposing the motor branch to masseter below the superolateral parotid. It is prudent to verify the presence of axonal tissue via a cross-sectional analysis at the time of surgery before committing to the use of the CFNG as the motor. Removal of excessive cheek fat and/or the buccal fat pad reduces unwanted bulk after muscle transfer. Meticulously placed anchoring sutures in the modiolus with subsequent, repeated manipulation allows for simulation of muscle action in anticipation of successful reinnervation weeks to months down the road. The precision of this step in achieving an aesthetically acceptable outcome cannot be overestimated.

Gracilis muscle harvest should include accurately measuring the length of the muscle with some degree of tension applied, removal of just enough length to approximate the preauricular to commissural distance with an additional centimeter on each end, conservative use of muscle width, and central placement of the neurovascular pedicle. Anchoring sutures should be placed in the distal end of the muscle transfer prior to harvest to assure solid purchase of the recipient bed correlate sutures. Once transplanted and revascularized, the neurorrhaphy must not be rushed. A precise end-to-end coaptation using the smallest and fewest number of sutures possible or tissue glue alone, done with particular attention being paid to size match as well as absence of tension, will maximize the chances for favorable restoration of function. The muscle must finally be secured to the preauricular malar fascia in the previously planned vector with the correct tension required to just perceptibly move the corner of the mouth. Postoperative care in the acute period is expectant. Patients and their families are encouraged to not expect evidence of function for at least 6 weeks and more often double that depending on the transfer. Functional recovery of a transplanted muscle has been seen up to 6 months after the initial transplantation.

The advantage of using the normal, contralateral facial nerve via CFNG as a donor rests in the potential for spontaneity and balanced nuance in motor control once function has been restored. While cranial nerve V, the motor branch to masseter, has been shown to be a stronger donor unit overall, the patient will require ongoing physical therapy to invoke a biting motion to activate the desired smile. Eventually, in the pediatric population most often, cortical plasticity allows for some degree of transference from a rote voluntary motion to a more inferred involuntary, subconscious motion with the trigger eventually becoming the intent to smile and not the cerebral dictate of biting for smiling. This may take some time and long periods of training, and is currently being scrutinized carefully in long-term studies.[20]

■ Elective Reconstruction: Eyelid

As noted, problems occurring with the periorbital structures in patients with congenital facial weakness include (1) drooping of the brow and upper lid because of lack of frontalis function, (2) inability to fully close the upper eyelid due to lack of orbicularis oculi function, and (3) sagging and eventual ectropion of the lower lid also because of periorbital muscle paresis. Fortunately, children are proportionately less affected by these issues than older adults who suffer from acquired forms of the disease such as Bell palsy and those sequelae associated with resection of

acoustic neuromas and other cerebral tumors. Lid closing can most elegantly be handled by the judicious placement of a gold weight in the upper lid whereas lower lid laxity may require a tarsal strip procedure and/or medial canthoplasty. Dynamic muscle transfers have been described but have limited application in this population.[21] Serial small procedures are the preferred method so that overcorrection be avoided. The selection, timing, and execution of these procedures should be done by only the most skilled oculoplastic surgeons who have demonstrated the skill and commitment to the community. Please refer to Chapters 21 and 22 of this book for a thorough discussion of this subject.

■ Conclusion

While the recognition and diagnosis of facial paralysis in the newborn presents an immediate crisis for the family, the large majority of patients will experience improvement and resolution of the abnormality. Consequently, the most important interdiction required of the physician is that of counseling and support while patient and thoughtful investigation of the causal basis proceeds. In the small number of cases mostly related to birth trauma that do not show improvement in the first few months, more comprehensive testing may be warranted. Early surgery for decompression, neuroma resection with direct neurorrhaphy, or interposition nerve grafting may play a limited role in a highly select group of patients. These decisions cannot be made lightly and should be discussed with surgeons who have developed a long-term understanding of early surgical intervention. Elective reconstruction does hold the promise of substantial restoration of function in either cases of hemifacial or bilateral paralysis.[22]

Reanimation for the purpose of smiling, recovery of oral competence, and improvement of speech may be expected with the appropriately chosen and executed motorized transfer as described previously. There is no greater satisfaction to the reconstructive surgeon and no deeper sense of appreciation and relief from the parents when a child afflicted with congenital facial weakness is successfully reintegrated into a more normal social discourse during early growth and development after motorized muscle transplantation.[23]

References

1. Schaitkin BM, Wiet RJ. Trauma to the facial nerve: external, surgical and iatrogenic. In: May M. The Facial Nerve: May's Second Edition. New York: Thieme Medical Publishers; 2000
2. Bergman I, May M, Wessel HB, Stool SE. Management of facial palsy caused by birth trauma. Laryngoscope 1986;96(4):381–384
3. House JW, Brackmann DE. Facial nerve grading system. Otolaryngol Head Neck Surg 1985;93(2):146–147
4. Ahrens A, Skarada D, Wallace M, Cheung JY, Neely JG. Rapid simultaneous comparison system for subjective grading scales grading scales for facial paralysis. Am J Otol 1999;20(5):667–671
5. Hughes CA, Harley EH, Milmoe G, Bala R, Martorella A. Birth trauma in the head and neck. Arch Otolaryngol Head Neck Surg 1999;125(2):193–199
6. Verzijl HT, van der Zwaag B, Cruysberg JR, Padberg GW. Möbius syndrome redefined: a syndrome of rhombencephalic maldevelopment. Neurology 2003;61(3):327–333
7. Carvalho GJ, Song CS, Vargervik K, Lalwani AK. Auditory and facial nerve dysfunction in patients with hemifacial microsomia. Arch Otolaryngol Head Neck Surg 1999;125(2):209–212

8. Puñal JE, Siebert MF, Angueira FB, Lorenzo AV, Castro-Gago M. Three new patients with congenital unilateral facial nerve palsy due to chromosome 22q11 deletion. J Child Neurol 2001; 16(6):450–452

9. Aramaki M, Udaka T, Kosaki R, et al. Phenotypic spectrum of CHARGE syndrome with CHD7 mutations. J Pediatr 2006;148(3): 410–414

10. Meyerson MD, Lewis E, Ill K. Facioscapulohumeral muscular dystrophy and accompanying hearing loss. Arch Otolaryngol 1984;110(4):261–266

11. Pastuszak AL, Schüler L, Speck-Martins CE, et al. Use of misoprostol during pregnancy and Möbius' syndrome in infants. N Engl J Med 1998;338(26):1881–1885

12. Ysunza A, Iñigo F, Rojo P, Drucker-Colin R, Monasterio FO. Congenital facial palsy and crossed facial nerve grafts: age and outcome. Int J Pediatr Otorhinolaryngol 1996;36(2):125–136

13. Harii K, Ohmori K, Torii S. Free gracilis muscle transplantation, with microneurovascular anastomoses for the treatment of facial paralysis. A preliminary report. Plast Reconstr Surg 1976; 57(2):133–143

14. Kumar PA, Hassan KM. Cross-face nerve graft with free-muscle transfer for reanimation of the paralyzed face: a comparative study of the single-stage and two-stage procedures. Plast Reconstr Surg 2002;109(2):451–462, discussion 463–464

15. O'Brien BM, Pederson WC, Khazanchi RK, Morrison WA, MacLeod AM, Kumar V. Results of management of facial palsy with microvascular free-muscle transfer. Plast Reconstr Surg 1990;86(1):12–22, discussion 23–24

16. Terzis JK, Noah ME. Analysis of 100 cases of free-muscle transplantation for facial paralysis. Plast Reconstr Surg 1997;99(7): 1905–1921

17. Koshima I, Tsuda K, Hamanaka T, Moriguchi T. One-stage reconstruction of established facial paralysis using a rectus abdominis muscle transfer. Plast Reconstr Surg 1997;99(1):234–238

18. Schaitkin BM. Nerve substitution techniques: XII–VII hook-up, XII–VII jump graft, and cross-facial graft. In: May M. The Facial Nerve: May's Second Edition. New York: Thieme Medical Publishers; 2000:611–633

19. Bae YC, Zuker RM, Manktelow RT, Wade S. A comparison of commissure excursion following gracilis muscle transplantation for facial paralysis using a cross-face nerve graft versus the motor nerve to the masseter nerve. Plast Reconstr Surg 2006;117(7):2407–2413

20. Lifchez SD, Matloub HS, Gosain AK. Cortical adaptation to restoration of smiling after free muscle transfer innervated by the nerve to the masseter. Plast Reconstr Surg 2005;115(6): 1472–1479, discussion 1480–1482

21. Frey M, Giovanoli P, Tzou CH, Kropf N, Friedl S. Dynamic reconstruction of eye closure by muscle transposition or functional muscle transplantation in facial palsy. Plast Reconstr Surg 2004; 114(4):865–875

22. Zuker RM, Goldberg CS, Manktelow RT. Facial animation in children with Möbius syndrome after segmental gracilis muscle transplant. Plast Reconstr Surg 2000;106(1):1–8, discussion 9

23. Rubin LR. The anatomy of a smile: its importance in the treatment of facial paralysis. Plast Reconstr Surg 1974;53(4):384–387

9 Bell Palsy and Ramsay Hunt Syndrome

Shingo Murakami

Bell palsy and Ramsay Hunt syndrome are two major causes of acute peripheral facial palsy, accounting for approximately two-thirds of all cases. Ramsay Hunt syndrome is caused by varicella zoster virus (VZV), while Bell palsy is defined as acute peripheral facial palsy of unknown cause. However, recent clinical and experimental studies have revealed that herpes simplex virus (HSV) type 1 is the major cause of Bell palsy. The clinical features and natural course of Bell palsy and Ramsay Hunt syndrome differ in several ways, perhaps reflecting the difference in behavior of HSV and VZV. First, while both show a unilateral facial palsy, Ramsay Hunt syndrome is differentiated by association with herpetic eruption on the pinna and vestibulocochlear dysfunction, such as hearing loss, tinnitus, and vertigo. Second, the severity of the facial paralysis is worse and its prognosis is poorer in Ramsay Hunt syndrome than in Bell palsy. Third, Bell palsy occasionally recurs, but Ramsay Hunt syndrome rarely does. This chapter summarizes current understanding of Bell palsy and Ramsay Hunt syndrome, and discusses some of the controversies surrounding these two common disorders of acute facial nerve paralysis.

■ Bell Palsy

Bell palsy is traditionally defined as idiopathic, acute unilateral peripheral facial palsy. Other symptoms of retroauricular pain, face and tongue numbness, taste disturbance, hyperacusis, and dry eye are occasionally present. Bell palsy is named after Sir Charles Bell (1774–1842), who described the seventh cranial nerve and its innervation patterns to the mimetic muscles,[1] and reported many cases of facial palsy.[2] Although Bell palsy is diagnosed by exclusion following a careful search for other causes, there are certain constant clinical features: (1) peripheral pattern of facial nerve paralysis with diffuse involvement of all branches; (2) sudden onset within 48 hours and a progressive course, reaching maximal weakness within a week; (3) absence of signs of central nervous system involvement; and (4) spontaneous functional recovery to some degree within 6 months.

Epidemiology

The incidence of Bell palsy varies between 20 and 30 per 100,000 people per year[3,4]; it accounts for ~60–75% of all acute peripheral facial palsy.[5] The male/female ratio for Bell palsy is approximately equal. The median age at onset is 40 years, but the disease may occur at any age.[6] The incidence is lowest in children under 10 years old and increases from the ages of 10 to 59 (**Fig. 9.1**). The left and right sides of the face are equally involved. There is no seasonal variation.[7] Bell palsy is occasionally complicated by diabetes mellitus or hypertension. In a report on 625 patients with Bell palsy, diabetes mellitus

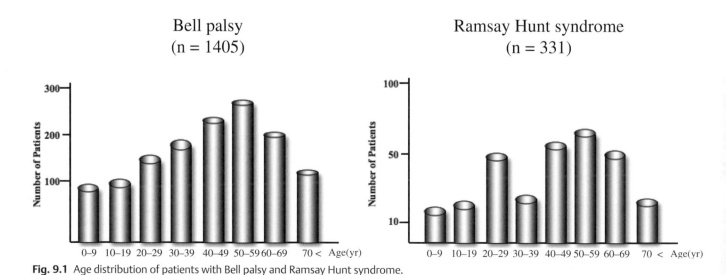

Fig. 9.1 Age distribution of patients with Bell palsy and Ramsay Hunt syndrome.

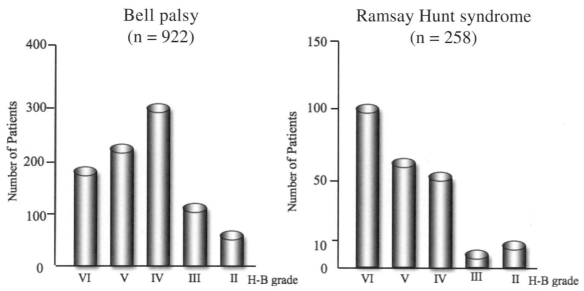

Fig. 9.2 Maximal degree of facial nerve paralysis in Bell palsy and Ramsay Hunt syndrome.

was associated in 7% and hypertension in 14.1%, respectively.[8] In another report, diabetes mellitus associated in 4.2–6.6% of Bell palsy, which is higher than the rate of 1.7–5.4% in the general population.[9]

Peitersen reported that 30% of patients had incomplete paralysis and 70% had complete paralysis; however, in 922 of our patients with Bell palsy, 5.4% had House-Brackmann grade II, 12.4% grade III, 34.4% grade IV, 26.3% grade V, and 21.7% grade VI (**Fig. 9.2**).[7]

Approximately 70% of patients with Bell palsy recover completely without treatment, but 20–30% may have permanent disfiguring facial weakness or other permanent sequelae, such as synkinesia and contracture, when medical treatment fails.[7] Compared with adults, the prognosis for facial nerve paralysis is generally favorable in children.[7,10] Poor prognostic factors are older age,[3] complete facial palsy, pain in the ear,[11] diabetes mellitus,[11] hypertension,[11] and/or impaired taste.[12]

Recurrence of Bell palsy occurs in 7.1–12% of patients,[13,14] with ipsilateral recurrence and contralateral involvement being roughly equal.[13] Patients with recurrences are more likely to have a family history of Bell palsy.[15] The incidence of diabetes mellitus in patients with recurrent Bell palsy is reported to be 2.5 times higher than that noted in nonrecurrent cases.[16]

Etiopathogenesis

Many hypotheses have been proposed for the cause of Bell palsy, including viral infection,[17] microcirculatory failure of the vasa nervorum,[18,19] ischemic neuropathy, and autoimmune reactions.[20,21] Of them, the viral inflammatory immune concept has gained the most support from clinical observations and experimental studies reported over the past 30 years.

Viral Etiology

Acute facial paralysis can occur as part of many viral diseases, such as infectious mononucleosis caused by the Epstein-Barr virus,[22] labial herpes (HSV),[23] chickenpox (VZV),[24] poliomyelitis (poliovirus),[25] mumps,[26] rubella,[27] adult T cell lymphoma,[28] and acquired immunodeficiency syndrome (human immunodeficiency virus).[29] Each viral disease has a unique presentation, but in many ways the facial paralysis is similar to that of Bell palsy: transient and with overall good outcome. This suggests that viral infection may cause facial nerve paralysis; however, patients with Bell palsy rarely have unique viral presentation other than facial nerve paralysis. Common cold sore virus HSV-1 is characterized by recurrent vesicular eruptions of the oral mucosa or lips. Primary HSV-1 infections usually occur in early childhood and are frequently asymptomatic, or may present as gingivostomatitis. The virus also has infectious affinity to the nerves, with latent infection in the neuronal cells and neuropathogenicity. These features of HSV-1 have suggested it as the most probable cause of Bell palsy.

In 1972, McCormick hypothesized that HSV is the cause of Bell palsy.[17] He suggested that HSV might be present in the geniculate ganglion of the facial nerve, where reactivation could cause a facial nerve neuropathy and infect the Schwann cells. Since then, many clinical and experimental studies have been attempted to obtain evidence for the HSV hypothesis. Serological studies were conducted by Adour et al[30] and Vahlne et al.[31] Using a complement fixation (CF) test, they demonstrated a higher prevalence of HSV antibodies in patients with Bell palsy than in the general population, suggesting previous exposure to HSV. However, they failed to find significant change in HSV antibody titers, or seroconversion, from the acute to convalescent phase, which would provide evidence for viral causality. This result is explained by the fact that reactivation of HSV-1, unlike VZV, can occur without a measurable antibody response. Nakamura et al[32] analyzed more sensitive and specific neutralization antibodies for HSV-1 and found 15% of patients with Bell palsy to be positive for these antibodies. Serological examination with CF and neutralization antibodies is an indirect test and does not provide direct evidence for the cause of Bell palsy.

Mulkens et al[33] first suggested a direct link between Bell palsy and HSV infection by cultivating HSV-1 from facial nerve epineurium obtained during decompression surgery. They isolated HSV from the specimens of one of two patients. On the other hand, Palva et al[34] failed to isolate the virus from cultivated neural tissue. Virus cultivation is specific but insensitive and inconsistent for identification of HSV. Murakami et al[35] used the powerful tool of polymerase chain reaction (PCR) to identify the HSV-1 and VZV genomes. They analyzed specimens of endoneurial fluid and postauricular muscle obtained during decompression surgery from patients with Bell palsy, Ramsay Hunt syndrome, and controls. The HSV-1 genome was detected specifically in 11 of 14 (79%) patients with Bell palsy, whereas the VZV genome was detected specifically in 8 of 9 (89%) patients with Ramsay Hunt syndrome. All controls tested negative for the HSV-1 and VZV genome. HSV-1 and VZV usually remain dormant in the geniculate ganglion of the facial nerve[36,37] and would probably not be detected in the endoneurial fluid or auricular muscle unless they were reactivated. Therefore, Murakami et al's study showed a direct association between Bell palsy and HSV-1 as well as Ramsay Hunt syndrome and VZV. Burgess et al[38] also amplified the HSV genome from the geniculate ganglion on the affected side of a patient who died 6 days after developing Bell palsy, lending further support to HSV etiology.

Animal experiments also support the HSV etiology of Bell palsy. Kumagami[39] made the first attempt to create an animal model of facial nerve paralysis using HSV. He injected HSV directly into the facial nerve at the stylomastoid foramen of the rabbit. He succeeded in causing facial nerve paralysis in 16 of the 19 animals within 6 days of virus inoculation. However, no animals except one showed improvement of the facial nerve paralysis in 223 days of follow-up. Thomander et al[40] inoculated two different neuropathogenetic strains of HSV-1 (KJ 502, F) into the tongues of mice and demonstrated virus antigens in various brainstem areas, including the facial motor nucleus, but they failed to create a model of facial nerve paralysis. Ishii et al[41,42] inoculated the Tomioka strain of HSV-1 into nasal mucosa, tongue, oral muscles, auricle, and intratemporal facial nerve of the mouse. They succeeded in inducing facial nerve paralysis only by inoculating the virus directly into the intratemporal facial nerve; inoculating the virus into the nasal mucosa, tongue, oral muscles, or auricle failed to produce paralysis. None of these attempts were successful in producing acute and transient facial paralysis resembling Bell palsy.

In 1995, Sugita et al[43] first succeeded in producing acute and transient facial paralysis in 57% of mice by inoculating the KOS strain of HSV-1 into the auricle of 4-week-old female mice. Facial nerve paralysis developed 6 to 9 days after virus inoculation, after which there was spontaneous recovery within 14 days. Histopathological findings of the facial nerve in this animal model resembled those seen in reports of patients with Bell palsy, with nerve swelling (**Fig. 9.3**), inflammatory cell infiltrates, and vacuolar degeneration.[43,44]

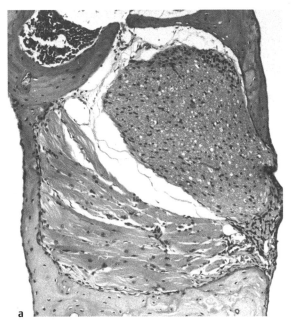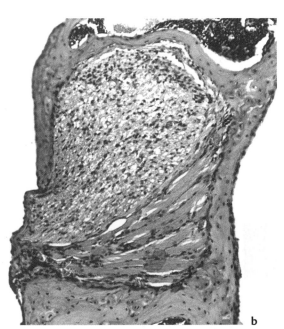

Fig. 9.3a, b Cross-section of the mouse intratemporal facial nerve. Note that sufficient space is seen between the facial nerve and facial canal in the unaffected side (**a**), but no space is seen in the affected side (**b**).

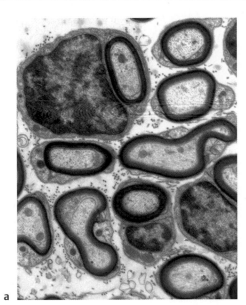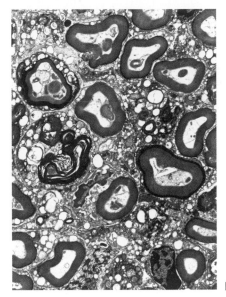

Fig. 9.4a, b Electron microscopic findings of the intratempotal mouse facial nerve. Note the varying kinds of nerve degeneration seen in the affected side (**a**) compared with unaffected side (**b**) of the facial nerve.

Honda et al[45] clarified the pathophysiology underlying facial nerve paralysis using electrical tests of the blink reflex and electroneurography with histopathological examinations. They confirmed that the basis of HSV-1 neuritis was mixed lesions of various nerve injuries (**Fig. 9.4**) and that recovery on electroneurography tended to be delayed compared with the recovery of the facial nerve paralysis. Murakami[46] and Hato[47] clarified the role of HSV-1 infection and immune functions in the pathogenesis of mouse facial nerve paralysis. They traced the migration route of the injected HSV from the auricle to the facial nerve and brainstem, and concluded that HSV infection in the facial nerve is a prerequisite for facial nerve paralysis. Hato's immunological experiment suggested that facial nerve paralysis is caused by direct viral injury rather than viral-induced cellular demyelination.[47] These murine models, however, are produced by primary infection with HSV-1, whereas Bell palsy is thought to be caused by reactivation of latent HSV-1 present in the geniculate ganglion. In 2001, Takahashi et al[48] developed the HSV-1 primary infection model into a reactivation model. They suppressed cell-mediated immunity using anti–cluster of differentiation 3 and then, 8 weeks after recovery from facial nerve paralysis, scratched auricular skin with a needle in the same area as the previous HSV-1 inoculation. In this experiment, facial nerve paralysis developed in 20% of the mice, whereas the HSV-1 genome was detected in 67% of facial nerves. This study confirmed that reactivation of HSV-1 can produce facial nerve paralysis similar to that in Bell palsy and also suggested that reactivation of HSV-1 in the geniculate ganglion does not always cause facial nerve paralysis, so-called asymptomatic or subclinical reactivation of HSV-1.

It is widely recognized that HSV in the trigeminal ganglion can produce dozens of episodes of labial herpes;

thus, one might wonder why, if HSV causes Bell palsy, the episodes are rarely repeated. The study by Takahashi et al[48] suggested an answer to this question by showing that facial nerve paralysis does not always appear even if HSV-1 is reactivated in the geniculate ganglion of the facial nerve. The manifestations and frequency of episodes developing in sensory and motor nerves seem somewhat different. Other factors, such as the anatomical structure of the facial canal, may be closely related to the pathomechanism of facial nerve paralysis.

Ischemia

Blood supply to the facial nerves derives from three arteries: the labyrinthine artery, middle meningeal artery, and stylomastoid artery. Microcirculatory failure of the vasa nervorum,[18,19] or ischemic neuropathy, is the most traditional hypothesis for the cause of Bell palsy. In 1944, Denny-Brown and Brenner[49] demonstrated that the demyelination and disruption of nerve fibers with loss of nerve conductivity was caused by ischemic injury from compression of arterial branches supplying the nerve, rather than by direct compression of axoplasmic flow. Hilger[18] postulated that Bell palsy is an ischemic neuritis resulting from segmental arteriolar spasm, based on clinical observations and Denny-Brown and Brenner's experimental study. Calcaterra et al[50] reported two cases of total unilateral facial paralysis after embolization of the middle meningeal artery, which suggested that ischemia of the tympanic portion of the facial nerve might be responsible for facial nerve paralysis. Kumoi et al[51] developed an animal model of ischemic facial palsy by embolization of internal and external maxillary arteries in cats. In this animal model, facial nerve paralysis developed immediately after embolization and recovered spontaneously after 2 months.

Autoimmune Injury

Autoimmune reaction against myelin components is a possible cause of peripheral nerve demyelination such as Guillan-Barré syndrome and multiple sclerosis. Abramsky et al[20] found that peripheral blood lymphocytes in patients with Bell palsy showed significant transformation in the presence of human basic protein from peripheral nerve myelin. McGovern et al[21] found that more profound facial nerve paralysis and severe histologic nerve damage developed in hyperimmune dogs than in nonsensitized dogs after injection of vasoconstrictors into the facial nerve. In further study, they found that cromolyn sodium, a mast cell degranulation inhibitor, prevented the neuropathic changes induced by horse serum injection into the perineurial space of the facial nerve. They concluded that degranulation of mast cells activated by complement or specific allergens may be the triggering mechanism that leads to nerve edema, ischemia, and paralysis.

Evidence for cellular and humoral autoimmune mechanisms of nerve injury has been reported in patients with Bell palsy. Jonsson et al[52] found an increase in levels of interferon-γ, but failed to find any change in interferon in the acute versus convalescent phases of facial nerve paralysis. They thought this increase of interferon may be representative of a chronic viral infection or reactivation. Yilmaz et al[53] examined serum cytokines in 23 patients with Bell palsy and found significantly higher levels of interleukin-6, interleukin-8, and tumor necrosis factor-α than in controls. They suggested that high serum interleukin-6 indicated enhanced repair of injury in astrocytes, and that high serum tumor necrosis factor-α level may have led to replication of HSV and an inflammatory process of virus-induced demyelination. In contrast, Bujía et al[54] found no difference in serum levels of soluble interleukin-2 receptors, which reflect T-lymphocyte activation, in patients with Bell palsy and age- and sex-matched controls. They concluded that T-cell activation was not a prominent feature in Bell palsy. Taking all of this into consideration, while immunological reaction may have important role in the pathogenesis of facial nerve paralysis, it is unlikely to be the primary cause of Bell palsy because autoimmune reactions occur regardless of whether they are triggered by antigens of virus, bacteria, parasites, or other foreign substances.

■ Ramsay Hunt Syndrome (Herpes Zoster Oticus)

Ramsay Hunt syndrome is the second most common cause of acute facial nerve paralysis. In 1907, James Ramsay Hunt reviewed 60 cases and suggested that their symptoms and signs resulted from geniculate ganglionitis of the facial nerve.[6] He classified clinical variations of this syndrome into the following four categories:

(1) Herpes auricularis; affecting the sensory portion of the seventh cranial nerve.
(2) Herpes auricularis with facial palsy; disease affecting the sensory and motor divisions of the facial nerve.
(3) Herpes auricularis with facial palsy and auditory symptoms; affecting sensory and motor divisions of the facial nerve with the vestibulocochlear nerve.
(4) In the more severe cases of type 3, symptoms of Ménière disease such as vertigo were also present.

Thus, the clinical symptoms and signs in Ramsay Hunt syndrome vary considerably. Ramsay Hunt was also the first to describe the relation between the geniculate ganglion and sensory function in the facial nerve. He also explained auditory and vestibular symptoms by the close proximity of the geniculate ganglion to the vestibulocochlear nerve within the bony facial canal.

Epidemiology

The incidence of Ramsay Hunt syndrome is approximately 2 to 5 per 100,000 people per year, accounting for 4.5–12% of acute facial palsies.[55,56] The rate is lower in children and increases dramatically at ages older than 40 (see **Fig. 9.1**). The increased incidence in the elderly is explained by an age-related decrease in cellular immune response to VZV.[57] Males/females and the left/right sides of the face are equally involved, and there is no seasonal variation. Recent studies suggest that immunization with zoster vaccine in elderly people and varicella vaccine in children reduces the incidence of herpes zoster as well as Ramsay Hunt syndrome.[58-60]

Etiopathogenesis

VZV causes two distinct diseases: chickenpox (varicella) and herpes zoster (shingles). A link between these two diseases has been suggested for over 100 years based on isolation of VZV from children with varicella who were exposed to adults with herpes zoster. These isolates have identical molecular profiles.[61] After primary infection of VZV, viruses cause skin lesions characterized by chickenpox and are transmitted retrogradely to the sensory ganglia via sensory nerves innervating the skin, then remain latent in the sensory ganglion cells. Primary VZV infection results in lifelong immunity. However, when VZV-specific cell-mediated immunity decreases, the latent viruses become reactivated and second episodes of herpes zoster or Ramsay Hunt syndrome appear.[62]

Symptoms and Signs

Ramsay Hunt syndrome is characterized by facial nerve paralysis, herpetic eruption on the auricle, and vestibulocochlear dysfunction. However, manifestations of these symptoms vary considerably and are inconsistent in the timing of appearance, severity, and prognosis. Only 64% of patients have all three symptoms, which appear mostly within 2 weeks.[63]

Herpetic Eruption

The most common site of herpetic eruption is the geniculate zone of the facial nerve: the concha of the auricle and a small part of the posteriomedial surface of the auricle (**Fig. 9.5**).[64] Other geniculate zones of the mucosa on the palate and the anterior two-thirds of the tongue are also involved.[64,65] In a large series of 325 patients with Ramsay Hunt syndrome, 8.3% of the patients developed herpetic eruption on the palate and the tongue (**Fig. 9.6**).[63] Herpetic eruption, however, may appear over the ear, face, neck, larynx, buccal mucosal, and/or other regions of lower cranial nerves IX, X, and XI in selected patients.[64,65] This indicates involvement of more than one ganglion.

Herpetic eruption appears in 87% of patients with Ramsay Hunt syndrome,[63] and it is the most important sign for diagnosis of the syndrome. However, its severity and timing of appearance are varied (see **Fig. 9.5**) and inconsistent, which sometimes leads to misdiagnosis in initial visits. In 66% of patients, herpetic eruption appears simultaneously or before development of facial palsy, but is delayed more than 2 days in 34% of patients.[60,63] Compared with adults, the herpetic eruptions in children are milder and tend to be delayed, with 50% of children and 31.9% of adults displaying vesicles after facial palsy.[60] Patients with delayed eruptions are often misdiagnosed with Bell palsy at initial presentation and occasionally fail to be treated with antiviral agents, leading to poor outcomes. Early diagnosis of VZV infection before appearance of herpetic eruption has been attempted by PCR. Murakami et al[66] examined skin exudates by scratching the geniculate zone of the auricle in patients with Ramsay Hunt syndrome before the appearance of herpetic eruption and identified VZV genome in five of seven patients (72%). Thus PCR will be a powerful tool for early diagnosis of VZV infection in acute facial palsy, although it is not yet available in office settings. Clinicians should be aware of this feature of delayed herpetic eruptions in Ramsay Hunt syndrome until such time that easy and rapid diagnosis of VZV infection becomes feasible.

Facial Nerve Paralysis

In Ramsay Hunt syndrome, the severity of facial nerve paralysis is worse and the prognosis poorer than in Bell palsy. Devriese and Moesker[55] reported that complete paralysis was twice as frequent as incomplete paralysis, and occurred more often in patients older than 50. In 322 of our patients, 5.8% had House-Brackmann grade II, 3.9% grade III, 24.5% grade IV, 25.6% grade V, and 40.2% grade VI (see **Fig. 9.2**). Peitersen[7] reported full recovery in only 22% of patients, and Devriese and Moesker[55] found complete recovery in only 16%.

Murakami et al[67] reported the results of treatment with the use of steroids and antiviral agent acyclovir in

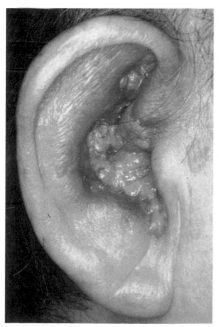
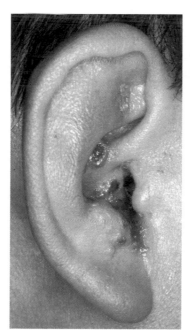
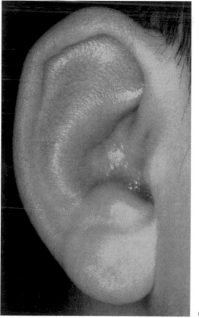

Fig. 9.5a–c Variations of herpetic eruption. Herpetic eruption in Ramsay Hunt syndrome varies considerably. (**a**) Severe eruptions with vesicles and swelling. (**b**) Moderate eruption. (**c**) Merely erythema.

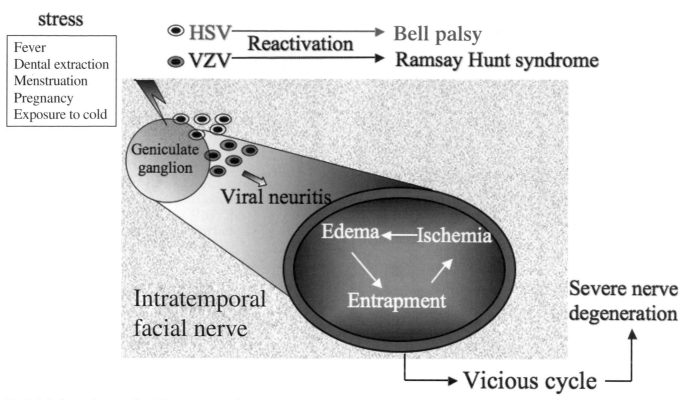

Fig. 9.9 Pathomechanism of viral facial nerve paralysis. Reactivation of herpes simplex virus (HSV) and varicella zoster virus (VZV) in the geniculate ganglion causes viral neuritis, producing a vicious cycle of edema, ischemia, and entrapment of the nerve in the bony facial canal that leads to severe nerve degeneration.

cellular immunity are thought to be important factors for viral reactivation.[79,80] The difference in the site of infection may also affect the frequency and spread of the viral reactivation.

Bell palsy and Ramsay Hunt syndrome may therefore be caused by reactivation of latent HSV and VZV, respectively, although the detailed mechanism of the virus reactivation is unclear. It could be viral neuropathy alone, ischemic neuropathy, or an autoimmune demyelination secondary to viral infection. Triggers known to be associated with Bell palsy and Ramsay Hunt syndrome are also known to reactivate herpes viruses. Preceding stress such as upper respiratory tract infection, fever, dental extraction, menstruation, or exposure to cold might reactivate latent herpes viruses in the geniculate ganglion. After the virus reactivates, it destroys ganglion cells and spreads into the endoneurial fluid.

The virus also infects Schwann cells, leading to demyelination and inflammation of the facial nerve.[81] This inflammatory response has been shown by gadolinium-enhanced magnetic resonance imaging in patients with Bell palsy and Ramsay Hunt syndrome.[82,83] Viral inflammation causes edema of the intratemporal facial nerve, which compresses itself in the bony facial canal, especially at the narrowest segment of the fundus of the internal auditory canal (meatal foramen)[84,85] or in the pyramidal portion[86,87] of the facial nerve. This is so-called entrapment. Nerve edema and entrapment has been demonstrated during decompression surgery.[86] Increased intraneural pressure blocks venous return, causing congestion of blood circulation. A vicious cycle of edema, compression, and ischemia of the nerve is an important factor associated with poor prognosis for facial nerve paralysis (**Fig. 9.9**).

References

1. Bell C. On the nerves. Giving an account of some experiments on their structure and functions, which leads to a new arrangement of the system. Philos Trans R Soc Lond 1821;3:398–428
2. The Nervous System of the Human Body. London: Longman, Rees, Orme, Brown, and Green; 1830
3. Hauser WA, Karnes WE, Annis J, Kurland LT. Incidence and prognosis of Bell's palsy in the population of Rochester, Minnesota. Mayo Clin Proc 1971;46(4):258–264
4. Yanagihara N. Incidence of Bell's palsy. Ann Otol Rhinol Laryngol Suppl 1988;137(supple 137):3–4
5. Adour KK, Byl FM, Hilsinger RL Jr, Kahn ZM, Sheldon MI. The true nature of Bell's palsy: analysis of 1,000 consecutive patients. Laryngoscope 1978;88(5):787–801
6. Katusic SK, Beard CM, Wiederholt WC, Bergstralh EJ, Kurland LT. Incidence, clinical features, and prognosis in Bell's palsy, Rochester, Minnesota, 1968-1982. Ann Neurol 1986;20(5):622–627

7. Peitersen E. The natural history of Bell's palsy. Am J Otol 1982;4(2):107–111

8. Yanagihara N, Hyodo M. Association of diabetes mellitus and hypertension with Bell's palsy and Ramsay Hunt syndrome. Ann Otol Rhinol Laryngol Suppl 1988;137:5–7

9. Asaki C, Ogiwara M, Kasama S, et al. Clinical study on recent Bell's palsy complicated with diabetes. J Pain Clin. 1995;147–151

10. May M, Fria TJ, Blumenthal F, Curtin H. Facial paralysis in children: differential diagnosis. Otolaryngol Head Neck Surg 1981;89(5):841–848

11. Adour KK, Wingerd J. Idiopathic facial paralysis (Bell's palsy): factors affecting severity and outcome in 446 patients. Neurology 1974;24(12):1112–1116

12. Diamant H, Ekstrand T, Wiberg A. Prognosis of idiopathic Bell's palsy. Arch Otolaryngol 1972;95(5):431–433

13. Pitts DB, Adour KK, Hilsinger RL Jr. Recurrent Bell's palsy: analysis of 140 patients. Laryngoscope 1988;98(5):535–540

14. May M. Differential diagnosis by history, physical findings and laboratory results. In: May M, ed. The Facial Nerve. New York: Thieme; 1986

15. Auerbach SH, Depiero TJ, Mejlszenkier J. Familial recurrent peripheral facial palsy. Observations of the pediatric population. Arch Neurol 1981;38(7):463–464

16. Graham MD, Kartush JM. Total facial nerve decompression for recurrent facial paralysis: an update. Otolaryngol Head Neck Surg 1989;101(4):442–444

17. McCormick DP. Herpes-simplex virus as a cause of Bell's palsy. Lancet 1972;1(7757):937–939

18. Hilger JA. The nature of Bell's palsy. Laryngoscope 1949;59(3):228–235

19. Devriese PP. Compression and ischaemia of the facial nerve. Acta Otolaryngol 1974;77(1):108–118

20. Abramsky O, Webb C, Teitelbaum D, Arnon R. Cellular immune response to peripheral nerve basic protein in idiopathic facial paralysis (Bell's palsy). J Neurol Sci 1975;26(1):13–20

21. McGovern FH, Estevez J, Jackson R. Immunological concept for Bell's palsy: further experimental study. Ann Otol Rhinol Laryngol 1977;86(3 Pt 1):300–305

22. Grose C, Feorino PM, Dye LA, Rand J. Bell's palsy and infectious mononucleosis. Lancet 1973;2(7823):231–232

23. Group P. Bell's palsy and herpes simplex infection. BMJ 1977;2(6090):829–830

24. McGovern FH. Bilateral Bell's palsy. Laryngoscope 1965;75:1070–1080

25. Yasui I, Miyasaki T. [Case of poliomyelitis due to virus type I manifested only by right facial paralysis]. Jpn J Infect Dis 1962;36:427–430

26. Beardwell A. Facial palsy due to the mumps virus. Br J Clin Pract 1969;23(1):37–38

27. Jamal GA, Al-Husaini A. Bell's palsy and infection with rubella virus. J Neurol Neurosurg Psychiatry 1983;46(7):678–680

28. Bartholomew C, Cleghorn F, Jack N, Edwards J, Blattner W. Human T-cell lymphotropic virus type I-associated facial nerve palsy in Trinidad and Tobago. Ann Neurol 1997;41(6):806–809

29. Schielke E, Pfister HW, Einhäupl KM. Peripheral facial nerve palsy associated with HIV infection. Lancet 1989;1(8637):553–554

30. Adour KK, Bell DN, Hilsinger RL Jr. Herpes simplex virus in idiopathic facial paralysis (Bell palsy). JAMA 1975;233(6):527–530

31. Vahlne A, Edström S, Arstila P, et al. Bell's palsy and herpes simplex virus. Arch Otolaryngol 1981;107(2):79–81

32. Nakamura K, Yanagihara N. Neutralization antibody to herpes simplex virus type 1 in Bell's palsy. Ann Otol Rhinol Laryngol Suppl 1988;137:18–21

33. Mulkens PS, Bleeker JD. Schroder, et al. Bell's palsy: a virus disease? An experimental study. In: Portmann M, ed. Facial Nerve. New York: Masson; 1985:248–252

34. Palva T, Hortling L, Ylikoski J, Collan Y. Viral culture and electron microscopy of ganglion cells in Meniere's disease and Bell's palsy. Acta Otolaryngol 1978;86(3–4):269–275

35. Murakami S, Mizobuchi M, Nakashiro Y, Doi T, Hato N, Yanagihara N. Bell palsy and herpes simplex virus: identification of viral DNA in endoneurial fluid and muscle. Ann Intern Med 1996;124(1 Pt 1):27–30

36. Furuta Y, Takasu T, Sato KC, Fukuda S, Inuyama Y, Nagashima K. Latent herpes simplex virus type 1 in human geniculate ganglia. Acta Neuropathol 1992;84(1):39–44

37. Takasu T, Furuta Y, Sato KC, Fukuda S, Inuyama Y, Nagashima K. Detection of latent herpes simplex virus DNA and RNA in human geniculate ganglia by the polymerase chain reaction. Acta Otolaryngol 1992;112(6):1004–1011

38. Burgess RC, Michaels L, Bale JF Jr, Smith RJH. Polymerase chain reaction amplification of herpes simplex viral DNA from the geniculate ganglion of a patient with Bell's palsy. Ann Otol Rhinol Laryngol 1994;103(10):775–779

39. Kumagami H. Experimental facial nerve paralysis. Arch Otolaryngol 1972;95(4):305–312

40. Thomander L, Aldskogius H, Vahlne A, Kristensson K, Thomas E. Invasion of cranial nerves and brain stem by herpes simplex virus inoculated into the mouse tongue. Ann Otol Rhinol Laryngol 1988;97(5 Pt 1):554–558

41. Ishii K, Kurata T, Nomura Y. Experiments on herpes simplex viral infections of the facial nerve in the tympanic cavity. Eur Arch Otorhinolaryngol 1990;247(3):165–167

42. Ishii K, Kurata T, Sata T, et al. An experimental model of type-1 herpes simplex virus infection of facial nerve. Eur Arch Otorhinolaryngol 1990;247(3):165–167

43. Sugita T, Murakami S, Yanagihara N, Fujiwara Y, Hirata Y, Kurata T. Facial nerve paralysis induced by herpes simplex virus in mice: an animal model of acute and transient facial paralysis. Ann Otol Rhinol Laryngol 1995;104(7):574–581

44. Wakisaka H, Hato N, Honda N, et al. Demyelination associated with HSV-1-induced facial paralysis. Exp Neurol 2002;178(1):68–79

45. Honda N, Hato N, Takahashi H, et al. Pathophysiology of facial nerve paralysis induced by herpes simplex virus type 1 infection. Ann Otol Rhinol Laryngol 2002;111(7 Pt 1):616–622

46. Murakami S, Hato N, Mizobuchi M, Doi T, Yanagihara N. Role of herpes simplex virus infection in the pathogenesis of facial paralysis in mice. Ann Otol Rhinol Laryngol 1996;105(1):49–53

47. Hato N, Hitsumoto Y, Honda N, Murakami S, Yanagihara N. Immunologic aspects of facial nerve paralysis induced by herpes simplex virus infection in mice. Ann Otol Rhinol Laryngol 1998;107(8):633–637

48. Takahashi H, Hitsumoto Y, Honda N, et al. Mouse model of Bell's palsy induced by reactivation of herpes simplex virus type 1. J Neuropathol Exp Neurol 2001;60(6):621–627

49. Denny-Brown D, Brenner C. Paralysis of nerve induced by direct pressure and by tourniquet. Arch Neurol Psychiatry 1944;51:1–26

50. Calcaterra TC, Rand RW, Bentson JR. Ischemic paralysis of the facial nerve: a possible etiologic factor in Bell's palsy. Laryngoscope 1976;86(1):92–97

51. Kumoi T, Iritani H, Nishimura Y, Minatogawa T. Animal model for ischemic facial nerve paralysis with selective vascular embolization. Ann Otol Rhinol Laryngol 1992;101(5):423–429

52. Jonsson L, Alm G, Thomander L. Elevated serum interferon levels in patients with Bell's palsy. Arch Otolaryngol Head Neck Surg 1989;115(1):37–40

53. Yilmaz M, Tarakcioglu M, Bayazit N, Bayazit YA, Namiduru M, Kanlikama M. Serum cytokine levels in Bell's palsy. J Neurol Sci 2002;197(1–2):69–72

54. Bujía J, Kim C, Bruegel F. Soluble interleukin 2 receptors in patients with Bell's palsy. Allergol Immunopathol (Madr) 1996; 24(3):112–115

55. Devriese PP, Moesker WH. The natural history of facial paralysis in herpes zoster. Clin Otolaryngol Allied Sci 1988;13(4):289–298

56. Robillard RB, Hilsinger RL Jr, Adour KK. Ramsay Hunt facial paralysis: clinical analyses of 185 patients. Otolaryngol Head Neck Surg 1986;95(3 Pt 1):292–297

57. Burke BL, Steele RW, Beard OW, Wood JS, Cain TD, Marmer DJ. Immune responses to varicella-zoster in the aged. Arch Intern Med 1982;142(2):291–293

58. Oxman MN, Levin MJ, Johnson GR, et al; Shingles Prevention Study Group. A vaccine to prevent herpes zoster and postherpetic neuralgia in older adults. N Engl J Med 2005;352(22): 2271–2284

59. Civen R, Chaves SS, Jumaan A, et al. The incidence and clinical characteristics of herpes zoster among children and adolescents after implementation of varicella vaccination. Pediatr Infect Dis J 2009;28(11):954–959

60. Hato N, Kisaki H, Honda N, Gyo K, Murakami S, Yanagihara N. Ramsay Hunt syndrome in children. Ann Neurol 2000;48(2): 254–256

61. Weller TH, Witton HM, Bell EJ. The etiologic agents of varicella and herpes zoster; isolation, propagation, and cultural characteristics in vitro. J Exp Med 1958;108(6):843–868

62. Miller AE. Selective decline in cellular immune response to varicella-zoster in the elderly. Neurology 1980;30(6):582–587

63. Murakami S, Hato N, Horiuchi J, et al. [Clinical features and prognosis of facial palsy and hearing loss in patients with Ramsay Hunt syndrome]. Nippon Jibiinkoka Gakkai Kaiho 1996;99(12): 1772–1779

64. Hunt JR. On herpetic inflammations of the geniculate ganglion: a new syndrome and its complications. J Nerv Ment Dis 1907; 34:73–96

65. Hunt JR. The symptom-complex of the acute posterior poliomyelitis of the geniculate, auditory, glossopharyngeal and pneumogastric ganglia. Arch Intern Med 1910;5:631–675

66. Murakami S, Honda N, Mizobuchi M, Nakashiro Y, Hato N, Gyo K. Rapid diagnosis of varicella zoster virus infection in acute facial palsy. Neurology 1998;51(4):1202–1205

67. Murakami S, Hato N, Horiuchi J, Honda N, Gyo K, Yanagihara N. Treatment of Ramsay Hunt syndrome with acyclovir-prednisone: significance of early diagnosis and treatment. Ann Neurol 1997; 41(3):353–357

68. Wayman DM, Pham HN, Byl FM, Adour KK. Audiological manifestations of Ramsay Hunt syndrome. J Laryngol Otol 1990; 104(2):104–108

69. Sweeney CJ, Gilden DH. Ramsay Hunt syndrome. J Neurol Neurosurg Psychiatry 2001;71(2):149–154

70. Aitken RS, Brain RT. Facial palsy and infection with zoster virus. Lancet 1933;I:19–22

71. Tomita H, Hayakawa W. Varicella-Zoster virus in idiopathic facial palsy. Arch Otolaryngol 1972;95(4):364–368

72. Lewis GW. Zoster sine herpete. BMJ 1958;2(5093):418–421

73. Furuta Y, Ohtani F, Kawabata H, Fukuda S, Bergström T. High prevalence of varicella-zoster virus reactivation in herpes simplex virus-seronegative patients with acute peripheral facial palsy. Clin Infect Dis 2000;30(3):529–533

74. Murakami S, Hato N, Horiuchi J, Honda N, Gyo K, Yanagihara N. Treatment of Ramsay Hunt syndrome with acyclovir-prednisone: significance of early diagnosis and treatment. Ann Neurol 1997; 41(3):353–357

75. Cawthorne T, Wilson T. Indications for intratemporal facial nerve surgery. Arch Otolaryngol 1963;78:429–434

76. Adour KK. Otological complications of herpes zoster. Ann Neurol 1994;35(Suppl):S62–S64

77. Croen KD, Ostrove JM, Dragovic LJ, Straus SE. Patterns of gene expression and sites of latency in human nerve ganglia are different for varicella-zoster and herpes simplex viruses. Proc Natl Acad Sci U S A 1988;85(24):9773–9777

78. Straus SE. Clinical and biological differences between recurrent herpes simplex virus and varicella-zoster virus infections. JAMA 1989;262(24):3455–3458

79. Sawtell NM, Poon DK, Tansky CS, Thompson RL. The latent herpes simplex virus type 1 genome copy number in individual neurons is virus strain specific and correlates with reactivation. J Virol 1998;72(7):5343–5350

80. Lekstram-Hines J, Pesnicak L, Straus SE. The quantity of latent viral DNA correlates with herpes simplex virus type I and 2 cause recurrent genital herpes outbreaks. J Virol 1998;72:2760–2764

81. Townsend JJ, Collins PK. Peripheral nervous system demyelination with herpes simplex virus. J Neuropathol Exp Neurol 1986;45(4):419–425

82. Daniels DL, Czervionke LF, Millen SJ, et al. MR imaging of facial nerve enhancement in Bell palsy or after temporal bone surgery. Radiology 1989;171(3):807–809

83. Jonsson L, Tien R, Engström M, Thuomas KA. Gd-DPTA enhanced MRI in Bell's palsy and herpes zoster oticus: an overview and implications for future studies. Acta Otolaryngol 1995;115(5):577–584

84. Fowler EP Jr. The pathologic findings in a case of facial paralysis. Acta Otolaryngol 1963;56:113–125

85. Fisch U, Esslen E. Total intratemporal exposure of the facial nerve. Pathologic findings in Bell's palsy. Arch Otolaryngol 1972; 95(4):335–341

86. Yanagihara N, Hato N, Murakami S, Honda N. Transmastoid decompression as a treatment of Bell palsy. Otolaryngol Head Neck Surg 2001;124(3):282–286

87. Nakashima S, Sando I, Takahashi H, Fujita S. Computer-aided 3-D reconstruction and measurement of the facial canal and facial nerve. I. Cross-sectional area and diameter: preliminary report. Laryngoscope 1993;103(10):1150–1156

10 Medical Treatment of Bell Palsy

Jeffrey T. Vrabec

Understanding the pathogenesis of a disease is fundamental in designing therapy. Preceding chapters have presented the differential diagnosis of acute facial paralysis and evidence linking reactivation of herpes simplex virus (HSV) with development of Bell palsy (BP). Therefore, this chapter begins with two assumptions: (1) that the diagnosis of BP implies an HSV-induced viral neuropathy and (2) that treatment must address the underlying viral illness or its consequences to alter the natural history of the disease.

■ Epidemiology

There have been many epidemiological studies intended to define the incidence of BP, with most estimates between 18 and 40 cases per 100,000 persons annually (**Table 10.1**).[1–8] Epidemiological studies may be based on a specific population or on encounters by a specific provider. Each type of study has its own inherent strengths and weaknesses. Population-based studies define the population at risk and survey all providers to generate incidence figures; however, the diagnosis is not independently confirmed. Practice-based studies have the advantage of a consistent diagnosis, while making the assumption that all of the population at risk are examined at a specific site. **Table 10.1** includes several large studies of each type, providing a consensus range for the annual incidence.

Several studies have examined annual incidence according to age, gender, ethnicity, climate, and season. There is some variability in the conclusions depending on the sample size and reliability of the correction of incidence figures to the control population. It is clear that BP is uncommon in children, with low incidence consistently reported in those under age 18. Incidence rates rapidly increase in the third decade to the overall population mean and then either reach a plateau or show a slight increase in the oldest age groups. The incidence of BP in women may be slightly greater. In reports that indicate a difference in incidence according to gender, women are universally cited as having the greater incidence. Likewise, there is some debate regarding seasonal variation of incidence figures. When seasonal variability is reported, the greater incidence is in the winter months. Campbell and Brundage show a modest increased risk in winter months with an odds ratio of 1.31 (95% confidence interval 1.13–1.51).[3]

Few studies examine ethnically heterogeneous populations. It is tempting to directly compare incidence figures between studies of geographically distinct populations, though it is not certain that the methodology is uniform. Slight differences in incidence among ethnic groups were encountered in a survey of U.S. military personnel, with the highest incidence in Hispanics.[3] Comparisons between surveys of predominantly Mexican Americans in Laredo, Texas, and predominantly Caucasians in Olmsted County, Minnesota, tend to support the assertion of a greater incidence in Hispanics.[2,6] However, these observations must be viewed within the context of HSV prevalence in the population.

Given the assumed role of HSV in the development of BP, it is useful to understand the epidemiology of HSV infection and basic virus physiology. HSV-1 is typically acquired via transmission of infected saliva. Introduction of the virus in the oral cavity allows retrograde uptake of the virus along sensory nerves, which can include branches of both the facial and trigeminal nerves. This results in establishment of a latent state of infection in sensory ganglia that is permanent. Viral replication is arrested by local and systemic immune responses primarily via CD8+ T cells, which also

Table 10.1 Incidence of Bell Palsy

Author	Country	Setting	N	Incidence/100,000	Race
Peitersen[1]	Denmark	Practice	1,701	32	Caucasian
Brandenburg and Annegers[2]	United States	Population	221	25	Hispanic
Campbell and Brundage[3]	United States	Population	1,181	40	Multiple
de Diego et al[4]	Spain	Practice	1,906	24	Caucasian
Hauser et al[5]	United States	Population	121	23	Caucasian
Katusic et al[6]	United States	Population	206	25	Caucasian
Yanagihara[7]	Japan	Population	1,663	30	Japanese
Adour et al[8]	United States	Practice	1,000	18	Caucasian

N, total cases in series.

remain permanently in the ganglion.[9,10] Presence of HSV in the geniculate ganglion is frequently documented in autopsy series, though the viral load is highly variable, indicating the significance of local cellular responses.[11,12] The virus is capable of reactivation, during which it uses host cellular enzymes, including ribonucleic acid polymerase II, and transcription factors for viral replication. The complete virion may spread to adjacent cells or is transported antegrade to peripheral tissues. The stimulus for reactivation of the virus is uncertain but may broadly involve intercellular signaling pathways including signal transduction and activators of transcription factors.[13] Following the stimulus for reactivation, it takes ~24 hours for viral synthesis to be completed. The process of viral replication results in lysis of many cell types, but this does not occur in neurons. The interaction between HSV, the host neuron, and the CD8+ T cell is incompletely understood, but predicts an ongoing process in which latency is maintained by successful arrest of intermittent viral synthesis and clinical reactivation is evident when the virus subverts CD8+ T cell–mediated suppression of viral synthesis.[9]

Prevalence of HSV infection increases with age, though the rate of acquisition varies substantially across different populations.[14] In general, the age at time of infection is greater in developed countries, implying an increased rate of infection in association with lower socioeconomic status. Seropositivity of HSV in the United States has been examined over time by the National Health and Nutrition Examination Survey (NHANES), conducted during the years 1976–1980, 1989–1994, and 1999–2004. The most recent NHANES III finds a decreasing seroprevalence in the past 30 years, with an overall prevalence of HSV-1 of 60% by age 49.[15]

Prevalence rates (in NHANES III) also vary according to ethnicity with the highest rates in Mexican-Americans (81%), intermediate in African-Americans (68%), and lowest in Caucasians (50% at age 49).[15] Similar trends are seen in a separate analysis of children under 13. In this group, Mexican-Americans born in Mexico have the highest prevalence rates, indicating earlier acquisition of HSV infection. Others born outside the United States had a greater prevalence than those born in the United States. The data also found correlation with socioeconomic status, as those children living in families with incomes below the poverty level had a greater prevalence of HSV-1 seropositivity (52% versus 24%; $p < 0.001$).[16]

The rate of acquisition of infection does vary by gender. Equal seroprevalence of HSV-1 is seen in children, emphasizing the role of intrafamilial spread of infection. Prevalence rates in women 14 to 29 years of age are significantly greater than men in each NHANES survey, though differences disappear with increasing age.[15] The faster rate of acquisition in women implies infection through sexual contacts and is mirrored in acquisition of HSV-2 infections. The data also implies young women have a greater probability of an older partner.

The declining rate of infection over time is attributed to rising socioeconomic status, smaller family sizes, and improved hygiene, and is mirrored in other developed countries.[17,18] This reasoning is confirmed by the higher prevalence in immigrant populations and greater decline in prevalence over time in individuals born in the United States. The strong trends linking HSV with socioeconomic status suggest that there may be little, if any, difference in susceptibility to HSV infection due to ethnicity. A difference in incidence of BP according to ethnicity was previously cited. Because none of the studies correct for seroprevalence of HSV, or socioeconomic status of the population of interest, differences in BP incidence are likely to be due to differences in HSV prevalence rather than a unique ethnic susceptibility to disease.

■ Natural History

The decision to prescribe treatment implies that there is benefit to the patient over nontreatment, creating a need for a thorough understanding of the natural history of the disease. Clinical observations and tests are used to classify patients according to severity with the intent to identify individuals with greater degrees of nerve degeneration. Several factors have a strong influence on the final outcome including degree of facial weakness, time to onset of recovery, degree of electrical degeneration, and age.

The largest series of untreated patients is described by Peitersen.[1] In this extensive series, recovery to normal function occurs in 71% of all patients. Twelve percent had minor sequelae that could include mild contracture. Thirteen percent had moderate sequelae, such as moderate weakness, obvious contracture, and synkinesis. Only 4% had severe residual weakness, disfiguring contracture, and marked synkinesis. In this series, 70% of patients developed complete paralysis and attained recovery to normal in 61%. Of those with incomplete paralysis, 94% eventually recovered to normal. The sooner signs of recovery began, the greater the probability of full recovery. Individuals with initial signs of recovery beginning after the second week had a significantly poorer probability of recovery to normal. However, 85% of all patients showed some signs of recovery within the first 3 weeks. There was a significant effect of age on recovery, as only 36% of individuals over age 60 attained full recovery versus 90% of those under 15. The most common associated symptoms were pain in 52%, dysgeusia in 34%, and hyperacusis in 14%.

Adour et al[8] reported a small series of 86 untreated patients seen within 5 days of onset. Of the entire group, 63% achieved return of normal function. Correction for degree of paralysis finds that complete recovery is seen in 72% of patients with incomplete paralysis, dropping to 40% if complete facial paralysis developed. Only 29% of their patients developed complete paralysis. Associated symptoms included pain in 62%, dysgeusia in 57%, and hyperacusis in 29%.

Devriese et al report an extensive series of 1,235 patients with BP, though treatment varied from none to medications or surgery.[19] The untreated patients constituted almost half of the series. Factors dictating no intervention included incomplete paralysis, medical contraindication, delay in diagnosis, and unknown reason. The 371 patients who retained some degree of facial function showed recovery to normal in 80%. The 98 patients in whom steroids were deemed contraindicated had unspecified medical conditions but had a mean age significantly greater (62.7 years) than those with incomplete paralysis. Consequently, recovery to normal in this untreated group was only 30%.

May et al reported a series of untreated patients (compared with transmastoid decompression) and supplemented this report with additional data supporting the wide difference in outcome depending on degree of weakness.[20] In the personal series of 405 untreated patients, 56% developed complete paralysis. Normal recovery was seen in 59% of these individuals compared with 97% in the patients with incomplete paralysis. Most of these patients had electroneuronography studies over a period of 14 days from the onset. The minimal electromyography amplitude was expressed as a percentage of the amplitude of the normal side. Individuals with < 10% function recovered to normal in only 13% of cases, while those with > 25% function attained a normal outcome 90% of the time.[21]

These reports are generally in agreement that those individuals with incomplete paralysis have a more favorable prognosis. The probability of normal recovery varies as does the incidence of complete paralysis in each series. Adour et al noted the lowest percentage of complete paralysis and the lowest probability of normal function in the incomplete group.[8] There are likely to be differences in how each group rates the degree of function, with Adour et al possibly being the most critical of small differences in facial function. Nonetheless, as recovery with incomplete paralysis is substantially better without treatment, these individuals must be accounted for in studies discussing efficacy of any proposed treatment. Differences in practice referral patterns or treatment philosophy over time and possibly intrarater variability may also influence reported results.

Insight into the natural history of HSV reactivation is gained by considering herpes labialis, a manifestation of reactivation from the trigeminal ganglion. Clinical features include characteristic vesicular lesions (from which HSV can be cultured) in a dermatomal pattern involving the perioral region or nasal cavity. A prodrome consisting of pain at the affected site, headache, and mild general malaise may begin 1 to 2 days prior to the development of cutaneous lesions. The vesicles are painful at onset and accompanied by local tissue edema that resolves as the lesions become crusted. The lesions typically heal completely in 7 to 10 days. Recurrences are triggered by stress, sun exposure, illness, and trauma.[22] Approximately 30% of the population has experienced recurrent herpes labialis,

with no differences according to gender or seasonality.[22,23] Those who experience recurrences report a frequency of once per year or less in 48% of cases, and four times per year or greater in only 16%.[23] The frequency and severity of recurrences tends to diminish with time.[24] Those with frequent recurrences display considerable variability in interval between recurrences, severity of lesions, and site (or side of face) involved.[25] The appearance of clinical lesions does not reflect the true frequency of viral reactivation. Sensitive methods of detection coupled with daily surveillance finds that > 90% of HSV-1 reactivation in the oral cavity is subclinical with 54% of episodes lasting < 24 hours.[26] These observations indicate that episodes of reactivation are not uniform at the molecular level and likely illustrate differing levels of viral synthesis prior to immune system intervention.

Obviously, there is a significant difference in the observed frequency of clinical reactivation of HSV from the geniculate and trigeminal ganglia. There are multiple potential explanations based on differences in local neuronal populations and their susceptibility to viral reactivation. In addition, it is likely that many instances of disturbed function limited to sensory branches of the facial nerve are unrecognized clinically. Finally, development of motor division paralysis (which is not observed in trigeminal nerve reactivation) is likely due to the unique anatomic relationship of the facial nerve to the meatal foramen, where it occupies ~98% of the available lumen.[27] The impact of developing intraneural edema will be manifest at the site where it is least tolerated.

■ Management

The list of therapies proposed for treatment of BP is as variable as it is long. Early therapies were presumably applied based on an assumed ischemic injury to the nerve. Thus, vasodilators such as histamine and nicotinic acid were promoted. Evolution to minimally invasive techniques included cervical sympathetic and stellate ganglion blocks, and steroid injections given intratympanically or to the stylomastoid foramen. Other more obscure therapies included radiation therapy, electrical stimulation, hyperbaric oxygen, and acupuncture. Support for any of these therapies is weak, including lack of controlled trials to address efficacy and an uncertain physiological mechanism to mitigate the disease development or progression.

The most commonly accepted clinical treatments include oral corticosteroids, antivirals, and topical eye care. Of these, eye care is the least controversial, and it is very important to prevent ocular complications such as corneal abrasion. Eye care usually consists of preservative-free artificial tears, a thicker ointment to be placed while sleeping, and possibly taping, patching, or use of a moisture chamber.

Steroids

Observations at surgery and histopathological examination of the facial nerve in BP have established that neural edema and inflammatory infiltrates are important features of the disorder.[28,29] Therefore, suppression of inflammation and reduction of edema are the primary treatment objectives to prevent nerve degeneration. Corticosteroids have been proposed for treatment of BP for over 60 years, but not without an ongoing debate as to their efficacy. Many early reports of efficacy have been criticized for nonrandomization, lack of placebo control, unvalidated measurement instrument, or inadequate power.[30] More controlled studies addressing the efficacy of steroid treatment for BP have been reported in the past 20 years, and when combined with techniques of meta-analysis, address earlier criticisms.

Recent large, randomized, controlled trials have produced greater evidence for the efficacy of oral steroids.[31,32] The two trials had a similar format in that individuals were enrolled within 72 hours of onset of the facial weakness and randomized to one of four groups: prednisone and placebo, antiviral and placebo, both active drugs, or two placebos. There are differences in the grading scales used, dosages of steroids and antivirals, persons involved in rating facial function, inclusion criteria (both do not exclude Lyme disease), and even patient contact (in person or a series of photographs). The groups were followed for 9 months or more and report similar findings. Patients receiving prednisone have a greater probability of achieving complete recovery of facial function compared with placebo.

Sullivan et al studied 551 patients in Scotland.[31] In this study, only three examiners rated all the patients; however, a series of four photographs was used for evaluation. The House-Brackmann scale was used for evaluation. The steroid treatment was prednisolone 500 mg (50 mg/day for 10 days) and the antiviral was acyclovir 2,000 mg/day for 10 days. In this study, 83% of patients displayed grade I function on the House-Brackmann scale at 3 months when treated with prednisone versus 64% in those not receiving prednisone ($p < 0.001$). At the last assessment at 9 months, 94% of patients receiving prednisone were judged to be grade I versus 82% of those not receiving steroids.

Engström et al analyzed a group of 839 patients in Sweden and Finland.[32] Up to 89 patients could have had Lyme disease, but they are included in the data assessment. The study used both the House-Brackmann scale and the Sunnybrook scale as rating instruments. The steroid treatment was prednisolone 450 mg (60 mg/day × 5, then taper by 10 mg/day) and the antiviral was valacyclovir 3,000 mg/day for 7 days. A large number of examiners (> 49) was used to record the data in this study. The study found 62% of patients receiving prednisone displayed normal function (Sunnybrook score of 100) at 3 months versus 51% in the patients not receiving prednisone ($p = 0.0007$). At 12 months, the comparable figures are 72% normal in the patients treated with prednisone versus 57% in those

without. At all time periods, normal function was more commonly achieved when using the House-Brackmann scale (grade I) versus the Sunnybrook scale (score of 100).

Subsequent meta-analyses including these studies confirm the utility of steroids in improving outcome in BP.[33,34] There are obvious methodological differences between these systematic reviews in trials included and data interpretation yet both conclude steroids are beneficial with a relative risk of 0.69 ($p = 0.001$) in the review by de Almeida et al and 0.71 ($p < 0.001$) in the review by Salinas et al.[33,34] Secondary analysis by de Almeida et al suggested that higher doses of prednisone (> 450 mg) are more effective.[33]

Antivirals

Antiviral medications including acyclovir and penciclovir are guanine analogs that lack a terminal hydroxyl group. When used as a substrate in deoxyribonucleic acid synthesis, this prevents further elongation of a growing chain.[35,36] The monophosphorylated form of each drug enters an infected cell where it is converted to a triphosphorylated form by viral thymidine kinase. Viral deoxyribonucleic acid polymerase has high affinity for the triphosphorylated drug, producing efficient and specific arrest of viral synthesis. Utility of these drugs requires an active process of viral replication, and they serve as an adjunct to the host immune response. A drawback of both drugs has been their poor oral bioavailability leading to the development of the prodrugs valacyclovir and famciclovir. Valacyclovir and famciclovir are metabolized in the liver to acyclovir and penciclovir, respectively. Safety of these agents is well documented and drug interactions are few.[37,38] Viral resistance to these agents is extremely rare in immunocompetent individuals, although occasionally seen in the immunocompromised. Alternative drugs targeting other steps in viral replication are under development.[39]

In general, antivirals would be predicted to have the greatest benefit when administered in advance of the stimulus for viral reactivation. For instance, antiviral prophylaxis is highly efficacious in preventing herpes labialis after dermabrasion.[40] When administered after the onset of clinical symptoms as in BP, the utility of the drug is reduced as viral replication is already under way. As time from onset of symptoms increases, so does the probability of successful arrest of viral replication by host immune responses. Thus, to produce any benefit, the antivirals must be administered as soon as possible and probably not after 72 hours.

The utility of antivirals in BP was first reported by Adour et al.[41] This double blind trial of 99 patients seen within 3 days of onset compared acyclovir 2 g/day to placebo, while all patients received prednisone (total dose of 450 mg over 10 days). Recovery to normal function was seen in 87% of patients treated with acyclovir and 72% of controls ($p = 0.06$). Approximately 20% of patients had complete paralysis. Hato et al examined efficacy of valacyclovir (1 g/day) versus placebo in a prospective manner in 221 patients treated within 7 days of onset, all of whom also received prednisolone.[42] Their definition of recovery included patients with some mild facial weakness. Using the same definition of recovery, the results were also similar in that 96.5% of antiviral group attained recovery compared with 90% in the placebo group ($p <$ 0.05). They did find the difference in prognosis to be more striking when comparing only those with complete paralysis: 90% recovery in the combined therapy group versus 75% in the steroid only group.

The outcomes of individuals treated only with antivirals, excluding concurrent use of steroid treatment, is unimpressive. De Diego et al report a randomized trial of acyclovir 2.4 g/day versus prednisone (1 mg/kg $\times$ 10 days with taper) in individuals enrolled within 4 days of onset of facial weakness.[43] Recovery in the 101 patients who completed the trial was defined as HB grade I or II, and was achieved in 94% of the steroid group and 78% of the antiviral group ($p = 0.002$). Similar findings are noted by Engström et al and Sullivan et al in which the antiviral-only arm of these trials does not differ from placebo.[31,32]

Recent meta-analyses report variable efficacy of antivirals in management of BP.[33,44] The inconsistency is not surprising considering each meta-analysis includes different studies and has a different definition of recovery. The studies conclude there is no benefit of antivirals alone versus placebo. However, when examining antivirals in combination with steroids, the relative risk of incomplete recovery reported by de Almeida et al is 0.75 ($p = 0.05$), compared with 0.71 ($p = 0.09$) reported by Lockhart et al.[33,44] The relative potency of antivirals used differs by a factor of 3 among trials, but secondary analysis by de Almeida et al did not find a significant difference in outcomes according to dosage.[33]

Summary of Management Recommendations

The previously discussed studies confirm the efficacy of steroids and suggest potential additional benefit of antivirals. However, the evidence regarding timing and dosage of these agents is less conclusive. Because the studies cited typically include only subjects enrolled early after onset of BP, one may rightfully assume that the effects of the medications are less when treatment is delayed. In addition, the severity of weakness at onset strongly influences recovery, thus those with mild and moderate degrees of weakness have less to gain with treatment. There is little evidence regarding recommended dosage as no studies examine different dosages of the active agent. Thus, the following recommendations are guidelines based on a combination of data and theoretical mechanisms of action.

Patients presenting within the first 72 hours are offered prednisone (total dose of 450 to 500 mg over 7 to 10 days) and valacyclovir (3 g/day over 5 days) or famciclovir (1 g/day over 5 days).[32] Lower doses of prednisone

may be less efficacious. Antiviral treatment should probably use higher doses than reported in most of the cited studies, as clinical differentiation between reactivation of HSV-1 and varicella zoster virus without associated skin lesions is difficult. Treatment of varicella zoster virus reactivation requires greater dosages of the antiviral agents for clinical benefit.[36,37] After 72 hours, the utility of antivirals would be questionable unless the patient was immunosuppressed.

Patients presenting after 1 week who retain some muscle function may not benefit from treatment. Counseling in this patient group should reflect on the high probability of recovery in view of the potential complications of treatment. The prognosis for those with complete paralysis is much poorer, and treatment is advocated even if presentation is delayed for more than 1 week. After 2 weeks from onset, it is unlikely that any treatment will have an impact on the recovery. Investigations of evoked electromyography data as a prelude to surgical decompression find that the outcome is largely determined by day 14. Individuals that did not show significant degeneration by this time enjoyed a good prognosis. In individuals with a poor prognosis, surgical intervention after 14 days did not influence recovery. By the same inference, a less aggressive intervention (i.e., medical therapy) would also not be expected to influence the recovery.[29,45]

■ Special Situations

Bell Palsy and Pregnancy

There is some controversy as to whether or not the etiology of Bell palsy occurring in pregnancy is the same or different than in patients who are not pregnant. This question has significant impact on management, as presumption of a different etiology would require a different treatment protocol. To address the question of etiology, relevant clinical observations of BP in pregnancy are reviewed.

The incidence of BP in pregnant women is no different than in all women of child-bearing age. In the United States (and other developed countries), a pregnancy rate of ~10% is observed. The reported prevalence of pregnant patients in clinical series of patients with BP is between 4 and 14%, thus not significantly deviating from expected.[46] The most widely cited report suggesting an increased incidence was given by Hilsinger et al.[47] However, our analysis finds the data in this paper is not consistent with national data on pregnancy rates in the United States.[46] This suggests the Hilsinger data reflects a population bias, such as active recruitment of pregnant patients with BP, or inaccurate calculation of the control population.

Nearly all reports of BP in pregnancy describe concentration of cases in the third trimester. The rarity of cases in early pregnancy may be a consequence of altered susceptibility of HSV reactivation. Both HSV-1 and HSV-2 display an increased incidence of recurrent lesions during the third trimester, and possibly, reduced incidence of recurrence (compared with nonpregnant women) during early pregnancy.[48,49]

Outcomes in pregnant patients are somewhat hard to evaluate given the small number of reports that directly address this question. If no treatment is given, poorer outcomes were observed in the pregnant patients.[1] However, when steroids were administered, no difference in outcome was observed.[47] Equivalent outcomes are also reported in pregnant patients with incomplete paralysis.[50] A nontreatment bias often exists, with pregnant patients frequently excluded, as seen in studies by Hilsinger et al and Gillman et al.[47,50]

Perceived differences in incidence or outcome of BP in pregnant patients likely reflect some selection bias in the study design. Without any substantial evidence to the contrary, it is unlikely that there is a different etiology for BP in pregnancy. Therefore, treatment is based on risk/benefit ratio of the drugs proposed for treatment. While the risks of steroids and antivirals have been outlined previously in this chapter, risks to the fetus must be considered. Steroids are associated with an increased risk of developmental defects when given in the first trimester.[51] However, steroids and antivirals are often administered in late pregnancy for both maternal and fetal disorders, and use in the setting of BP is justified after the first trimester.

Recurrent/Bilateral Bell Palsy

Any recurrence of acute facial weakness or bilateral involvement must arouse suspicion of a more ominous diagnosis than Bell palsy, including neoplasm, neurodegenerative disease, or chronic intracranial infection.[52,53] There is a clear distinction between bilateral sequential and bilateral simultaneous facial palsy. If the interval between onset of weakness on one side of face and the other is very short (i.e., less than a few weeks), the probability of a systemic process is enhanced. Alternatively, intervals exceeding several months allow consideration of independent reactivation of HSV from each geniculate ganglion. The differential diagnosis presented in **Table 10.2** is considered in bilateral and recurrent cases, though shorter intervals between episodes, associated neurological symptoms,

Table 10.2 Differential diagnosis of recurrent/bilateral facial paralysis

Facial nerve neoplasm, benign or malignant, primary or metastatic
Melkersson Rosenthal syndrome
Intracranial infectious diseases
Carcinomatous meningitis
Neurosarcoidosis
Gullain-Barré syndrome
Lyme disease
Aural tuberculosis
Skull base osteitis

Table 10.3 Recurrence rate of Bell Palsy

Author	Year	Nrec	Total	Rate (%)
Park and Watkins[55]	1949	31	440	7
Yanagihara et al[56]	1984	117	2,390	4.9
Pitts et al[57]	1988	140	1,980	7
Devriese et al[19]	1990	104	1,212	8.5
Peitersen[1]	2002	115	1,701	6.8

Nrec, number of recurrent cases observed.

and physical exam findings influence the diagnostic approach (see also Chapter 7 for differential diagnosis). The most useful tests for diagnosis in recurrent/bilateral facial weakness include imaging and lumbar puncture. Unique magnetic resonance imaging findings can be diagnostic for many of the conditions outlined in **Table 10.2**, while cerebrospinal fluid analysis may allow diagnosis of many infectious diseases or malignant neoplasms.[54]

Recurrent episodes of BP are uncommon, occurring in ~7% of patients (**Table 10.3**).[1,19,55–57] Recurrences can affect either side of the face: the side paralyzed initially or the previously uninvolved side, with equal probability. An individual that has experienced a recurrence may have an increasing probability of subsequent recurrence, though these data are based on a very small number of subjects. However, less than 1 in 1,000 individuals having BP experience more than three episodes. Some cases occur within 1 year, though most occur after 5 years, producing a mean interval between recurrences of 6 to 13 years.[57,58]

There does not appear to be any difference in prognosis for individuals with recurrent BP, even when correcting for recurrent ipsilateral versus contralateral paralysis.[57,58] In view of this observation, management should follow the same protocol outlined previously. Some have advocated decompression of the labyrinthine segment for recurrent cases. Given the low probability of ipsilateral recurrence and the similar outcome with medical treatment, it would be very difficult to prove efficacy in a randomized clinical trial of prophylactic decompression.

Familial Bell Palsy

The observance of BP in families has been described on many occasions (**Table 10.4**).[1,8,59–62] Most reports describe

Table 10.4 Prevalence of affected family members by history

Author	Year	Total	+FH	%
Alter[59]	1963	105	30	28.5
Willbrand et al[60]	1974	230	14	6
Adour et al[8]	1978	1,048	84	8
Alonso-Vilatela et al[61]	1979	115	35	30.5
Yanagihara et al[62]	1988	625	26	4
Peitersen[1]	2002	1,701	NS	4

+FH, cases with a positive family history; NS, not stated in manuscript.

a limited number of affected individuals (often only two) across two or three generations. There are two basic study designs: those that include examination of all affected family members and those which rely on the patient's recall without actual confirmation of the diagnosis. Most published reports are of the latter type, which leads to substantial variability and uncertainty in the data obtained. The reported prevalence of BP in family members ranges from 2–30%, with the highest incidence in the smaller studies. Possibly, selection bias influences the prevalence figures in these reports. Only a single study reports a control group, finding a family history of BP in 30% of those with a history of BP versus 4% in those individuals without a history of BP.[61] Common features of familial cases include a very high incidence of recurrent palsy, estimated to be between 20 and 30%, and a young age of onset, typically in the teens.

Multiple different modes of inheritance have been proposed, which is not surprising given the variability in the reported prevalence rate. An autosomal dominant pattern is most frequently described, though penetrance is very low. This suggests that any familial tendency may be multifactorial. The probability of some genetic contribution to the disease is strengthened by a study of hospital admission data for BP in Sweden over a 15-year interval.[63] An increased risk of developing BP was seen in siblings but not in spouses, implying that host genetic factors are important in determining disease susceptibility. The specific genetic predisposition is uncertain but anatomical factors such as a narrow meatal foramen or increased susceptibility to viral infections are possible. Genetic determinants of HSV reactivation could include a permissive cellular environment for establishment of infection and/or reactivation from latency.[23,64] Once again, the limited data available do not indicate a different prognosis in familial cases. Therefore, no alterations in management are recommended.

Several reported pedigrees of familial facial paralysis include individuals that suffer from oculomotor nerve palsies in association with the facial palsy, a clinical finding that is not associated with BP.[65,66] Melkersson Rosenthal syndrome, with its associated facial edema, represents another distinct example of familial recurrent facial palsy.[67] The etiology of multiple cranial neuropathy or facial palsy with facial edema is obscure and likely to be different than BP. Speculation as to the underlying cause for these other forms of familial facial palsy might include brainstem ischemia/infarction, multiple sclerosis, metabolic dysfunction, migraine, and any chronic granulomatous process.[68]

References

1. Peitersen E. Bell's palsy: the spontaneous course of 2,500 peripheral facial nerve palsies of different etiologies. Acta Otolaryngol Suppl 2002(549):4–30

2. Brandenburg NA, Annegers JF. Incidence and risk factors for Bell's palsy in Laredo, Texas: 1974–1982. Neuroepidemiology 1993;12(6):313–325

3. Campbell KE, Brundage JF. Effects of climate, latitude, and season on the incidence of Bell's palsy in the US Armed Forces, October 1997 to September 1999. Am J Epidemiol 2002;156(1):32–39

4. De Diego JI, Prim MP, Madero R, Gavilán J. Seasonal patterns of idiopathic facial paralysis: a 16-year study. Otolaryngol Head Neck Surg 1999;120(2):269–271

5. Hauser WA, Karnes WE, Annis J, Kurland LT. Incidence and prognosis of Bell's palsy in the population of Rochester, Minnesota. Mayo Clin Proc 1971;46(4):258–264

6. Katusic SK, Beard CM, Wiederholt WC, Bergstralh EJ, Kurland LT. Incidence, clinical features, and prognosis in Bell's palsy, Rochester, Minnesota, 1968–1982. Ann Neurol 1986;20(5):622–627

7. Yanagihara N. Incidence of Bell's palsy. Ann Otol Rhinol Laryngol Suppl 1988;137(137):3–4

8. Adour KK, Byl FM, Hilsinger RL Jr, Kahn ZM, Sheldon MI. The true nature of Bell's palsy: analysis of 1,000 consecutive patients. Laryngoscope 1978;88(5):787–801

9. Divito S, Cherpes TL, Hendricks RL. A triple entente: virus, neurons, and CD8+ T cells maintain HSV-1 latency. Immunol Res 2006;36(1–3):119–126

10. Arbusow V, Derfuss T, Held K, et al. Latency of herpes simplex virus type-1 in human geniculate and vestibular ganglia is associated with infiltration of CD8+ T cells. J Med Virol 2010;82(11):1917–1920

11. Vrabec JT, Alford RL. Quantitative analysis of herpes simplex virus in cranial nerve ganglia. J Neurovirol 2004;10(4):216–222

12. Arbusow V, Schulz P, Strupp M, et al. Distribution of herpes simplex virus type 1 in human geniculate and vestibular ganglia: implications for vestibular neuritis. Ann Neurol 1999;46(3):416–419

13. Kriesel JD. The roles of inflammation, STAT transcription factors, and nerve growth factor in viral reactivation and herpes keratitis. DNA Cell Biol 2002;21(5–6):475–481

14. Smith JS, Robinson NJ. Age specific prevalence of infection with herpes simplex virus types 2 and 1: a global review. J Infect Dis 2002;186(Suppl 1):S3–S28

15. Xu F, Sternberg MR, Kottiri BJ, et al. Trends in herpes simplex virus type 1 and type 2 seroprevalence in the United States. JAMA 2006;296(8):964–973

16. Xu F, Lee FK, Morrow RA, et al. Seroprevalence of herpes simplex virus type 1 in children in the United States. J Pediatr 2007;151(4):374–377

17. Pebody RG, Andrews N, Brown D, et al. The seroepidemiology of herpes simplex virus type 1 and 2 in Europe. Sex Transm Infect 2004;80(3):185–191

18. Hashido M, Kawana T, Matsunaga Y, Inouye S. Changes in prevalence of herpes simplex virus type 1 and 2 antibodies from 1973 to 1993 in the rural districts of Japan. Microbiol Immunol 1999;43(2):177–180

19. Devriese PP, Schumacher T, Scheide A, de Jongh RH, Houtkooper JM. Incidence, prognosis and recovery of Bell's palsy. A survey of about 1000 patients (1974–1983). Clin Otolaryngol Allied Sci 1990;15(1):15–27

20. May M, Klein SR, Taylor FH. Idiopathic (Bell's) facial palsy: natural history defies steroid or surgical treatment. Laryngoscope 1985;95(4):406–409

21. May M, Schaitkin BM. The Facial Nerve. May's Second Edition. New York: Thieme; 2000:352–353

22. Spruance SL. The natural history of recurrent oral-facial herpes simplex virus infection. Semin Dermatol 1992;11(3):200–206

23. Young TB, Rimm EB, D'Alessio DJ. Cross-sectional study of recurrent herpes labialis. Prevalence and risk factors. Am J Epidemiol 1988;127(3):612–625

24. Ship II, Miller MF, Ram C. A retrospective study of recurrent herpes labialis (RHL) in a professional population, 1958–1971. Oral Surg Oral Med Oral Pathol 1977;44(5):723–730

25. Davis LE, Redman JC, Skipper BJ, McLaren LC. Natural history of frequent recurrences of herpes simplex labialis. Oral Surg Oral Med Oral Pathol 1988;66(5):558–561

26. Mark KE, Wald A, Magaret AS, et al. Rapidly cleared episodes of herpes simplex virus reactivation in immunocompetent adults. J Infect Dis 2008;198(8):1141–1149

27. Eicher SA, Coker NJ, Alford BR, Igarashi M, Smith RJ. A comparative study of the fallopian canal at the meatal foramen and labyrinthine segment in young children and adults. Arch Otolaryngol Head Neck Surg 1990;116(9):1030–1035

28. Liston SL, Kleid MS. Histopathology of Bell's palsy. Laryngoscope 1989;99(1):23–26

29. Fisch U, Esslen E. Total intratemporal exposure of the facial nerve. Pathologic findings in Bell's palsy. Arch Otolaryngol 1972;95(4):335–341

30. Stankiewicz JA. A review of the published data on steroids and idiopathic facial paralysis. Otolaryngol Head Neck Surg 1987;97(5):481–486

31. Sullivan FM, Swan IR, Donnan PT, et al. Early treatment with prednisolone or acyclovir in Bell's palsy. N Engl J Med 2007;357(16):1598–1607

32. Engström M, Berg T, Stjernquist-Desatnik A, et al. Prednisolone and valaciclovir in Bell's palsy: a randomised, double-blind, placebo-controlled, multicentre trial. Lancet Neurol 2008;7(11):993–1000

33. de Almeida JR, Al Khabori M, Guyatt GH, et al. Combined corticosteroid and antiviral treatment for Bell palsy: a systematic review and meta-analysis. JAMA 2009;302(9):985–993

34. Salinas RA, Alvarez G, Daly F, Ferreira J. Corticosteroids for Bell's palsy (idiopathic facial paralysis). Cochrane Database Syst Rev 2010;(3):CD001942

35. Rolan P. Pharmacokinetics of new antiherpetic agents. Clin Pharmacokinet 1995;29(5):333–340

36. Beutner KR. Valacyclovir: a review of its antiviral activity, pharmacokinetic properties, and clinical efficacy. Antiviral Res 1995;28(4):281–290

37. Simpson D, Lyseng-Williamson KA. Famciclovir: a review of its use in herpes zoster and genital and orolabial herpes. Drugs 2006;66(18):2397–2416

38. Tyring SK, Baker D, Snowden W. Valacyclovir for herpes simplex virus infection: long-term safety and sustained efficacy after 20 years' experience with acyclovir. J Infect Dis 2002;186(Suppl 1):S40–S46

39. Dropulic LK, Cohen JI. Update on new antivirals under development for the treatment of double-stranded DNA virus infections. Clin Pharmacol Ther 2010;88(5):610–619

40. Wall SH, Ramey SJ, Wall F. Famciclovir as antiviral prophylaxis in laser resurfacing procedures. Plast Reconstr Surg 1999;104(4):1103–1108, discussion 1109

41. Adour KK, Ruboyianes JM, Von Doersten PG, et al. Bell's palsy treatment with acyclovir and prednisone compared with prednisone alone: a double-blind, randomized, controlled trial. Ann Otol Rhinol Laryngol 1996;105(5):371–378

42. Hato N, Yamada H, Kohno H, et al. Valacyclovir and prednisolone treatment for Bell's palsy: a multicenter, randomized, placebo-controlled study. Otol Neurotol 2007;28(3):408–413

43. De Diego JI, Prim MP, De Sarriá MJ, Madero R, Gavilán J. Idiopathic facial paralysis: a randomized, prospective, and controlled study using single-dose prednisone versus acyclovir three times daily. Laryngoscope 1998;108(4 Pt 1):573–575

44. Lockhart P, Daly F, Pitkethly M, Comerford N, Sullivan F. Antiviral treatment for Bell's palsy (idiopathic facial paralysis). Cochrane Database Syst Rev 2009;(4):CD001869

45. Gantz BJ, Rubinstein JT, Gidley P, Woodworth GG. Surgical management of Bell's palsy. Laryngoscope 1999;109(8):1177–1188

46. Vrabec JT, Isaacson B, Van Hook JW. Bell's palsy and pregnancy. Otolaryngol Head Neck Surg 2007;137(6):858–861

47. Hilsinger RL Jr, Adour KK, Doty HE. Idiopathic facial paralysis, pregnancy, and the menstrual cycle. Ann Otol Rhinol Laryngol 1975;84(4 Pt 1):433–442

48. Scott D, Moore S, Ide M, Coward P, Baylis R, Borkowska E. Recrudescent herpes labialis during and prior to early pregnancy. Int J Gynaecol Obstet 2003;80(3):263–269

49. Harger JH, Amortegui AJ, Meyer MP, Pazin GJ. Characteristics of recurrent genital herpes simplex infections in pregnant women. Obstet Gynecol 1989;73(3 Pt 1):367–372

50. Gillman GS, Schaitkin BM, May M, Klein SR. Bell's palsy in pregnancy: a study of recovery outcomes. Otolaryngol Head Neck Surg 2002;126(1):26–30

51. Park-Wyllie L, Mazzotta P, Pastuszak A, et al. Birth defects after maternal exposure to corticosteroids: prospective cohort study and meta-analysis of epidemiological studies. Teratology 2000;62(6):385–392

52. Teller DC, Murphy TP. Bilateral facial paralysis: a case presentation and literature review. J Otolaryngol 1992;21(1):44–47

53. Keane JR. Bilateral seventh nerve palsy: analysis of 43 cases and review of the literature. Neurology 1994;44(7):1198–1202

54. Ramsey KL, Kaseff LG. Role of magnetic resonance imaging in the diagnosis of bilateral facial paralysis. Am J Otol 1993;14(6):605–609

55. Park HW, Watkins AL. Facial paralysis; analysis of 500 cases. Arch Phys Med Rehabil 1949;30(12):749–762

56. Yanagihara N, Mori H, Kozawa T, Nakamura K, Kita M. Bell's palsy. Nonrecurrent v recurrent and unilateral v bilateral. Arch Otolaryngol 1984;110(6):374–377

57. Pitts DB, Adour KK, Hilsinger RL Jr. Recurrent Bell's palsy: analysis of 140 patients. Laryngoscope 1988;98(5):535–540

58. Devriese PP, Pelz PG. Recurrent and alternating Bell's palsy. Ann Otol Rhinol Laryngol 1969;78(5):1091–1104

59. Alter M. Familial aggregation of Bell's palsy. Neurology 1973;23:503–505

60. Willbrand JW, Blumhagen JD, May M. Inherited Bell's palsy. Ann Otol Rhinol Laryngol 1974;83(3):343–346

61. Alonso-Vilatela M, Bustamante-Balcárcel A, Figueroa-Tapia HH. Family aggregation in Bell's palsy. Acta Otolaryngol 1979;87(3-4):413–417

62. Yanagihara N, Yumoto E, Shibahara T. Familial Bell's palsy: analysis of 25 families. Ann Otol Rhinol Laryngol Suppl 1988;137:8–10

63. Hemminki K, Li X, Sundquist K. Familial risks for nerve, nerve root and plexus disorders in siblings based on hospitalisations in Sweden. J Epidemiol Community Health 2007;61(1):80–84

64. Vrabec JT, Liu L, Li B, Leal SM. Sequence variants in host cell factor C1 are associated with Ménière's disease. Otol Neurotol 2008;29(4):561–566

65. Aldrich MS, Beck RW, Albers JW. Familial recurrent Bell's palsy with ocular motor palsies. Neurology 1987;37(8):1369–1371

66. Sørensen TT. Familial recurrent cranial nerve palsies. Acta Neurol Scand 1988;78(6):542–543

67. Rogers RS III. Melkersson-Rosenthal syndrome and orofacial granulomatosis. Dermatol Clin 1996;14(2):371–379

68. Brazis PW. Isolated palsies of cranial nerves III, IV, and VI. Semin Neurol 2009;29(1):14–28

11 Surgical Treatment of Bell Palsy

Sarah E. Mowry and Bruce J. Gantz

Symmetric movement of the facial features is an integral part of how humans communicate. Loss of facial symmetry results in difficulty with communication and social stigma. Patients who suffer from facial asymmetry have difficulty communicating because the listener focuses on the asymmetry rather than what the speaker is saying. Furthermore, a small percentage of patients will have eye exposure; exposure keratitis is painful and might result in blindness. While any operation for idiopathic facial paralysis is normally a cosmetic procedure, the impact of restoring facial symmetry is much more far reaching.

The majority of patients with idiopathic facial palsy, Bell palsy, will resolve with conservative treatment, but there remains a subgroup of patients who continue to have poor facial nerve outcomes despite medical treatment. Between 10 and 15% of patients will have residual deficits in facial function without treatment.[1] The difficulty is in identifying in a timely fashion the patients who will benefit from surgical decompression. This chapter includes a review of surgical intervention for Bell palsy, the indications for surgery, and a technique for facial nerve decompression.

■ Historical Perspective

The first facial nerve decompression for Bell palsy was described by Balance and Duel in 1932.[2] They advocated decompression of only the distal 1 cm of the mastoid segment for cases of Bell palsy. The prevailing sentiment at the time was compression of the vascular supply to the nerve at the stylomastoid foramen resulted in the facial paralysis; therefore, further exposure of the nerve was not necessary to improve the vascular supply to the nerve. They did not speculate on the cause of the vascular compression. Interestingly, these authors also remarked on inflammation of the geniculate ganglion seen in some of their cases but attribute this finding only to cases of Ramsay Hunt syndrome. They did recommend decompression of the geniculate ganglion in patients with Ramsay Hunt syndrome when faradic stimulation was lost, but cautioned that outcomes are guarded. They did not recommend decompression of the geniculate ganglion in Bell palsy.

Between the 1930s and the 1950s, surgical decompression involved more proximal portions of the mastoid segment but did not involve the entire facial nerve. In Kettel's 1963 monograph on "Pathology and surgery of Bell palsy,"

he ascribed the facial weakness to autonomic dysregulation of the vascular supply of the nerve at the stylomastoid foramen.[3] He recommended distal decompression of the nerve when the patient demonstrated a complete paralysis and electromyography (EMG) showed no voluntary activity. He also noted that surgical intervention for Bell palsy was a controversial issue, as indeed it remains today.

There was much debate about both the cause of Bell palsy and the location of the lesion between the 1930s and the 1970s. Several authors felt the lesion was located at the origin of the chorda tympani.[4,5] Blatt and Freeman favored chorda tympani neurectomy as treatment for Bell palsy, although this procedure was not widely adopted.[6] Another group of surgeons advocated for transmastoid decompression.[7,8] This decompression extended from the geniculate ganglion or distal labyrinthine segment to the stylomastoid foramen. It did not involve the meatal foramen or address the full length of the labyrinthine segment. In the procedure described by Yanagihara et al in 1979, the incus is removed and the supralabyrinthine air cells are removed to gain access to the geniculate ganglion and the tympanic segment of the nerve. The incus is then replaced at the end of the decompression and secured in place with fibrin glue.[8] In one of the largest series of surgically treated patients, Yanagihara and colleagues evaluated 101 patients with Bell palsy who met the following criteria: age > 16 years, House-Brackmann (HB) grade V or VI, > 95% degeneration on evoked EMG, failed medical therapy, and with no severe systemic illness.[9] Patients were offered surgery within 3 months of the onset of paralysis. Of these 101 patients, 58 opted for transmastoid decompression and the remaining 43 patients refused surgical intervention. In general, those patients who underwent surgery achieved normal or near-normal facial function at a higher rate than those who only received steroids. There were two factors that negatively impacted on long-term facial function: age > 50 and prolonged time to surgical intervention. However, the authors noted that although patients with these factors had worse outcomes in general, surgical intervention improved the long-term outcome when compared with steroids alone. In the patients > 50 years, the overall recovery rate to HB grades I or II was > 25% for those who underwent surgery and < 20% for those who used steroids alone. Although patients operated on after 30 days of paralysis had worse overall recovery rates, those who underwent surgery between 31 and 60 days had a better chance of HB grade I or II function (38%) compared with those who did not have surgery

(23%). Unfortunately, no statistical analysis was provided for these subgroups.

May also performed transmastoid decompression of the facial nerve[7] but failed to find significant benefit. Although he originally advocated for facial nerve decompression, after evaluating his case series, May retracted his endorsement of surgery.[10,11] He felt the risks of the operation did not outweigh the benefits because he had found no difference in outcomes between surgical and nonsurgical patients. May's retraction was highly influential, and many surgeons stopped recommending operative intervention to patients with Bell palsy. However, a few case series have been published since then, most notably the case controlled series by Gantz et al as described subsequently.[12] Several other groups have reported on small numbers of patients operated within variable time intervals and with mixed results.[13,14]

The electrical testing of the facial nerve has also undergone a variety of changes since the 1920s. Prior to the 1960s, electrical testing relied on faradic (short duration direct current or alternating current) and galvanic (high voltage direct current of long duration) stimulation. Response to the stimulation was assessed by visual inspection. Routine use of EMG began in the 1960s and provided clinicians with a more sensitive, although still indirect, method to evaluate the integrity of the facial nerve. Fisch and Esslen popularized the term electroneuronography (ENoG), which has been shortened to electroneurography in the literature. Whereas EMG uses penetrating needle electrodes, ENoG uses surface electrodes and an external electric stimulus to assess the status of the nerve. Despite the fact that ENoG may be somewhat less sensitive when compared with EMG, ENoG is the preferred method of facial nerve testing in the literature. ENoG demonstrates degeneration of the nerve fibers within 3 to 5 days. However, the presence of fibrillation potentials, diagnostic of severe denervation, take between 10 and 25 days to develop on EMG. Prior to the development of fibrillation potentials, the percentage of denervated motor action units is not clear on EMG.[15]

Other testing used in the past to identify the site of the lesion of the nerve include Schirmer lacrimation testing, electrical taste testing, and stapedial reflex testing. Many patients present with normal lacrimation testing and abnormal stapedial reflex testing or abnormal taste testing. Prior to routine electrical testing, this topognostic testing was used by many authors to justify distal decompression. Later work revealed that topognostic testing is insensitive to identify the site of the lesion. Gantz et al performed intraoperative evoked EMG (EEMG) and compared the results to preoperative Schirmer lacrimation testing in 13 patients undergoing subtemporal decompression.[16] They found that 4 of 12 patients with normal Schirmer tests had lesions proximal to the geniculate ganglion and that the 1 patient with a lesion of the mastoid segment of the nerve had an abnormal

lacrimation test. Schirmer test correctly identified the site of lesion in only 61% of patients.

■ Rationale for Subtemporal Decompression

In 1961, House described the middle fossa approach to the internal auditory canal.[17] He advocated use of this procedure in several situations: acoustic tumor removal, facial nerve surgery, and vestibular nerve section for intractable Ménière disease. House and Crabtree in 1965[18] and Pulec in 1966[19] described total facial nerve decompression using the middle fossa transmastoid approach. The middle cranial fossa (MCF) approach provides access to the facial nerve from the brainstem to the tympanic segment of the facial nerve. The MCF approach allows for auditory and vestibular function preservation. Prior to 1961, full access to the nerve required a translabyrinthine approach, sacrificing hearing and balance function, neither of which is acceptable for a patient with a 50% chance of good functional recovery.

As more subtemporal decompressions were performed, information regarding pathologic findings in the facial nerve was reported. In 1972, Fisch and Esslen reported on a series of 12 patients who underwent total facial nerve decompression via the middle fossa approach. In 11 of the 12 patients, the nerve was found to have "pronounced [edema], red swelling ... with marked vascular injection ... proximal to the geniculate ganglion."[20] Eight of these eleven patients had involvement of the nerve within the internal auditory canal. Five of the eleven patients had swelling within the nerve distal to the geniculate ganglion. To identify the site of the conduction abnormality, Fisch and Esslen performed serial intraoperative EEMG starting from the stylomastoid foramen and ascending to the internal auditory canal. In the three patients tested in this manner, the conduction abnormality was located proximal to the geniculate ganglion and within the internal auditory canal (IAC).

Gantz et al also reported this proximal conduction abnormality.[16] Eighteen patients with between 90 and 98% degeneration on preoperative ENoG underwent decompression. In two patients, intraoperative EEMG could not be performed for technical reasons. Of the remaining 16 patients, 15 (94%) demonstrated conduction blocking proximal to the geniculate ganglion. One patient had a conduction block at the origin of the chorda tympani. According to these data, the vast majority of patients will have a conduction block proximal to the geniculate ganglion. Decompression should therefore involve the bony canal proximal to the geniculate ganglion.

There is anatomic data to corroborate the intraoperative conduction findings. The fallopian canal in the labyrinthine segment is particularly narrow: 0.69 mm in diameter on average.[21] There is also a tight arachnoid band at the opening of the fallopian canal in the fundus (meatal foramen).[21,22] These two anatomic "bottlenecks" do not allow room for edema of the nerve without compromise of the nerve fibers.

Taken together, the anatomic findings with the intraoperative electrical testing suggest the pathology in Bell palsy is localized to the distal IAC or labyrinthine segment of the nerve. If the patient is to be offered a decompression surgery, the operation should involve the entire labyrinthine segment with lysis of the arachnoid band within the fundus. Exposure to this area is best achieved via the MCF approach.

■ Indications for Surgical Intervention

While there are many clinicians who endorse surgical intervention in a selected patient population,[9,12,22] there are others who feel surgery is never indicated in Bell palsy.[10,23] At the present time, the evidence in the literature regarding facial nerve decompression is primarily from case series. There are no meta-analyses of surgical intervention, and a Cochrane Review of surgical therapy for early treatment of Bell palsy has been proposed but has not been completed.[24] Nor is there any formally randomized controlled trial for any surgical intervention for Bell palsy. May et al calculated the number of patients needed to adequately power a randomized trial for surgical intervention.[11] Using a Chi-squared test with type I error of 0.05, 716 patients would need to be enrolled.[11] Given the rarity of surgical necessity and the ethical dilemmas surrounding randomization in a surgical study, a truly randomized trial is unlikely to occur. A decision for surgery is therefore based on the available information regarding patient outcomes and a frank discussion with the patient.

Patients presenting within 14 days of the onset of Bell palsy who have complete facial paralysis are encouraged to undergo electrical testing. Electrical testing should not be performed in the first 3 to 5 days because wallerian degeneration of the severely affected nerve fibers has not occurred. Electrical testing is used to determine the percentage of nerve fibers that have undergone conduction blockade. Nerve fibers that remain intact but have axonoplasm flow blockade (neuropraxia) can be electrically stimulated distal to the site of conduction blockade. Fibers undergoing wallerian degeneration as a result of injury to the axon (axonomesis) or the entire neural tubule (neurotmesis) cannot be stimulated distal to the site of injury. When the neural tubule remains intact, the axon can regenerate to its original motor unit; in neurotmesis, axonal regrowth can result in aberrant innervation and synkinesis. Current testing can distinguish neuropraxia from axonomesis/neurotmesis but cannot differentiate between types of wallerian degeneration. However, the rate of degeneration can give insight as to the degree of axonal injury; rapid denervation is associated with

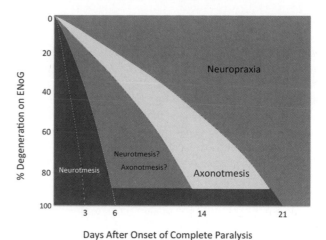

Fig. 11.1 The rate of degeneration indicates the level of neural injury. Nerves undergoing complete neurotmesis rapidly reach maximal degeneration. Those undergoing axonomesis take considerably longer to totally degenerate. In Bell palsy, the fibers undergo a combination of neurotmesis and axonomesis. (Used with permission from Gantz BJ, Rubinstein JT, Gidley P, Woodworth GG. Surgical management of Bell Palsy. Laryngoscope. 1999;109:1180.)

neurotmesis whereas slower degeneration is seen in axonomesis (**Fig. 11.1**). Currently, two electrical tests are in use to determine the extent of nerve degeneration and surgical candidacy: ENoG and voluntary EMG.

EMG allows for evaluation of spontaneous motor unit potentials of the facial muscles. During a voluntary EMG, no external electric stimulus is applied to the nerve. However, the patient may stimulate the muscle voluntarily. Transcutaneous needle electrodes measure electric activity within the muscle. The presence of a compound motor action potential response on voluntary EMG indicates early deblocking of neuropraxic fibers. ENoG measures the compound muscle action potential of the nerve at the nerve terminus after a maximal electrically evoked stimulus. ENoG allows for a comparison between the two sides of the face. The response of the weakened side of the face is reported as a percentage of the response of the normal side. Whereas EMG records the action potential in a small number of muscle fibers around the needle electrode, the ENoG records activity from the whole muscle because the electrodes are placed over the surface.

Patients with < 90% nerve degeneration on ENoG have a good prognosis (recovery to HB I or II). Those with > 90% nerve degeneration have a less optimistic prognosis. When ENoG demonstrates > 95% degeneration within 2 weeks of the onset of the paralysis, there is only a 40 to 50% chance of recovery to HB I or II.[22] Patients who progress to 90% degeneration will have further degeneration to the 95% level 90% of the time. Therefore, to prevent the progression to the 95% degeneration level, Fisch recommended decompression when the patient reaches 90% degeneration on ENoG.[22]

Fisch advocated daily testing between the sixth and fourteenth day or 90% degeneration is reached. Serial testing provides information about the rate of denervation; those that rapidly progress to the 90% level have more severe neural injury (neurotmesis) and thus are less likely to have return to normal facial function.[25] Because testing on a single day does not provide information about the velocity of the degeneration, patients with complete paralysis should undergo serial testing.

Patients who demonstrate no function on ENoG should also undergo voluntary EMG. The addition of voluntary EMG allows identification of motor unit potential with voluntary movement of the facial muscles. The presence of voluntary motor unit potentials indicates a good prognosis for return of facial function. The presence of voluntary motor unit potentials excludes the patient from surgery. Many studies in the literature do not use voluntary EMG and rely solely on ENoG to assess for surgical candidacy.[10,11,23] These authors saw no difference in recovery of function following surgery in patients with ENoG denervation > 90% when compared with steroids alone. It is likely that these patients who had full recovery of function despite the poor ENoG findings had early deblocking of the nerve and would have had a positive voluntary EMG, and thus a good prognosis for recovery. These patients should

have been excluded from surgical decompression in the first place.

Intervention is required before day 14 after the onset of complete paralysis. In the controlled series published by Gantz et al, those patients operated on after day 14 had no improvement in facial nerve function when compared with nonsurgical control patients who received steroids.[12] Fisch also advocated early surgical intervention based on the presumed pathophysiology of nerve damage.[25] Neurotmesis (disruption of both the axon and the endoneurium) results in rapid loss of neural response. With loss of both the axon and the endoneurium, regrowth of the nerve results in aberrant innervation with resulting weakness and synkinesis. Axonomesis (loss of the axon with preservation of the endoneurium) progresses more slowly, so that although there is near total denervation, the neural pathways remain. In the latter situation, as the axon regrows, it can innervate the appropriate muscle and results in good functional recovery (**Fig. 11.2**).

Fisch noted that patients who progress to > 95% degeneration after 4 weeks of paralysis have good spontaneous return of function (93%). Those with degeneration within the first 3 weeks did not (64% with good recovery). The cause of the difference in recovery rates relates to the degree of the neural injury.[22]

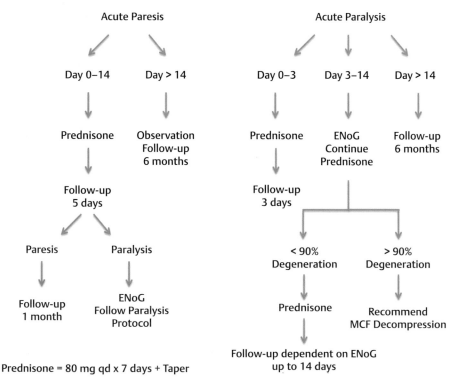

Fig. 11.2 Algorithm for surgical decision making. EMG, electromyography; ENoG, electroneuronography; MCF, middle cranial fossa. (Used with permission from Gantz BJ, Rubinstein JT, Gidley P, Woodworth GG. Surgical management of Bell Palsy. Laryngoscope. 1999;109:1181.)

Finally, the patient must be willing to undergo a surgical procedure. The operation is performed via a middle fossa approach and has associated risks. Decompression of the labyrinthine segment requires drilling near the cochlea and superior semicircular canal, and there is a risk of hearing loss or vestibular dysfunction. Other risks include meningitis, temporal lobe edema resulting in temporary aphasia, seizure, stroke, and death. Given these risks, some patients choose not to undergo surgery. However, other patients are willing to accept those surgical risks for the opportunity to maximize their recovery potential. A detailed and thorough discussion of the procedure and its risks and benefits should be had with any surgical candidate.

These surgical criteria were validated in the case-controlled study by Gantz et al.[12] Thirty patients were enrolled over a 15-year period at the University of Iowa. To qualify for the surgical arm of the study, patients had to present within 14 days of the onset of complete paralysis (grade VI) as measured by the HB scale, have > 90% degeneration on ENoG, and no voluntary EMG activity. Patients were allowed to choose between the treatment groups: surgical ($n = 19$) or nonsurgical ($n = 11$). Patients electing oral steroid treatment were considered nonsurgical controls. A second group of patients ($n = 7$) was operated on early in the study period between days 14 and 28 of paralysis, as originally recommended by Fisch. This group of patients represented a surgical control group as they were treated past the 14-day criteria. Surgical patients underwent decompression of the distal IAC, meatal foramen, labyrinthine segment, geniculate ganglion, and tympanic segment via a middle fossa exposure. No patient in the steroid control group achieved a grade I at 7 months of follow-up. In the nonsurgical control group, 4 of 11 patients achieved a grade II facial weakness and 7 of 11 (64%) patients were grade III, considered a poor outcome. In the surgical control group, two patients had good outcome (HB grade II), whereas the remaining five had a poor outcome (HB grade III). Among patients undergoing decompression within 14 days, 18 of 19 patients had a good outcome (HB I or II), and only 1 patient had a grade III outcome. The statistical comparison of these three groups was significant in favor of early surgical decompression ($p = 0.0001$). To date, this is the only study in the literature with rigorous inclusion criteria and both medical and surgical controls. The decisive results of this study validate the following criteria for decompression (see **Fig. 11.2**):

- Complete facial paralysis, grade VI on the HB scale[26]
- Decompression must occur within 14 days of the onset of complete paralysis
- ENoG findings of > 90% nerve degeneration
- No voluntary EMG motor action potentials
- Patient desires to undergo surgical intervention

■ Description of Procedure

Based on the previously mentioned anatomic and physiologic findings in severe Bell palsy, patients are recommended for exposure and decompression of the nerve via a middle fossa approach. This approach affords access to the IAC, meatal foramen, labyrinthine segment, geniculate ganglion, and the proximal tympanic segment of the nerve.

Following endotracheal intubation, the bed is turned 180 degrees to provide complete access to the head. The skin incision is designed in a 6 × 8–cm rounded box shape based posteriorly with the inferior limb curving post auricular. The incision must not be placed anterior to the temporal hairline to prevent injury to the temporal branch of the facial nerve (**Fig. 11.3**).

The temporoparietal fascia is left attached to the skin flap. The temporalis muscle is reflected anteriorly after harvesting a large piece of the fascia for later use. The craniotomy is performed to center the bone flap over the zygomatic root. The bony window should measure 4 × 5 cm. The vertical sides of the bone flap should be parallel to facilitate placement of the House-Urban retractor (**Fig. 11.4**).

Once the bony flap is removed, the dura is elevated off the floor of the middle fossa under magnification. The limits of exposure are the middle meningeal artery anteriorly and the petrous ridge posteriorly. This can be a difficult maneuver and care must be taken when elevating the dura around the greater superficial petrosal nerve to prevent its avulsion from the geniculate ganglion, which is dehiscent

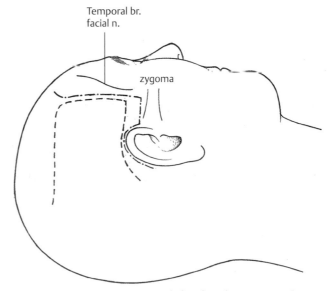

Fig. 11.3 Patient positioning and skin flap design. Note the incision is kept behind the hairline to prevent injury to the temporal branch of the facial nerve. The image is shown from the surgeon's perspective.

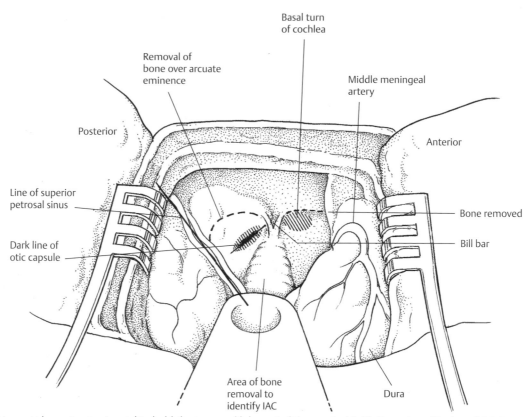

Left Ear

Basal turn
of cochlea

Removal of
bone over arcuate
eminence

Middle meningeal
artery

Posterior

Anterior

Line of superior
petrosal sinus

Bone removed

Dark line of
otic capsule

Bill bar

Area of bone
removal to
identify IAC

Dura

Fig. 11.4 The House-Urban retractor is used to hold the temporal lobe out of the surgical field. Correct positioning of this instrument places the blade under the petrous ridge at the location of the porus acousticus. This position can be approximated by a line placed 60 degrees from the superior semicircular canal and toward the greater superficial petrosal nerve. IAC, internal auditory canal.

5–15% of the time.[18,27] Dural reflections are frequently encountered in the petrosquamous suture line; they should be cauterized with a bipolar forceps and then transected sharply. The House-Urban retractor is then positioned to retract the temporal lobe (see **Fig. 11.4**).

Identification of the IAC then proceeds by first identifying the superior semicircular canal. Although the arcuate eminence is a general landmark for the superior semicircular canal, the semicircular canal should be identified by drilling down the eminence. A preoperative Stenver view plain radiograph is useful to determine the amount of bone that overlies the otic capsule. The superior semicircular canal will be perpendicular to the petrous ridge and at a 60-degree angle to the IAC (**Fig. 11.5**).[28]

The IAC is then skeletonized at the porus. The IAC should be skeletonized for 180 degrees of its circumference at the porus. As the dissection proceeds laterally, the IAC moves both laterally and cephalad. In the mid and lateral portion of the IAC, only ~120 degrees of the canal can be dissected. The entirety of the bone from the porus to Bill bar should be removed. Once the meatus of the labyrinthine segment has been identified at Bill bar, the bony canal should be

removed from the meatal foramen to the geniculate ganglion. The bony removal over the labyrinthine segment is ~90 degrees of the canal. This allows for decompression but avoids inadvertent injury to the basal turn of the cochlea, which is < 1 mm anterior and inferior to the labyrinthine segment of the nerve. The ganglion must then be unroofed. Finally, the fallopian canal is followed into the tympanic segment (**Fig. 11.6**). This necessitates opening the epitympanum. Care should be taken to not injure the ossicles during this dissection.

The fallopian canal should be opened as far as the cochleariform process. A very thin layer of bone should be left over the course of the nerve until the entire nerve is exposed. This bony layer is then removed with small right angle hooks. After the bone has been removed from the nerve, the dura of the IAC should be opened away from the facial nerve and out to the distal IAC using a microscalpel (Beaver no. 59–10). The tight arachnoid band at the meatal foramen must then be incised. The epineurium/periosteum of the labyrinthine segment should be opened to the geniculate ganglion. The epineurium from the cochleariform process back to the geniculate ganglion should also be opened.

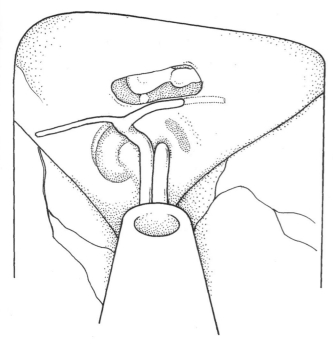

Fig. 11.5 View of the middle fossa floor. The internal auditory canal is skeletonized medially 180 degrees. Laterally, the internal auditory canal exposure is limited to 120 degrees. The labyrinthine segment is fully exposed from the meatal foramen to the geniculate ganglion. The cochlea is <1 mm anterior and inferior to the labyrinthine segment.

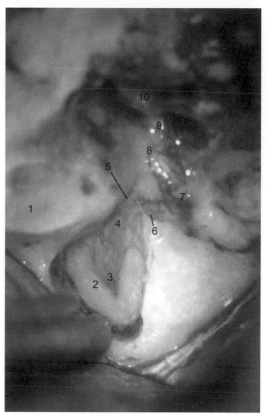

Fig. 11.6 Completed exposure. An intraoperative image taken of a right middle fossa facial nerve decompression. The superior semicircular canal has been blue-lined (*1*). The internal auditory canal (IAC) is identified medially (*2*), and the lateral portion of the IAC dura is fully decompressed (*3*). The facial nerve within the distal IAC (*4*), meatal foramen (*5*), and labyrinthine segment (*6*) is very edematous. The geniculate ganglion (*7*) has also been unroofed. The tympanic segment (*8*) is decorticated to the level of the cochleariform process (*9*). The ossicles have been unroofed to facilitate this exposure (*10*).

Once the nerve is exposed, intraoperative EEMG is performed. The facial nerve stimulator, such as a Prass probe or Parsons-McCabe facial nerve stimulator, is used. The tympanic segment is stimulated first to ensure that a signal can be obtained distally. The labyrinthine or fundal segment is then stimulated. In > 90% of the patients, the conduction block will be located within the labyrinthine segment or the geniculate ganglion.

Following the exposure of the nerve, a free muscle graft from the under surface of the temporalis muscle is harvested. This muscle is used to plug the dural defect. The previously harvested fascia graft is then brought to cover the IAC and epitympanic defects. The inner table of the calvarium is then harvested to resurface the epitympanic defect (**Fig. 11.7**).

The House-Urban retractor is removed, and hemostasis is confirmed around the area of the middle meningeal artery. Two dural elevation sutures are placed inferiorly in the craniotomy window and tacked to the temporalis muscle. These sutures help to close the space between the dura and the bone flap. The bone flap is then replaced in the window, but it is not necessary to secure it with miniplates. The temporalis muscle is then closed in a watertight fashion with interrupted absorbable suture. The subdermal layer is closed with the galea/temporoparietal fascia in an interrupted fashion. The skin is closed with interrupted nylons suture. A pressure dressing should be applied to the wound.

■ Postoperative Care

Patients should be monitored in the intensive care unit overnight with frequent neurological checks. Due to the temporal lobe elevation, the patient should be maintained on a 2 L/24 hours fluid restriction after arrival to the intensive care unit. This is continued for 48 hours. The pressure dressing is changed every day to assess the skin and check for hematoma or cerebrospinal fluid effusion. Pain control can be adequately maintained with oral narcotics and judicious use of intravenous narcotics for breakthrough pain. Patients are maintained nil per os until postoperative day 1. Eye care should be continued through the postoperative period. Steroids (hydrocortisone or dexamethasone) should also be continued for 48 hours.

There are exceptional reports of patients experiencing immediate improvement in facial nerve function following decompression.[8,29] However, patients should expect a slow recovery of function and should be counseled to expect 3 to 6 months before they experience signs of

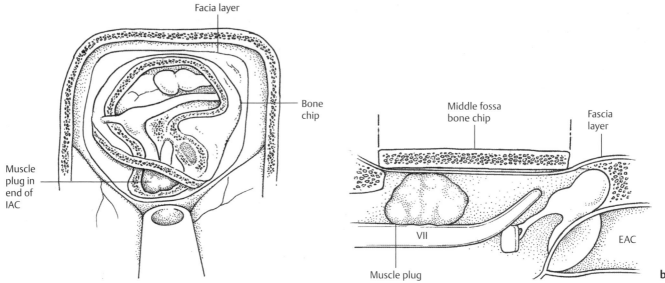

Fig. 11.7a, b Epitympanic repair. A muscle plug is harvested from the temporalis and used to seal the distal end of the internal auditory canal (IAC). A temporalis fascia graft is then placed between the bone graft and dura to complete the repair. The inner table of the calvarium is removed from the bone window and used to repair the epitympanic bony dehiscence.

recovery. Synkinesis can develop up to 12 months following injury as fibers regenerate to the periphery.

■ Complications and Pitfalls

The most likely serious complications involve injury to the basal turn of the cochlea or injury to the facial nerve. Pulec reported 200 cases of decompression with no change in sensorineural hearing levels. Four patients had conductive hearing loss of < 10 dB. One patient developed serous otitis media and reported a conductive hearing loss of 30 dB.[30] Bleeding from the anterior inferior cerebellar artery, which frequently loops into the proximal anterior inferior cerebellar artery, can be catastrophic. The MCF approach does not provide adequate access for exposure and control of the artery and its accompanying veins. Control can be accomplished with a retrosigmoid or suboccipital craniotomy. Injury to this vessel results in infarction of the brainstem, cerebellum, and inner ear.

Other complications are those associated with the MCF approach. Temporary aphasia from temporal lobe retraction of the dominant language center is more common in older patients with left-sided surgery. Other risks include meningitis, cerebrospinal fluid leak (2–6%),[31] seizure, stroke, or hematoma (epidural/subarachnoid/parenchymal). Due to

exposure of the epitympanum, there is the possibility of temporal lobe encephalocele; resurfacing the tegmen with the inner table of the calvarial bone flap diminishes the risk of this problem. Manipulation of the ossicles may result in conductive hearing loss; accidental drilling of the ossicles may result in a vibratory injury to the inner ear.

■ Conclusion

Recent data regarding the use of steroids and antivirals for the treatment of Bell palsy suggest that prompt medical treatment may improve outcomes and reduce the risk of poor function in the long term. Medical therapy is preferable as it is less invasive and carries less risk. However, there remain a small number of patients who continue to have poor outcomes despite maximal medical therapy. Due to the small number of patients who meet surgical criteria as well as the ethical problems of a true randomized trial, the full benefit/efficacy of early surgical decompression may never be known. However, the current data in the literature demonstrate that when identified early, patients with complete facial paralysis benefit from surgical decompression. Prompt surgical intervention may prevent the devastating long-term sequelae of facial asymmetry and improve the patient's quality of life.

References

1. Peitersen E. The natural history of Bell's palsy. Am J Otol 1982; 4(2):107–111
2. Balance C, Duel AB. The operative treatment of facial palsy: by the introduction of nerve grafts into the fallopian canal and by other intratemporal methods. Arch Otolaryngol 1932;15:1–70
3. Kettel K. Pathology and surgery of Bell's Palsy. Laryngoscope 1963;73:837–849
4. May M, Schlaepfer WM. Bell's palsy and the chorda tympani nerve: a clinical and electron microscopic study. Laryngoscope 1975;85(12 pt 1):1957–1975
5. Gussen R. Pathogenesis of Bell's palsy. Retrograde epineurial edema and postedematous fibrous compression neuropathy of the facial nerve. Ann Otol Rhinol Laryngol 1977;86(4 Pt 1): 549–558

6. Blatt IM, Freeman JA. Chorda tympani neurectomy: a simple nerve decompression operation for the cure of Bell's palsy. J La State Med Soc 1968;120(4):197–201

7. May M. Total facial nerve exploration: transmastoid, extralaby-rinthine, and subtemporal indications and results. Laryngoscope 1979;89(6 Pt 1):906–917

8. Yanagihara N, Gyo K, Yumoto E, Tamaki M. Transmastoid decompression of the facial nerve in Bell's palsy. Arch Otolaryngol 1979; 105(9):530–534

9. Yanagihara N, Hato N, Murakami S, Honda N. Transmastoid decompression as a treatment of Bell palsy. Otolaryngol Head Neck Surg 2001;124(3):282–286

10. May M, Klein SR, Taylor FH. Indications for surgery for Bell's palsy. Am J Otol 1984;5(6):503–512

11. May M, Klein SR, Taylor FH. Idiopathic (Bell's) facial palsy: natural history defies steroid or surgical treatment. Laryngoscope 1985; 95(4):406–409

12. Gantz BJ, Rubinstein JT, Gidley P, Woodworth GG. Surgical management of Bell's palsy. Laryngoscope 1999;109(8): 1177–1188

13. Bodénez C, Bernat I, Willer JC, Barré P, Lamas G, Tankéré F. Facial nerve decompression for idiopathic Bell's palsy: report of 13 cases and literature review. J Laryngol Otol 2010;124(3): 272–278 10.1017/S0022215109991265

14. Takeda T, Takebayashi S, Kakigi A, Nakatani H, Hamada M. Total decompression of the facial nerve - superior prelabyrinthine cell tracts approach. ORL J Otorhinolaryngol Relat Spec 2010;71(Suppl 1):112–115

15. Rapper AH, Samuels MA. Electrophysiologic and Laboratory Aids in the Diagnosis of Neuromuscular Disease. In: Rapper AH, Samuels MA, eds. Adams and Victor's Principles of Neurology, 9th ed [e-book]. New York: McGraw-Hill; 2009. Available from www.accessmedicine.com

16. Gantz BJ, Gmür A, Fisch U. Intraoperative evoked electromyography in Bell's palsy. Am J Otolaryngol 1982;3(4):273–278

17. House WF. Surgical exposure of the internal auditory canal and its contents through the middle, cranial fossa. Laryngoscope 1961; 71:1363–1385

18. House WF, Crabtree JA. Surgical exposure of the petrous portion of the 7th nerve. Arch Otolaryngol 1965;81:506–507

19. Pulec JL. Total decompression of the facial nerve. Laryngoscope 1966;76(6):1015–1028

20. Fisch U, Esslen E. Total intratemporal exposure of the facial nerve. Arch Otolaryngol 1972;95:335–341

21. Ge XX, Spector GJ. Labyrinthine segment and geniculate ganglion of facial nerve in fetal and adult human temporal bones. Ann Otol Rhinol Laryngol suppl 1981;90(4 Pt 2, Suppl85)1–12

22. Fisch U. Surgery for Bell's palsy. Arch Otolaryngol 1981;107(1):1–11

23. Adour KK. Decompression for Bell's palsy: why I don't do it. Eur Arch Otorhinolaryngol 2002;259(1):40–47

24. McAllister K, Walker D, Donnan PT, Swan I. Surgical interventions for the early management of Bell's palsy. Cochrane Database Syst Rev 2011; (2):CD007468 10.1002/14651858.CD007468.pub2

25. Fisch U. Prognostic value of electrical tests in acute facial paralysis. Am J Otol 1984;5(6):494–498

26. House JW, Brackmann DE. Facial nerve grading system. Otolaryngol Head Neck Surg 1985;93(2):146–147

27. Rhoton AL Jr, Pulec JL, Hall GM, Boyd AS Jr. Absence of bone over the geniculate ganglion. J Neurosurg 1968;28(1):48–53

28. Kartush JM, Kemink JL, Graham MD. The arcuate eminence. Topographic orientation in middle cranial fossa surgery. Ann Otol Rhinol Laryngol 1985;94(1 Pt 1):25–28

29. McCabe BF. Some evidence for the efficacy of decompression for Bell's palsy: immediate motion postoperatively. Laryngoscope 1977;87(2):246–249

30. Pulec JL. Early decompression of the facial nerve in Bell's palsy. Ann Otol Rhinol Laryngol 1981;90(6 Pt 1, 6 Part I):570–577

31. Weber PC, Gantz BJ. Results and complications from acoustic neuroma excision via middle cranial fossa approach. Am J Otol 1996;17(4):669–675

12 Traumatic Facial Nerve Management

J. Walter Kutz Jr., Brandon Isaacson, and Peter S. Roland

Trauma is second to idiopathic facial paralysis (Bell palsy) as the most common cause of facial paralysis. The course of the facial nerve is complex with intracranial, intratemporal, and extratemporal segments. The nerve is at risk for injury along any of these segments from external, surgical, or iatrogenic trauma. Management of facial nerve trauma is often challenging as spontaneous recovery cannot be predicted and is often satisfactory without intervention. The two most important factors predicting recovery and potential intervention include onset and degree of paralysis. In this chapter, the evaluation and management of traumatic facial nerve paralysis is discussed.

■ External Trauma

Temporal bone fractures occur in 4.4–9.4% of patients presenting with head injuries and in up to 40% of patients with basilar skull fractures, especially those associated with motor vehicle accidents.[1,2] Approximately 14–22% of patients with skull fractures will have an associated temporal bone fracture.[3] Patients with temporal bone fractures often present with other severe and life-threatening issues that appropriately take precedence with respect to diagnosis and management.

Evaluation

A careful history and physical exam can often confirm the presence or absence of hearing loss, vertigo, facial paralysis, cerebrospinal fluid leak, and in some cases a vascular injury in patients with a basilar skull fracture. Patients with otorrhea or hemotympanum will at a minimum have some conductive hearing loss. Fractures that traverse the otic capsule will almost always result in a significant sensorineural hearing loss. A simple tuning fork test will confirm the type of hearing loss present, which is of critical importance if surgery is being considered to address a persistent cerebrospinal fluid leak or facial paralysis.

Evaluation of facial nerve function during the initial examination is crucial when predicting recovery and the need for surgical intervention. In the setting of external trauma, facial function should be assessed as soon as possible. Eyewitness accounts from the scene of the accident should be interpreted with caution; however, useful information may be obtained. Many patients have severe concomitant injuries and arrive intubated and sedated, making the initial evaluation of facial function difficult.

Painful stimuli such as a sternal rub or pressure under the superior orbital rim may stimulate facial movement. Despite the examiner's best efforts, often an adequate exam may not be possible and the patient will need to be reassessed once his or her condition has stabilized.

Onset and Degree of Paralysis

Sudden and Complete

Facial paralysis that is sudden and complete portends a worse prognosis with only 36% of patients making a full recovery in a recent large meta-analyses.[4] The challenge is to differentiate which patients will have poor recovery from those that will experience good recovery. A combination of imaging and electrical testing will determine if surgical exploration is warranted.

Delayed or Incomplete

Delayed paralysis confirms the continuity of the facial nerve and occurs due to edema of the facial nerve in the fallopian canal, especially around the meatal foramen.[5] If the paresis does not progress to complete paralysis, management is always expectant and full recovery is almost certain. If the paralysis progresses to complete, electrical testing may be performed. Surgical decompression is rarely indicated because > 90% of patients will have full recovery of facial function.[3,6–8] Surgery may be considered if electric testing places the patient in a poor prognostic category. Many surgeons use the same electrophysiological criteria as in Bell palsy when determining if facial nerve decompression is warranted (see Chapter 11).

Unclear Onset

Often the onset of paralysis cannot be determined due to confounding factors such as neurological status or other life-threatening injuries. In these cases, the onset of paralysis is questionable and these patients should be classified as acute onset. Electrical testing is paramount in these circumstances if surgical exploration is considered.

Classification of Temporal Bone Fractures

Temporal bone fractures have historically been categorized according to their orientation with respect to the petrous ridge (longitudinal, oblique, transverse).[9] Defining the

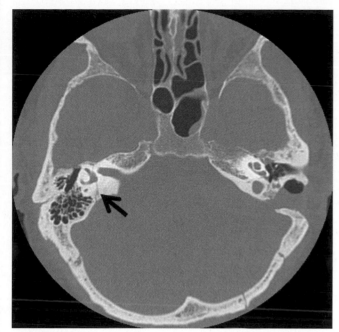

Fig. 12.1 Axial computed tomography scan demonstrating an otic capsule fracture crossing though the common crus and medial vestibule that resulted in an immediate and complete facial paralysis.

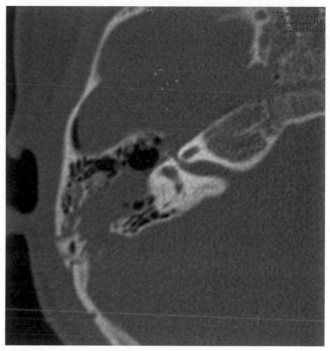

Fig. 12.2 Axial computed tomography scan demonstrating a right longitudinal temporal bone fracture involving the perigeniculate region.

fracture according to involvement of the otic capsule has become the preferred classification scheme as it has been shown to be a better prognostic indicator of intratemporal complications including facial paralysis.[2] Otic capsule–sparing fractures occur far more frequently (> 94%) than fractures that traverse the otic capsule (< 6%).[2,3] Facial paralysis is twice as common in otic capsule–involving fractures where the tympanic facial nerve is the most commonly injured segment.[2,10] **Fig. 12.1** demonstrates an otic capsule fracture crossing the common crus and medial vestibule resulting in a facial paralysis. Six percent to 14% of otic capsule–sparing fractures are associated with facial paralysis that usually involves the perigeniculate portion of the facial nerve.[2,3,10]

Diagnostic Testing

Thin-cut computed tomography (CT) is the mainstay of radiographic assessment of the patient with traumatic facial nerve injury. CT can demonstrate a skull base fracture in almost all cases. Images must be carefully examined to make sure all fracture lines are identified as multiple fractures are often present. While many fractures conform to one of the types described previously ("longitudinal" or "transverse"), others do not. Most fractures associated with facial paralysis will involve the area of the geniculate ganglion and/or labyrinthine segment of the facial nerve. **Fig. 12.2** demonstrates a longitudinal fracture affecting the perigeniculate region resulting in facial paralysis. If facial paralysis is complete, an attempt should be made to assess

the extent of displacement and/or fragmentation of the fallopian canal to estimate the likelihood that the nerve is transected or that the facial nerve is compressed by bone fragments. In the face of complete facial paralysis and/or a poor prognosis from electrodiagnostic testing, image findings of severe injury as suggested by the CT scan would encourage surgical exploration.

If the fracture involves the petrous carotid canal, a CT or magnetic resonance angiogram is essential. The most common location for a basilar skull fracture to involve the carotid canal is at the lacerum-cavernous junction.[11] An unrecognized carotid injury may result in stroke or death if not promptly diagnosed.

If the paralysis is of immediate onset, electrodiagnostic testing can be very useful in determining the extent of injury. While both electroneuronography (evoked electromyography) and maximal stimulation testing can provide useful information, electroneuronography is more precise and provides an objective record of the evaluation. Absent response on the injured side on electroneuronography suggests transection of the nerve. A full description of electrodiagnostic testing can be found in Chapter 5. Electrodiagnostic test results should be considered together with CT findings.

Management

Several controversies exist with respect to the management of facial paralysis secondary to a temporal bone fracture. The timing and degree of facial paralysis is of critical importance with respect to prognosis and management. Patients with immediate onset complete paralysis with poor prognostic electrodiagnostic testing are candidates for surgical exploration of the facial nerve. Most reports agree that surgical intervention 14 days after the injury is rarely indicated; however, several authors suggest that late facial nerve exploration may have some benefit in cases where an impinging bone fragment or transection of the nerve is suspected.[4,12,13] The surgical approach for facial nerve exploration primarily depends on the hearing status and location of the fracture. Patients with anacusis or otic capsule–involving fractures are typically managed with a translabyrinthine approach.[12] A middle fossa possibly combined with a transmastoid approach is utilized in patients with intact hearing and fractures that involve the perigeniculate and more distal segments of the facial nerve.[12]

Outcomes

Facial paralysis resulting from blunt trauma has a favorable outcome in most cases.[4] A recent review of the literature demonstrated that 82% of patients with a partial paralysis who were observed achieved complete recovery. Administration of steroids seemed to result in improved outcomes over those patients observed, resulting in normal function in 95% of patients with partial facial paralysis. With respect to onset of paralysis ~80% of patients with delayed paralysis who underwent no intervention recovered normal function. It is well known that traumatic complete facial paralysis has a worse outcome than in those individuals with partial or incomplete paralysis. In a pooled series of 480 patients with complete paralysis, 57% of patients who were observed, 44% of the patients who were administered steroids, and 21% of patients undergoing decompression demonstrated complete recovery of function. Complete lack of recovery was observed in 1.7% of patients as compared with 10% of patients undergoing decompression. No patients who were administered steroids developed a complete long-term facial paralysis.[4]

Extratemporal Facial Nerve Trauma

The most common cause of extratemporal facial nerve injury is from penetrating trauma or iatrogenic injury. A careful examination of all branches of the facial nerve is warranted in cases of external penetrating facial trauma. Ideally, penetrating facial injuries with resultant facial weakness should be explored immediately, provided the patient is medically stable. Transected branches can usually be identified through the existing facial laceration. A facial nerve integrity monitor can be used to identify distal facial nerve branches if the exploration can be performed within 72 hours from the time of injury prior to the onset of wallerian degeneration. The main trunk of the facial nerve can be identified at the stylomastoid foramen or in the mastoid fallopian canal if localization of the proximal branches is difficult. The nerve

can then be traced to the pes anserinus and from there to the proximal transected end of the facial nerve.

Primary repair of the facial nerve without mobilization is associated with improved outcomes as opposed to rerouting or grafting. Improved outcomes are also seen when fewer branches are injured.[14]

Ballistic Trauma

Injuries from periauricular gunshot wounds can result in significant morbidity and not infrequently mortality. **Fig. 12.3** demonstrates a CT of a gunshot wound to the temporal bone resulting in transection of the mastoid segment of the facial nerve. These patients often present with altered mental status and may have other injuries requiring prompt evaluation and management. Ballistic injuries to the skull base as opposed to blunt trauma more commonly result in lower cranial nerve injuries, hearing loss, cerebrospinal fluid leaks, vascular, and intracranial injuries.[15] The largest series of temporal bone gunshot wounds reported the outcomes of 43 patients; 22 patients presented with facial paresis or paralysis. Fifteen of these twenty-two patients presented with complete paralysis in all branches. Twelve patients underwent surgical exploration, and 75% of those were found to have complete disruption of the facial nerve. The most common sites of facial nerve injuries were the vertical, tympanic, and proximal extratemporal main trunk. Surgical exploration with decompression and cable grafting when indicated is recommended in patients with complete paralysis and when imaging evidence of nerve disruption or impingement exists.

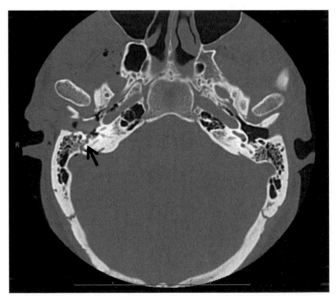

Fig. 12.3 Axial computed tomography scan of a patient who sustained a gunshot wound to the face where the bullet impacted on the tympanic bone and mastoid tip. The patient was noted to have an immediate complete facial paralysis. Air is seen in the infratemporal fossa. There is an otic capsule sparing fracture that traverses the mastoid fallopian canal (*arrow*).

■ Surgical Trauma

Cerebellopontine Angle

Facial nerve injury at the cerebellopontine angle most commonly occurs during removal of a vestibular schwannoma. Larger tumors have a higher incidence of long-term facial nerve dysfunction.[16,17] Intraoperative facial nerve monitoring during tumor removal has become standard and has been shown to result in improved long-term facial nerve outcomes.[17–19] Adequate exposure, copious irrigation during drilling, and careful suctioning and dissecting will minimize facial nerve trauma. Tos et al demonstrated that the most common site of injury is at the porus acousticus, and suctioning and thermal drill injury are the most common mechanisms resulting in facial nerve injury.[20]

The use of steroids is common after the removal of a vestibular schwannoma to minimize edema and possible facial nerve dysfunction. If the facial nerve paresis is incomplete in the immediate postoperative period, the prognosis for an excellent recovery is good. If a complete paralysis occurs immediately after surgery, the long-term prognosis is poorer.[21] Facial nerve stimulation after tumor removal can predict long-term facial function.[22–24] Neff et al showed that 85% of patients recovered to House–Brackmann grade I or II if the minimum stimulus was 0.05 mA or less and the response amplitude was 240 microV or greater.[25]

Management of facial paresis or paralysis with an intact nerve is expectant and includes the use of steroids. If recovery does not occur within a year, other reanimation procedures such as a XII–VII graft or a muscle transfer should be considered. If the nerve was severed during tumor resection, multiple techniques exist to repair the nerve. If there is an adequate stump of the facial nerve at the brainstem, a cable graft using the sural or greater auricular nerve should be considered. Anastomosis using fibrin glue is as successful as suture repair and is technically less demanding and time-consuming.[26] If a proximal facial nerve stump cannot be identified, other reanimation techniques such as a XII–VII graft should be considered.

Intratemporal

Facial nerve injury involving the tympanic and mastoid segments may occur during any otologic procedure. The mechanism of injury is different with the tympanic segment injured more often during dissection and the mastoid segment injured during drilling. Green et al reviewed 22 patients with iatrogenic facial nerve injuries from otologic surgery. The most common procedure was a mastoidectomy; however, facial nerve injury was also reported during tympanoplasty and canalplasty. Furthermore, 79% of injuries were not identified at the time of surgery.[27]

If the nerve is exposed but not transected, the condition of the nerve should be inspected. The first step is to decompress and expose the nerve proximal and distal to the injured segment. Whether to open the nerve sheath is controversial. If intraneural hemorrhage is identified, the epineurium should be opened and the blood evacuated. **Fig. 12.4** illustrates an intraneural hematoma with

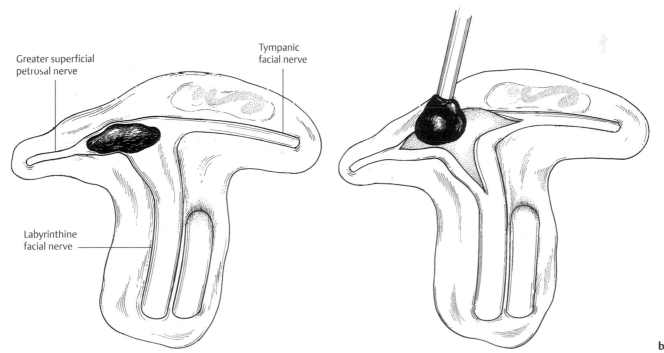

Fig. 12.4a, b (**a**) An intraneural hematoma involving the facial nerve in the region of the geniculate ganglion. (**b**) Evacuation of an intraneural hematoma after the epineurium has been opened.

subsequent evacuation. If the facial nerve is transected, the ends may be approximated. If the ends cannot be approximated without tension, a cable graft should be used. If the facial nerve is partially transected, the options include interposition of a partial graft, keeping the preserved portion intact and placing a tubule around the nerve, or placing a nerve graft. Bento et al compared the three techniques in a retrospective review of 42 patients and determined the most favorable results were in patients who received a completed transection and nerve graft.[28] Green et al recommend completed transection and repair if the extent of injury to the facial nerve is difficult to determine because underestimation of injury is common.[29]

Middle Ear

Surgical trauma may occur during middle ear dissection. The tympanic facial nerve is dehiscent in 18–30% of patients with cholesteatoma, with the most common segment superior to the oval window.[30,31] When the dehiscent facial nerve is covered with granulation tissue or cholesteatoma matrix, dissection from the nerve may result in injury. This can be avoided by meticulous technique and the identification of the facial nerve using intraoperative facial nerve stimulation. Important surgical landmarks include the cochleariform process and the tensor tympani canal, which are often the last structures to be eroded by a cholesteatoma. The Jacobson nerve can be identified coursing over the promontory and followed superiorly to identify the cochleariform process.

The tympanic facial nerve has been shown to be dehiscent over the oval window in 3–8% of patients undergoing a stapedectomy. A dehiscent facial nerve is not a contraindication for a stapedectomy; however, removal of scutal bone and identification of the facial nerve is essential before a stapedectomy is performed. A prolapsed facial nerve may prevent visualization of the footplate, leading to abortion of the procedure. Facial nerve anomalies can also be encountered with the nerve overlying the promontory, bifurcating around the footplate, or passing through the arch of the stapes. The operation can continue if the nerve can be avoided during instrumentation.

Mastoid Segment

The facial nerve is rarely dehiscent in the mastoid segment but is more commonly injured during drilling. The most common segment injured during a mastoidectomy is just distal to the second genu. The inferior vertical facial nerve is at risk during canalplasty because the nerve may course lateral to the annulus. Intraoperative facial nerve monitoring may be helpful to avoid facial nerve injury but is not a substitute for a thorough understanding of the surgical anatomy. Drilling in the direction of the nerve and the use of copious irrigation are techniques that will minimize the possibility of facial nerve trauma. Often, granulation tissue

may be difficult to differentiate from the facial nerve. The facial nerve will "spring back" when palpated. The use of an intraoperative facial nerve stimulator may be needed in difficult cases.

Extratemporal

Extratemporal trauma may occur during parotidectomy, rhytidectomy, submandibular gland excision, neck dissection, and other approaches involving the extratemporal facial nerve. These injuries may be categorized as transection, stretch, or crush injuries.

The facial nerve branches at the pes anserinus soon after exiting the stylomastoid foramen. During a parotidectomy, the main trunk and the peripheral branches of the facial nerve are at risk. The risk for facial nerve injury increases with malignant tumors, total parotidectomy, and revision surgery.[32–35] If the nerve was unintentionally severed, primary anastomosis should be performed. Branches medial to a line through the lateral canthus do not need repair because the expected deficit is minimal. If the facial nerve is repaired, evidence of recovery may be seen as early as 4 months and should be apparent by 8 months.

Facial nerve injury may occur during a rhytidectomy procedure, although the reported incidence of permanent facial paresis is 0.1% in experienced hands.[36,37] The frontal branch is at greatest risk due to the superficial course as the nerve passes over the zygomatic arch. Avoiding deep-plane dissection superior to the zygomatic arch or anterior to the temporal hairline can minimize facial nerve injury. The marginal mandibular branch is also at risk, especially if the flap is elevated in a subplatysmal plane. If the patient wakes with facial paralysis, time should be given for the effects of local anesthetics to wear off. Other mechanisms of injury to consider include stretch injury, compression from tight dressings, electrocautery trauma, suture, or hematoma.

■ Iatrogenic Trauma

Iatrogenic injuries to the facial nerve may occur from multiple causes including direct trauma resulting in transection, compression, stretch injury, crush injury, or thermal injury from drilling or electrocautery. A thorough knowledge of the anatomy, identification of the facial nerve, and meticulous surgical technique can minimize the chance of injury.

Transection

Iatrogenic transection may occur along any segment of the facial nerve and can be caused by sharp transection, drill injury, or avulsion. Repair should be performed when the injury is identified. Direct anastomosis may be performed if it is tension-free; however, a cable graft will usually be

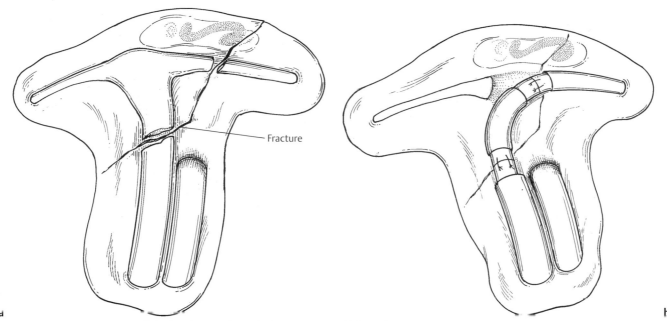

Fig. 12.5a, b (**a**) Transection of the facial nerve through the tympanic and labyrinthine segments of the facial nerve. (**b**) A cable graft is used to repair the severed nerve.

required. **Fig. 12.5** shows a transected facial nerve through the tympanic and labyrinthine segments repaired with a cable graft. The greater auricular, medial antebranchial cutaneous, or sural nerve may be used. In the cerebellopontine angle, a single suture or fibrin glue is adequate. If the transection occurs along the intratemporal portion of the nerve, the fallopian canal can be used to support the nerve and graft.

Compression

Compression injury most commonly involves the intratemporal segment of the facial nerve. Intraneural edema, hemorrhage between the fallopian canal and facial nerve, bone fragments, or aggressive packing may cause compression injury. Identification of these problems at the time of surgery will minimize the chance of a compressed nerve. **Fig. 12.6** demonstrates bony fragments compressing the facial nerve with subsequent removal of the impinging fragments. Facial paralysis may be progressive in these cases, and management is dependent on the possible mechanisms of compression that were encountered during the operation. Re-exploration may be indicated if complete paralysis occurs and electrophysiological testing suggests degeneration. Cases with delayed but incomplete paresis can be managed expectantly with excellent recovery likely.

Stretch

Stretch injury may occur during removal of a cerebellopontine angle tumor or in the extratemporal segment.

Mechanisms include direct stretching of the facial nerve during tumor dissection or while using retractors. If the nerve is intact, no further treatment is indicated and recovery should be expected. Occasionally, the recovery may be incomplete and synkinesis may develop. If the nerve is partially avulsed, direct repair without tension or a cable graft may be indicated depending in the extent of injury.

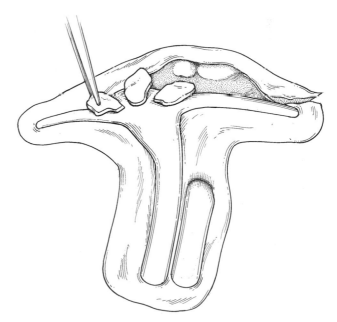

Fig. 12.6 Bony fragments impinging the facial nerve in the region of the geniculate ganglion. The bony fragments are carefully removed to relieve pressure on the facial nerve.

Crush

Crush injury may occur from instrumentation, such as a misplaced hemostat, retraction, or trauma. Recent animal studies have demonstrated that crush injury to the intratemporal facial nerve results in facial motor nuclei cell loss. In contrast, facial motor nuclei cell loss was not seen in extratemporal crush injuries.[38,39] If a crush injury is identified, the decision to resect and repair the damaged segment is based on clinical judgment. Most animal studies demonstrate complete recovery of crushed motor nerves.[40,41] If the nerve is not repaired at the time of the crush injury, re-exploration should be considered if no evidence recovery has occurred after 4 months.

■ Conclusion

Traumatic facial nerve injury is a common problem encountered in a busy otologic practice. The onset and degree of paralysis are the most important aspects of the history to prompt possible surgical intervention and to determine prognosis for recovery. Patients with delayed or incomplete paralysis have an excellent prognosis, and surgical intervention is rarely indicated. In patients with acute or complete paralysis, imaging and electrophysiological testing are useful to determine which patients will have a poor prognosis and may be considered for surgical exploration.

References

1. Exadaktylos AK, Sclabas GM, Nuyens M, et al. The clinical correlation of temporal bone fractures and spiral computed tomographic scan: a prospective and consecutive study at a level I trauma center. J Trauma 2003;55(4):704–706

2. Dahiya R, Keller JD, Litofsky NS, Bankey PE, Bonassar LJ, Megerian CA. Temporal bone fractures: otic capsule sparing versus otic capsule violating clinical and radiographic considerations. J Trauma 1999;47(6):1079–1083

3. Brodie HA, Thompson TC. Management of complications from 820 temporal bone fractures. Am J Otol 1997;18(2):188–197

4. Nash JJ, Friedland DR, Boorsma KJ, Rhee JS. Management and outcomes of facial paralysis from intratemporal blunt trauma: a systematic review. Laryngoscope 2010;120(Suppl 4):S214

5. Fisch U. Facial paralysis in fractures of the petrous bone. Laryngoscope 1974;84(12):2141–2154

6. McKennan KX, Chole RA. Facial paralysis in temporal bone trauma. Am J Otol 1992;13(2):167–172

7. Turner JWA. Facial palsy in closed head injuries. Lancet 1944;246:756–757

8. Maiman DJ, Cusick JF, Anderson AJ, Larson SJ. Nonoperative management of traumatic facial nerve palsy. J Trauma 1985;25(7):644–648

9. Nosan DK, Benecke JE Jr, Murr AH. Current perspective on temporal bone trauma. Otolaryngol Head Neck Surg 1997;117(1):67–71

10. Darrouzet V, Duclos JY, Liguoro D, Truilhe Y, De Bonfils C, Bebear JP. Management of facial paralysis resulting from temporal bone fractures: Our experience in 115 cases. Otolaryngol Head Neck Surg 2001;125(1):77–84

11. Resnick DK, Subach BR, Marion DW. The significance of carotid canal involvement in basilar cranial fracture. Neurosurgery 1997;40(6):1177–1181

12. Chang CY, Cass SP. Management of facial nerve injury due to temporal bone trauma. Am J Otol 1999;20(1):96–114

13. Quaranta A, Campobasso G, Piazza F, Quaranta N, Salonna I. Facial nerve paralysis in temporal bone fractures: outcomes after late decompression surgery. Acta Otolaryngol 2001;121(5):652–655

14. Frijters E, Hofer SO, Mureau MA. Long-term subjective and objective outcome after primary repair of traumatic facial nerve injuries. Ann Plast Surg 2008;61(2):181–187

15. Shindo ML, Fetterman BL, Shih L, Maceri DR, Rice DH. Gunshot wounds of the temporal bone: a rational approach to evaluation and management. Otolaryngol Head Neck Surg 1995;112(4):533–539

16. Brackmann DE, Cullen RD, Fisher LM. Facial nerve function after translabyrinthine vestibular schwannoma surgery. Otolaryngol Head Neck Surg 2007;136(5):773–777

17. Lalwani AK, Butt FY, Jackler RK, Pitts LH, Yingling CD. Facial nerve outcome after acoustic neuroma surgery: a study from the era of cranial nerve monitoring. Otolaryngol Head Neck Surg 1994;111(5):561–570

18. Kileny P, Kemink J, Tucci D, Hoff J. Neurophysiologic intraoperative facial and auditory function in acoustic neuroma surgery. In: Tos M, Thomsen J, eds. Acoustic Neuroma: Proceedings of the First International Conference on Acoustic Neuroma. Amsterdam/New York: Kugler Publications, 1992:569–574

19. Isaacson B, Kileny PR, El-Kashlan H, Gadre AK. Intraoperative monitoring and facial nerve outcomes after vestibular schwannoma resection. Otol Neurotol 2003;24(5):812–817

20. Tos M, Youssef M, Thomsen J, Turgut S. Causes of facial nerve paresis after translabyrinthine surgery for acoustic neuroma. Ann Otol Rhinol Laryngol 1992;101(10):821–826

21. Arriaga MA, Luxford WM, Atkins JS Jr, Kwartler JA. Predicting long-term facial nerve outcome after acoustic neuroma surgery. Otolaryngol Head Neck Surg 1993;108(3):220–224

22. Goldbrunner RH, Schlake HP, Milewski C, Tonn JC, Helms J, Roosen K. Quantitative parameters of intraoperative electromyography predict facial nerve outcomes for vestibular schwannoma surgery. Neurosurgery 2000;46(5):1140–1146, discussion 1146–1148

23. Nissen AJ, Sikand A, Curto FS, Welsh JE, Gardi J. Value of intraoperative threshold stimulus in predicting postoperative facial nerve function after acoustic tumor resection. Am J Otol 1997;18(2):249–251

24. Prasad S, Hirsch BE, Kamerer DB, Durrant J, Sekhar LN. Facial nerve function following cerebellopontine angle surgery: prognostic value of intraoperative thresholds. Am J Otol 1993;14(4):330–333

25. Neff BA, Ting J, Dickinson SL, Welling DB. Facial nerve monitoring parameters as a predictor of postoperative facial nerve outcomes after vestibular schwannoma resection. Otol Neurotol 2005;26(4):728–732

26. Bacciu A, Falcioni M, Pasanisi E, et al. Intracranial facial nerve grafting after removal of vestibular schwannoma. Am J Otolaryngol 2009;30(2):83–88

27. Green JD Jr, Shelton C, Brackmann DE. Iatrogenic facial nerve injury during otologic surgery. Laryngoscope 1994;104(8 Pt 1):922–926

28. Bento RF, Salomone R, Brito R, Tsuji RK, Hausen M. Partial lesions of the intratemporal segment of the facial nerve: graft versus partial reconstruction. Ann Otol Rhinol Laryngol 2008;117(9): 665–669

29. Green JD Jr, Shelton C, Brackmann DE. Surgical management of iatrogenic facial nerve injuries. Otolaryngol Head Neck Surg 1994;111(5):606–610

30. Selesnick SH, Lynn-Macrae AG. The incidence of facial nerve dehiscence at surgery for cholesteatoma. Otol Neurotol 2001; 22(2):129–132

31. Moody MW, Lambert PR. Incidence of dehiscence of the facial nerve in 416 cases of cholesteatoma. Otol Neurotol 2007;28(3): 400–404

32. Koch M, Zenk J, Iro H. Long-term results of morbidity after parotid gland surgery in benign disease. Laryngoscope 2010;120(4): 724–730

33. Yuan X, Gao Z, Jiang H, et al. Predictors of facial palsy after surgery for benign parotid disease: multivariate analysis of 626 operations. Head Neck 2009;31(12):1588–1592

34. Upton DC, McNamar JP, Connor NP, Harari PM, Hartig GK. Parotidectomy: ten-year review of 237 cases at a single institution. Otolaryngol Head Neck Surg 2007;136(5):788–792

35. Bron LP, O'Brien CJ. Facial nerve function after parotidectomy. Arch Otolaryngol Head Neck Surg 1997;123(10):1091–1096

36. McCollough EG, Perkins SW, Langsdon PR. SASMAS suspension rhytidectomy. Rationale and long-term experience. Arch Otolaryngol Head Neck Surg 1989;115(2):228–234

37. Baker DC, Conley J. Avoiding facial nerve injuries in rhytidectomy. Anatomical variations and pitfalls. Plast Reconstr Surg 1979;64(6):781–795

38. Marzo SJ, Moeller CW, Sharma N, Cunningham K, Jones KJ, Foecking EM. Facial motor nuclei cell loss with intratemporal facial nerve crush injuries in rats. Laryngoscope 2010;120(11): 2264–2269

39. Sharma N, Cunningham K, Porter RG Sr, Marzo SJ, Jones KJ, Foecking EM. Comparison of extratemporal and intratemporal facial nerve injury models. Laryngoscope 2009;119(12): 2324–2330

40. Chen LE, Seaber AV, Glisson RR, et al. The functional recovery of peripheral nerves following defined acute crush injuries. J Orthop Res 1992;10(5):657–664

41. Hadlock TA, Heaton J, Cheney M, Mackinnon SE. Functional recovery after facial and sciatic nerve crush injury in the rat. Arch Facial Plast Surg 2005;7(1):17–20

13 Facial Weakness as a Complication of Otologic Diseases

Thomas E. Linder

The facial nerve is quite resistant to infectious lesions within the temporal bone. In an Australian database of 1,074 patients with facial palsy, only 29 individuals (3%) were identified with acute otitis media (AOM; $n = 10$); cholesteatoma ($n = 10$ [7 acquired; 3 congenital]); mastoid cavity infections ($n = 2$); malignant otitis externa ($n = 2$); noncholesteatomatous chronic suppurative otitis media ($n = 2$); tuberculous mastoiditis ($n = 1$); suppurative parotitis ($n = 1$); and chronic granulomatosis ($n = 1$).[1] Early medical treatment of acute otitis media, proper drainage of acute mastoiditis, timely diagnosis of acquired cholesteatomas, and the rarity of temporal bone involvement of systemic diseases (e.g., Wegener granulomatosis) reduce the incidence of acute or chronic lesions of the facial nerve. The fallopian canal is a bony protection of the facial nerve within the temporal bone with few spontaneous dehiscences. These involve mainly the tympanic segment close to the oval window and the geniculate ganglion toward the middle cranial fossa dura. Facial weakness may be the first presenting sign of the disease in supralabyrinthine cholesteatomas or may worsen the prognosis of the underlying pathology as in necrotizing otitis media. This chapter summarizes infectious lesions within the temporal bone leading to facial palsy.

■ Acute Otitis Media

The overall incidence of intratemporal complications of AOM has decreased and the need for operative treatment is declining during the antibiotic era. Newer attempts of withholding antibiotics for 24 to 48 hours have not increased the incidence of acute mastoiditis, estimated at 1.2 to 4.2 cases per 100,000 per year. Most episodes of AOM occur in children; therefore, the prevalence of AOM with subsequent facial palsy is more frequent in children than in adults. Fischer et al published one of the largest series of 61 patients with facial nerve paralysis associated with acute suppurative otitis media.[2] Most publications report on 10 to 20 patients within 5 to 10 years observation time. Patients with incomplete palsy (facial nerve paresis) may not be referred to larger centers as their outcome is excellent and surgery rarely indicated. Acute facial palsy may be the first symptom of AOM or may accompany acute mastoiditis as a complication of bacterial otitis media.[3] The same organisms causing AOM alone have been associated with AOM with facial palsy, although factors such as virulence of the organism, host resistance, or a higher incidence

of spontaneous fallopian canal dehiscences have been postulated. Pressure-induced lesions, venous congestion with subsequent swelling of the nerve, and toxic irritations have been implicated in the pathophysiology. Computed tomography (CT) scans are highly recommended to verify the severity of the AOM (subperiosteal abscess, coalescent mastoiditis, sigmoid sinus thrombosis) and to evaluate the course of the fallopian canal (search for dehiscences), as well as to exclude other pathology (e.g., indirect signs of an underlying cholesteatoma). In acute suppurative otitis media with purulent discharge, it is difficult to exclude an underlying cholesteatoma otoscopically at the first visit.

Surgical decompression has been previously recommended but randomized clinical trials do not exist and the overall excellent prognosis has questioned the beneficial role of surgery. Antibiotic treatment should always be initiated. Steroids may be added, but evidence for their effectiveness is lacking.[4] The author favors myringotomy (for bacterial cultures) with ventilations tubes (to allow drainage through the middle ear). Mastoidecomy is indicated in cases of acute mastoiditis and/or subperiosteal abscess formation. However, the author does not advocate facial nerve exploration and decompression. A review of the literature does not support facial nerve decompression in AOM with facial palsy. Exploration of the facial nerve from the stylomastoid foramen to the geniculate ganglion in case of acute suppurative infection (e.g., bleeding granulation tissue, fibrinous adhesions in the middle ear) is technically demanding and superfluous.

Patients with incomplete palsy do have a very favorable prognosis with full recovery within a short time period of a few days to 3 weeks. Patients with complete paralysis during AOM also have a good prognosis, though with a prolonged time to maximum improvement of a few weeks to months.[5] Most studies confirm complete recovery of facial nerve function in all cases.[6] Few reports reveal incomplete recovery of House-Brackmann (HB) II in 3–15% or HB III in 3%[2,7]; however, unsatisfactory outcomes (HB IV-VI) have not been reported. Adults rarely present with AOM and therefore present a low risk of developing facial palsy during a course of AOM. Studies with adults are rare and confirm the excellent prognosis.[8]

■ Necrotizing External Otitis

Necrotizing external otitis may also be called malignant external otitis because it is a devastating and potentially

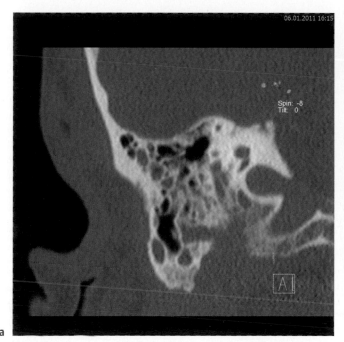
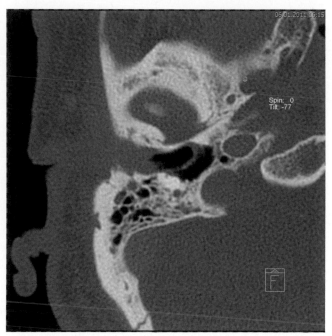

Fig. 13.1a, b Axial (**a**) and coronal (**b**) computed tomography scans of a patient with necrotizing otitis externa with minimal opacification of well-developed mastoid air cells and suspected small bony erosions along the floor of the external ear canal and the mastoid tip. The fallopian canal is barely reached.

lethal disease. Elderly and diabetic male patients seem to be at higher risk. *Pseudomonas aeruginosa* as the main infectious agent may spread through the fissures of Santorini and the tympanomastoid suture to induce a severe skull base osteomyelitis with further involvement of the infratemporal fossa and the jugular foramen. Patients often complain of pain in the early morning hours, awakening at night. Initially, the otoscopic finding is rather unspectacular with resistant granulation tissue at the bony-cartilaginous junction of the external ear canal. The close proximity of the mastoid segment of the facial nerve to the origin of the infection and the vicinity of the stylomastoid foramen to the extension of the infection toward the jugular bulb predisposes the facial nerve to become involved. Facial nerve and lower cranial nerve palsies can be the first alarming symptom and guide the physician to order CT *and* magnetic resonance imaging (MRI) scans, revealing evidence for osteomyelitis and spread of the infection along the skull base. On CT scans, limited opacification of mastoid air cells along with a thickening of the external ear canal skin may be the first faint signs of this devastating infection (**Fig. 13.1**). MRI, however, reveals the true extent of the infection along the skull base into the soft tissues of the infratemporal fossa and toward the neural elements of the jugular foramen (**Fig. 13.2**).

Involvement of the facial nerve is a poor prognostic sign.[9] Further progression with involvement of the lower cranial nerves (IX-XII) or extension toward the petrous apex (VI palsy) precede a lethal outcome. The treatment

of suspected or confirmed (radiologically or via biopsy) necrotizing external otitis has evolved from primarily surgical to a prolonged medical treatment using a combination of intravenous antibiotics against *P. aeruginosa* over 2 to 4 months. Ciprofloxacin as a single agent readily induces resistant strains and may worsen the outcome. Bacterial cultures from the external ear canal or the mastoid are suggested but may be negative due to previous antibiotic treatment. Controversies still exist regarding surgical debridement and facial nerve decompression.[10] Reviewing the literature, the main treatment

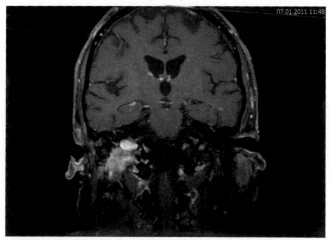

Fig. 13.2 Magnetic resonance imaging of the same patient in **Fig. 13.1** with marked inflammatory reaction (gadolinium enhancement) on T1 extending along the skull base into the infratemporal fossa.

remains medical with intravenous antibiotic therapy. Mastoidectomy with surgical drainage of coalescent otomastoiditis seems appropriate in cases of disease progression (e.g., sigmoid sinus thrombosis, lower cranial nerve palsies, or facial nerve paralysis[10] with radiographic signs of osteolysis). Facial nerve decompression with opening of the epineurium has not been widely performed and may not improve the outcome overall. It appears that full recovery of the infectious disease does not necessarily correlate with full recovery of facial function.[10,11]

■ Chronic Otitis Media

Facial palsy with chronic suppurative otitis media without cholesteatoma primarily affects adults or adolescents and rarely pediatric patients. An underlying cholesteatoma has to be excluded by otoscopy and imaging (CT and eventually non–echo-planar imaging diffusion MRI). Other differential diagnoses include tuberculosis, Wegener disease, or histiocytosis X. Dry perforations do not impair facial function; however, intermittent or chronic draining (suppurative) perforations may be complicated by acute or slowly progressive facial palsy. Facial palsy may not be the only symptom of a hostile environment. Vertigo, labyrinthitis, and sensorineural hearing loss with tinnitus are other symptoms of progressive middle ear infection. Imaging using CT scans is mandatory to evaluate the extent of the disease within the temporal bone and to check for dehiscences along the fallopian canal. Immediate broad spectrum intravenous antibiotics and steroids are routinely administered. Incomplete facial palsy (paresis) and early cessation of the drainage are in favor of a rapid recovery of normal facial function. Surgery to cure the underlying disease can then be postponed and electively planned. Progression to facial nerve paralysis requires surgical intervention at the earliest possible moment. Electrical testing prior to surgery (electroneuronography in acute or subacute paralysis, electromyography in long-standing facial paralysis) determines the extent of neural damage and has a prognostic implication. Total loss of electrical response may have a worse outcome. The type of surgical approach is dictated by the extent of the disease and the exposure required to follow the course of the facial nerve. In a well pneumatized temporal bone, a closed cavity setting with posterior tympanotomy and epitympanotomy/-ectomy can be sufficient; otherwise, an open mastoidoepitympanectomy allows complete exposure of the facial nerve from the geniculate ganglion to the stylomastoid foramen.[12]

The facial nerve should be explored throughout the middle ear and mastoid. In case of early surgery and acute facial paralysis, intraoperative facial nerve stimulation may enable the surgeon to verify the lesion site (often along the tympanic, dehiscent segment). Distal stimulation in these instances may still be possible (reaction audible at the monitor), whereas proximal stimulation does not reveal any reaction. The segment identified can then be exposed and decompressed distally and proximally. In most instances, intraoperative stimulation is no longer possible (due to the length and severity of facial nerve damage) and the facial nerve needs to be skeletonized from the stylomastoid foramen to the geniculate ganglion. If no lesion is identified, total facial nerve decompression does not seem to be necessary and may be an overtreatment.[13] Early decompression and removal of the pathology within the middle ear does have a favorable prognosis, reaching normal or near-normal (HB II) function within a few months. In cases of long-standing facial paralysis or patients revealing no response on preoperative electric testing, the final outcome may be unsatisfactory.[14]

A postmortem study by Schuknecht revealed an osteolytic inflammatory lesion in an elderly diabetic patient with a large focus of osteitis invading the fallopian canal, compressing the nerve, and inflammatory cells had infiltrated the degenerated facial nerve.[15] It therefore appears prudent to explore the facial nerve at surgery and to remove any lytic granulation tissue and osteitic bony debris. Fortunately, these types of lesions in patients with noncholesteatomatous chronic middle ear infections are becoming quite rare in Western countries.

Chronic Otitis Media with Cholesteatoma

Acquired and congenital cholesteatomas may both involve the facial nerve and induce facial palsies. The location and presenting signs are different and the surgical approach must be tailored to the pathology.

Acquired Cholesteatoma of the Temporal Bone

Chronic otitis media with cholesteatoma formation (primary or secondary acquired cholesteatomas) may cause facial palsy by extraneural compression or even completely destroy the nerve itself. An anatomical study revealed spontaneous fallopian canal dehiscences in almost 30% of regular autopsies. One-third (15/44) of the individuals affected displayed bilateral findings, thus resulting in 19.7% (59/300) of temporal bones affected, typically at the oval window niche.[16] In a clinical study of 67 patients, 33% revealed bony dehiscences, underscoring the high risk of injury to the facial nerve by the extension of a cholesteatoma toward the epitympanum and by the surgeon dissecting near the facial nerve when removing the cholesteatoma matrix.[17]

Patients presenting with acute facial palsy and an underlying middle ear cholesteatoma should be treated as an emergency. In most instances, compression of the nerve requires immediate decompression to achieve

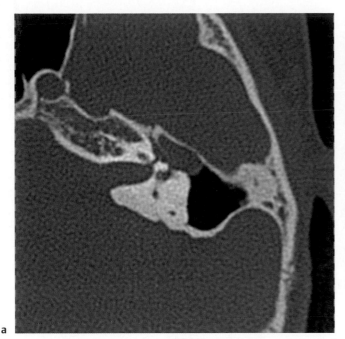
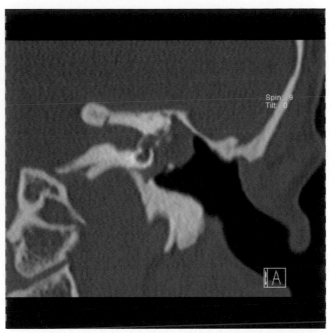

a
b

Fig. 13.3a, b Axial (**a**) and coronal (**b**) computed tomogrpahy scan of patient with acute facial palsy due to recurrent cholesteatoma along the tympanic segment of the exposed facial nerve without supralabyrinthine extension. Release of cholesteatoma content under local anesthesia and total removal a few days later improved facial function from House-Brackmann V to House-Brackmann II within 1 month.

prompt recovery. In a study by Quaranta et al, a significant difference could be identified between patients operated within 7 days (full recovery) versus delayed interventions with variable outcome.[18] It may also be justified to open the cholesteatoma sac and release the keratin content as an emergency intervention and to plan the complete removal of the cholesteatoma and facial nerve decompression a few days later (**Fig. 13.3**). Patients may also present late, suffering from partial palsy over a few months before referral to the ear, nose, and throat department. In case of partial palsy, improvement of facial function can be expected, although a normal outcome cannot be guaranteed even if surgery is performed as soon as possible.[19] An open mastoidoepitympanectomy with full access to the facial nerve from the geniculate ganglion to the stylomastoid segment is the primary approach. The surgeon should not limit him- or herself by trying to preserve the canal wall or maintain the anatomy of the external ear canal. The lesion most often involves the tympanic and pyramidal segment of the facial nerve, and the stapes suprastructure is frequently destroyed. Therefore, reconstruction of the ossicular chain does not have the first priority. Patients presenting with a long-standing total nerve paralysis do not have a favorable outcome. In most instances, the integrity of the facial nerve can be preserved, whereas in few occasions, the nerve may be thoroughly compressed to a thin layer of a few fibers or even be totally destroyed. In these cases, facial nerve

grafting should improve the final outcome from HB VI to HB IV or rarely HB III after 8 to 20 months.

Petrous Apex and Facial Palsy

Petrous bone cholesteatomas are considered a special entity of either congenital or acquired cholesteatomas extending into the petrous apex. Even at larger tertiary referral centers, these cholesteatomas are rare with about two to four new cases every year. They can be subdivided into supra- and infralabyrinthine cholesteatomas depending on their route of extension. The majority of apical cholesteatomas are of supralabyrinthine extension.[20] Acquired forms are petrous bone cholesteatomas arising within the middle ear space and invading the anterior region of the petrous bone through the anterior epitympanum and follow the facial nerve medially to the geniculate ganglion.[21] They may be missed at the first surgery if the clinician does not pay sufficient attention to the initial CT scans. These residual cholesteatomas then present with a progressive facial palsy (**Fig. 13.4**) and require revision surgery (**Fig. 13.5**).

The extension and invasion of these apical cholesteatomas determine their first presenting symptoms. In half of all cases in recent reviews and also in our own experience, one of the most frequent symptoms is progressive or recurrent facial palsy even to the extent of a total paralysis (HB VI).[22,23] Invasion into the cochlea or internal auditory canal may lead to sensorineural hearing loss up to total deafness. Vertigo is a rather infrequent finding. On CT scans,

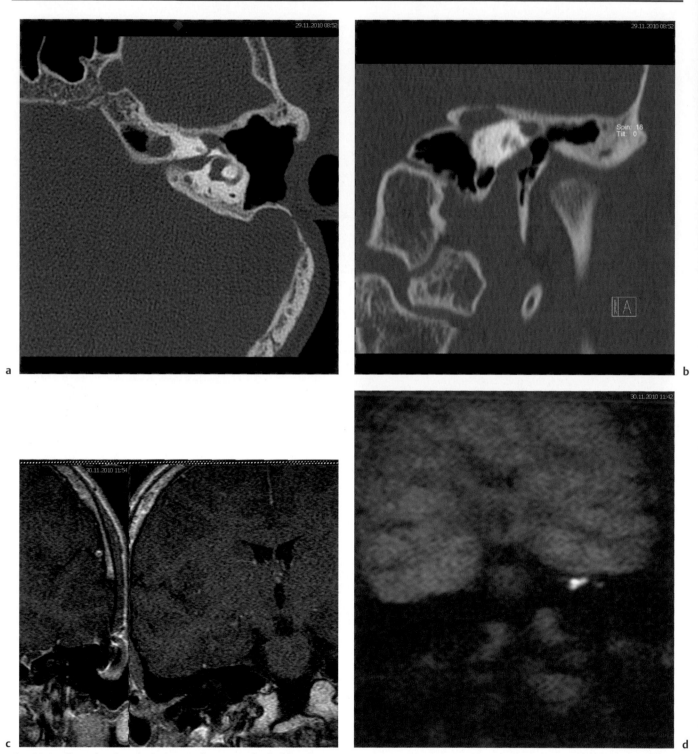

Fig. 13.4a–d Axial and coronal computed tomography (**a, b**) and magnetic resonance imaging scans (**c**, T1; **d**, non–echo-planar imaging diffusion sequence) of supralabyrinthine extension of a middle ear cholesteatoma operated previously with insufficient removal. Residual growth led to a facial paralysis that recovered completely upon total removal of the cholesteatoma using a combined approach. (**a, b**) Enlarged geniculate ganglion and a lesion in an apical cell after previous open cavity surgery. (**c, d**) Coronal magnetic resonance imaging scans typical for the supralabyrinthine extension of the cholesteatoma above the geniculate ganglion and cholesterol within the apical cell.

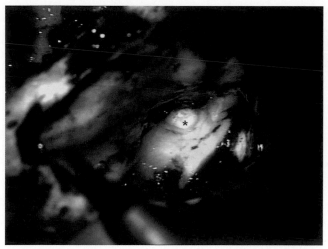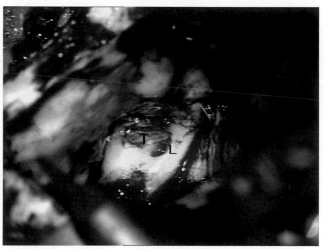

Fig. 13.5a, b Intraoperative (middle fossa) view of cholesteatoma pearl pushing onto the geniculare ganglion before (**a**) and after (**b**) removal. The asterisk indicates a white cholesteatoma pearl before removal. L, labyrinthine segment; T, tympanic segment of facial nerve after removal of the cholesteatoma with immediate improvement of facial function.

these lesions appear as sharp-cut erosions of bone medial to the superior semicircular canal, adjacent to the geniculate ganglion and superior to the internal auditory meatus. Non–echo-planar imaging diffusion MRI sequences (see **Fig. 13.4d**) allow a proper diagnosis and distinguish these lesions from cholesterol granulomas of the petrous apex, hemangiomas of the geniculate ganglion, or other rare lesions involving the geniculate and labyrinthine segment of the facial nerve. The awareness of these lesions and easy access to CT and MRI scanners have improved the diagnostic work-up and have led to an earlier diagnosis of smaller lesions.[23]

The challenge of these lesions is (1) the surgical approach and (2) the management of the facial nerve. The supralabyrinthine extension of these cholesteatomas does not allow sufficient view through a mastoidectomy and epitympanectomy approach such as in temporal bone cholesteatomas limited to the middle ear and antrum. A pure lateral approach requires the partial or total removal of the labyrinth and—depending on the anterior extension—also of the cochlea. Because total deafness does result, a subtotal petrosectomy with transotic removal of the cholesteatoma (**Fig. 13.6**) and fat obliteration of the surgical cavity will provide sufficient and safe exposure of the lesion.[24] An extension into an infratemporal fossa approach type B is used in cases of cholesteatoma involvement along the horizontal segment of the carotid artery into the petrous apex, and an infratemporal fossa approach type A may be required in cases of jugular bulb infiltration.[24,25] In all these instances, hearing preservation is not an option. Fistulas into the labyrinth or cochlea are often already present prior to surgery, and the patient is habituated to moderate or severe hearing loss prior to surgery. In case of limited cholesteatoma extension just medial to the geniculate ganglion and superior to the internal auditory canal

with only minimal hearing loss, a combined approach may be selected: The transmastoid-supralabyrinthine approach (or mastoidectomy/middle-fossa approach) allows two viewing positions (see **Fig. 13.5**): (1) the lateral view onto the tympanic and geniculate segment of the facial nerve through the mastoidoepitympanectomy, and (2) the craniotomy over the root of the zygoma and the limited extradural retraction of the temporal lobe allows the superior view over the middle cranial fossa and the geniculate, labyrinthine, and intrameatal segments of the facial nerve within a 60-degree angle anterior to the superior semicircular canal and just posterior to the cochlea.[21,24,25] The experience of the surgeon, the meticulous analysis of the preoperative CT and MRI scans, and the preoperative facial nerve and hearing status of the patient determine the access route.

The facial nerve can usually be preserved in patients with incomplete or short-term facial palsy. The cholesteatoma matrix needs to be carefully dissected free along the involved segments and along the dura with preservation of its integrity. Opening the dura over the internal auditory canal may lead to a temporary cerebrospinal fluid leak. Intraoperative facial nerve stimulation distal to the compression site is possible, and proximal stimulation may improve immediately once the cholesteatoma is removed. In patients with recent preoperative facial weakness, the facial function will improve rapidly within a few days and return to normal or near-normal (HB I-II) within 2 to 4 months.

The bigger surgical challenge is faced in patients with a long standing facial paralysis or an almost complete facial palsy (HB V) over several weeks to months as well as in patients after previous surgery and facial paralysis. In these patients, hearing preservation or staged hearing reconstruction is not a primary issue.[26] Decompression of a tiny

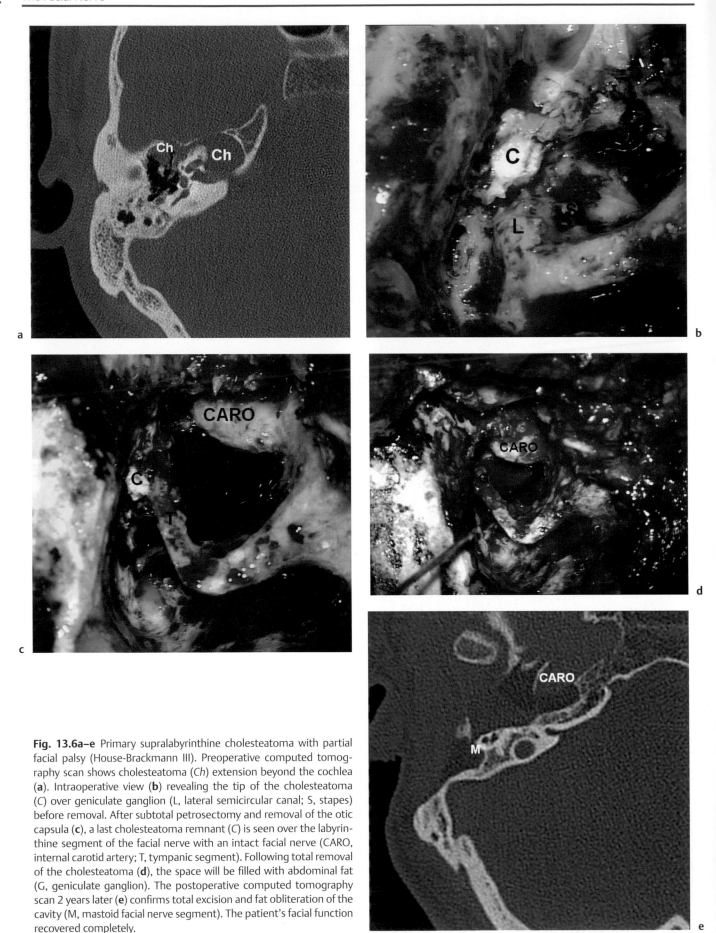

Fig. 13.6a–e Primary supralabyrinthine cholesteatoma with partial facial palsy (House-Brackmann III). Preoperative computed tomography scan shows cholesteatoma (*Ch*) extension beyond the cochlea (**a**). Intraoperative view (**b**) revealing the tip of the cholesteatoma (*C*) over geniculate ganglion (L, lateral semicircular canal; S, stapes) before removal. After subtotal petrosectomy and removal of the otic capsula (**c**), a last cholesteatoma remnant (*C*) is seen over the labyrinthine segment of the facial nerve with an intact facial nerve (CARO, internal carotid artery; T, tympanic segment). Following total removal of the cholesteatoma (**d**), the space will be filled with abdominal fat (G, geniculate ganglion). The postoperative computed tomography scan 2 years later (**e**) confirms total excision and fat obliteration of the cavity (M, mastoid facial nerve segment). The patient's facial function recovered completely.

and thinned out facial nerve segment may not improve the facial function at all or remain at a final result of a HB grade IV. The surgeon has to decide whether he or she transects the compressed (and sometimes infiltrated) nerve segment and grafts the lesion site with a greater auricular or sural nerve graft. The final outcome should be a HB IIIa or Fisch score of 60–75%. A hypoglossal-facial nerve anastomosis is rarely required. With proper exposure, the rate of residual cholesteatoma should be an exception. In case of obliteration of the cavity (subtotal petrosectomy) or in case of a combined approach a follow-up CT and non–echo-planar imaging diffusion MRI should be performed after 1 and 3 years to verify complete eradication of the lesion. These petrous bone supralabyrinthine cholesteatomas are challenging lesions and should be referred to experienced centers to avoid residual or recurrent pathologies.

■ Other Inflammatory Lesions of the Middle Ear and Mastoid

Wegener Granulomatosis

Wegener granulomatosis is a systemic disease characterized by a necrotizing vasculitis of small-sized vessels and the formation of granulomatous lesions classically in the upper and lower respiratory tracts and kidneys. The prevalence of ear involvement varies from 20–50% and depends also on the delay until diagnosis and treatment. Otologic involvement may occasionally be the first presentation of Wegner disease and often poses a diagnostic dilemma. Our personal experience and the published case reports are all quite consistent: adult patients without previous ear disease present with subacute otitis media (initially unilateral with subsequent bilateral involvement) with effusion (OME). Patients suffer from otalgia and marked hearing loss. Audiometry often reveals a combined hearing loss with rapid deterioration, which may rarely lead to total deafness.[27] CT scans are nonspecific and reveal partial or total opacification of the middle ear and mastoid without bony erosion (**Fig. 13.7**).

Many patients undergo myringotomy, ventilation tube placement, and mastoid drainage. Intraoperatively, the mastoid cells are filled with swollen mucosa, the antrum is blocked, and the tympanic membrane and the middle ear mucosa are thickened with some degree of serous effusion. Bacteriological cultures are negative and, unfortunately, mucosal biopsies show only nonspecific inflammatory changes. Surgery does not improve the patient's condition and often does not help in the diagnosis, because the biopsies are not typical for Wegener disease. Laboratory tests in this localized and limited form of Wegener granulomatosis may also be nonspecific in the beginning with elevated erythrocyte sedimentation rates and increased levels of C-reactive protein. The specific cytoplasmic immunofluorescence staining pattern of antineutrophil

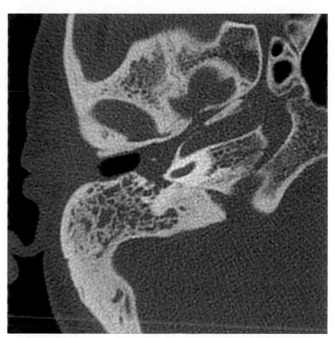

Fig. 13.7 Computed tomography scan of patient with bilateral mixed hearing loss and confirmed Wegener granulomatosis with marked mucosal swelling and inflammatory changes with limited effusion prior to medical treatment.

cytoplasmic antibiodies (c-ANCA) is often negative in the beginning.[28] It has been estimated that for active locoregional disease, the sensitivity drops to 60%, whereas in the generalized form it approaches over 90%.[29] Therefore, c-ANCA titers should be ordered repeatedly over the course of the disease.

Facial palsy in association with temporal bone involvement of Wegener disease is rare but may further delay the proper diagnosis and lead to unnecessary surgery. Most case reports describe uni- and rarely bilateral rapid progressive facial palsy up to total paralysis. The correct diagnosis of Wegener disease is made weeks to months after onset of the otitis media with effusion and facial palsy either by a positive chest CT revealing multiple nodular lesions (initially missed on a regular chest X-ray), by positive biopsies from nasopharyngeal lesions, by detection of c- or p-ANCA titers along the course of the disease, or by rapid deterioration of the patient's general condition and detection of renal involvement. Therefore, a high index of suspicion is necessary. The standard medical treatment using a combination of immunosuppressants (cyclophosphamide) and prednisolone, occasionally also with trimethoprim/sulfamethoxazole may improve the middle ear inflammation, but may not necessarily improve the sensorineural hearing loss (although we had observed a marked improvement in a recent patient). Most case reports describe an improvement in facial nerve function, but complete recovery is not expected. Therefore, diagnosis should be suspected early and treatment should be initiated before facial nerve involvement. Mastoid surgery does not improve the outcome and can be avoided.

Systemic Necrotizing Vasculitides

Among the other systemic necrotizing vasculitides with a potential lethal outcome are polyarteritis nodosa, microscopic polyangiitis, and the Churg-Strauss syndrome. They very rarely are accompanied with facial nerve palsy due to middle ear pathology. The vasculitis is pathologically often indistinguishable from the vasculitis of Wegener granulomatosis, and they are also associated with circulating ANCA autoantibodies. Polyarteritis nodosa is a multisystemic disease characterized by necrotizing inflammatory lesions of medium and small muscular arteries leading to microaneurysms with hemorrhage. It affects preferentially skin, joints, gut, and the kidney, but may also manifest itself along peripheral nerves. Uni- and bilateral facial nerve involvement has been described clinically[30] and by human temporal bone studies.[31] Histologically, the middle ear mucosa showed chronic inflammatory cell infiltration and granulation tissue with seropurulent effusion, and the arteritis was more obvious in the vessels accompanying the facial nerve along the fallopian canal.[31] These findings were observed in both temporal bones although the facial palsy was unilateral and had partially recovered. Microscopic polyangiitis causes a pulmonary-renal vasculitic syndrome with involvement of capillaries and venules and sometimes lacks arterial involvement. Churg-Strauss syndrome is associated with asthma and eosinophilia and the most common ear, nose, and throat manifestations are allergic rhinitis and nasal polyposis with only one case of facial palsy being reported.[32]

Differential Diagnosis of Systemic Inflammatory Diseases

Systemic infections such as human immunodeficiency virus may lead to middle ear disease and facial palsy.[33] The same holds true for otosyphilis. The lesion site is infranuclear and may be due to encephalomyelitis or a lymphocyte infiltration and involves the facial nerve segment in the cerebellopontine angle and internal auditory canal rather than along the intratemporal fallopian canal.

These patients may also develop middle ear tuberculosis. Tuberculous otitis media is now rarely seen in Western countries and is more frequently reported out of Africa and Asia. In a retrospective study in Korea, 5 of 52 patients had developed facial palsy during the course of otitis media due to *Mycobacterium tuberculosis*.[34] These patients present with chronic otorrhea resistant to conventional therapy and may reveal multiple tympanic membrane perforations and bone resorption on CT scans, contrary to the vasculitic etiology described previously.

Treatment is predominantly medical, and surgery is rarely indicated. Abscess formation may require surgical drainage; however, facial nerve decompression is not warranted.

References

1. Makeham TP, Croxson GR, Coulson S. Infective causes of facial nerve paralysis. Otol Neurotol 2007;28(1):100–103
2. Fischer FT, Chandler JR, May M, Schaitkin BM. Infection: Otitis media, cholestatoma, necrotizing external otitis, and other inflammatory disorders. In: May M, Schaitkin B.M. The Facial Nerve. New York: Thieme; 2000: 383–385
3. Wang CH, Chang YC, Shih HM, Chen CY, Chen JC. Facial palsy in children: emergency department management and outcome. Pediatr Emerg Care 2010;26(2):121–125
4. Evans AK, Licameli G, Brietzke S, Whittemore K, Kenna M. Pediatric facial nerve paralysis: patients, management and outcomes. Int J Pediatr Otorhinolaryngol 2005;69(11):1521–1528
5. Popovtzer A, Raveh E, Bahar G, Oestreicher-Kedem Y, Feinmesser R, Nageris BI. Facial palsy associated with acute otitis media. Otolaryngol Head Neck Surg 2005;132(2):327–329
6. Leskinen K, Jero J. Complications of acute otitis media in children in southern Finland. Int J Pediatr Otorhinolaryngol 2004;68(3):317–324
7. Yonamine FK, Tuma J, Silva RF, Soares MC, Testa JR. Facial paralysis associated with acute otitis media. Braz J Otorhinolaryngol 2009;75(2):228–230
8. Redaelli de Zinis LO, Gamba P, Balzanelli C. Acute otitis media and facial nerve paralysis in adults. Otol Neurotol 2003;24(1):113–117
9. Lee S, Hooper R, Fuller A, Turlakow A, Cousins V, Nouraei R. Otogenic cranial base osteomyelitis: a proposed prognosis-based system for disease classification. Otol Neurotol 2008;29(5):666–672
10. de Ru AJ, Aarts MCJ, van Benthem PPG. Malignant external otitis: changing faces. Int Adv Oto. 2010;6:274–276
11. Franco-Vidal V, Blanchet H, Bebear C, Dutronc H, Darrouzet V. Necrotizing external otitis: a report of 46 cases. Otol Neurotol 2007;28(6):771–773
12. Fisch U, May JS, Linder T. Tympanoplasty, Mastoidectomy, and Stapes Surgery. New York: Thieme; 2008
13. Ozbek C, Somuk T, Ciftçi O, Ozdem C. Management of facial nerve paralysis in noncholesteatomatous chronic otitis media. B-ENT 2009;5(2):73–77
14. Yetiser S, Tosun F, Kazkayasi M. Facial nerve paralysis due to chronic otitis media. Otol Neurotol 2002;23(4):580–588
15. Schuknecht HF. Pathology of the Ear. Cambridge, MA; Harvard University Press; 1974: 429
16. Di Martino E, Sellhaus B, Haensel J, Schlegel JG, Westhofen M, Prescher A. Fallopian canal dehiscences: a survey of clinical and anatomical findings. Eur Arch Otorhinolaryngol 2005;262(2):120–126
17. Selesnick SH, Lynn-Macrae AG. The incidence of facial nerve dehiscence at surgery for cholesteatoma. Otol Neurotol 2001; 22(2):129–132
18. Quaranta N, Cassano M, Quaranta A. Facial paralysis associated with cholesteatoma: a review of 13 cases. Otol Neurotol 2007;28(3):405–407
19. Siddiq MA, Hanu-Cernat LM, Irving RM. Facial palsy secondary to cholesteatoma: analysis of outcome following surgery. J Laryngol Otol 2007;121(2):114–117
20. Fisch U. 'Congenital' cholesteatomas of the supralabyrinthine region. Clin Otolaryngol Allied Sci 1978;3(4):369–376
21. Steward DL, Choo DI, Pensak ML. Selective indications for the management of extensive anterior epitympanic cholesteatoma

via combined transmastoid/middle fossa approach. Laryngoscope 2000;110(10 Pt 1):1660–1666

22. Omran A, De Denato G, Piccirillo E, Leone O, Sanna M. Petrous bone cholesteatoma: management and outcomes. Laryngoscope 2006;116(4):619–626

23. Magliulo G. Petrous bone cholesteatoma: clinical longitudinal study. Eur Arch Otorhinolaryngol 2007;264(2):115–120

24. Fisch U, Mattox D. Microsurgery ofthe Skull Base. New York: Thieme; 1988

25. Sanna M, Pandya Y, Mancini F, Sequino G, Piccirillo E. Petrous bone cholesteatoma: classification, management and review of the literature. Audiol Neurootol 2011;16(2):124–136

26. Linder T, Fisch U. Facial Nerve Disorders. In: Kirtane M.V., Brackmann D., Borkar D.M., de Souza Ch. Comprehensive textbook of otology. Mumbai, India: Bhalani Publishing House; 2010:417–437

27. Bohne S, Koscielny S, Burmeister HP, Guntinas-Lichius O, Wittekindt C. [Bilateral deafness and unilateral facial nerve palsy as presenting features of Wegener's granulomatosis: a case report]. HNO 2010;58(5):480–483

28. Banerjee A, Armas JM, Dempster JH. Wegener's granulomatosis: diagnostic dilemma. J Laryngol Otol 2001;115(1):46–47

29. Bibas A, Fahy C, Sneddon L, Bowdler D. Facial paralysis in Wegener's granulomatosis of the middle ear. J Laryngol Otol 2001;115(4):304–306

30. Vathenen AS, Skinner DW, Shale DJ. Treatment response with bilateral mixed deafness and facial palsy in polyarteritis nodosa. Am J Med 1988;84(6):1081–1082

31. Joglekar S, Deroee AF, Morita N, Cureoglu S, Schachern PA, Paparella M. Polyarteritis nodosa: a human temporal bone study. Am J Otolaryngol 2010;31(4):221–225

32. Bacciu A, Bacciu S, Mercante G, et al. Ear, nose and throat manifestations of Churg-Strauss syndrome. Acta Otolaryngol 2006;126(5):503–509

33. Linstrom CJ, Pincus RL, Leavitt EB, Urbina MC. Otologic neurotologic manifestations of HIV-related disease. Otolaryngol Head Neck Surg 1993;108(6):680–687

34. Cho YS, Lee HS, Kim SW, et al. Tuberculous otitis media: a clinical and radiologic analysis of 52 patients. Laryngoscope 2006;116(6):921–927

14 Facial Nerve Tumors

Michael Hoa, Eric P. Wilkinson, and Derald E. Brackmann

Tumors of the facial nerve are rare causes of facial paralysis. Nonetheless, the possibility of neoplastic involvement of the facial nerve should be considered in every patient with facial nerve–related symptoms. Of facial nerve tumors, facial nerve schwannomas (FNSs), considered to be intrinsic facial nerve tumors, and facial nerve hemangiomas (FNHs), which are extraneural in origin, are the most common. In this chapter, the authors focus on the presentation, evaluation, and management of these tumors.

■ Facial Nerve Schwannomas

FNSs are uncommon tumors of the temporal bone. First described by Schmidt in 1930, FNSs remain uncommon with no more than 500 cases described in the literature.[1,2] The reported incidence ranges from 0.8–1.9%.[3–5]

Tumor Anatomy, Pathology, and Pathogenesis

FNSs arise sporadically from the Schwann cell sheaths. They may involve any area of the facial nerve, but have a predilection for the perigeniculate area, the tympanic segment, and the mastoid segment (**Fig. 14.1**).[6,7] Skip lesions,

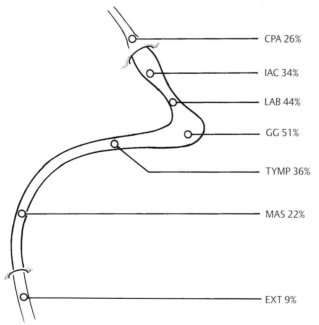

Fig. 14.1 Nerve segment involvement by facial nerve schwannomas. CPA, cerebellopontine angle; EXT, extratemporal; GG, geniculate ganglion; IAC, internal auditory canal; LAB, labyrinthine; MAS, mastoid; TYMP, tympanic.

CPA 26%

IAC 34%

LAB 44%

GG 51%

TYMP 36%

MAS 22%

EXT 9%

or multiple segments of involvement, are not infrequent. Despite having the appearance of multiple discrete tumors on a nerve, histopathological studies have noted discrete intraneural connections between separate portions of the lesion.[8] Their gross appearance is that of a diffuse bulging of the facial nerve, sometimes over several segments. The tumors are relatively homogeneous tan to gray in color, with larger tumors exhibiting areas of cystic formation. Microscopically, intact nerve fibers can permeate a tumor and thus biopsy of these lesions may precipitate a facial paralysis.[8] Typically, the tumors are well encapsulated and consist of two distinct histological patterns. Antoni A areas show broad interlacing ribbons of spindle cells with elongated nuclei, generally arranged in wave or whirl patterns. Verocay bodies, which are zones where the cells are arranged in palisades at either end of a bundle of parallel fibers, can be seen in the Antoni A regions. Antoni B areas are composed of a loose tissue arrangement that is often described as stellate and pleomorphic cells embedded in a myxoid ground substance with occasional multinucleated giant cells.

Clinical Presentation

As with other schwannomas, FNSs typically grow slowly over time. FNSs usually do not cause symptoms until they are fairly large and may manifest initially with hearing symptoms. Symptoms include slowly progressive facial paresis or paralysis and hearing loss, though tinnitus, pain, vestibular symptoms, or an ear canal mass may be present.[9] In the presence of a middle ear or ear canal mass, biopsy must not be performed because of the likelihood of resulting facial paralysis. Lipkin and colleagues, in their review of 238 cases, found patient age ranged from 4 to 81 years, with a mean age of 39 years.[9] Gender and sidedness were equally distributed. The most common symptoms were facial paralysis (73%), hearing loss (50%), tinnitus (13%), and ear canal mass (13%). Patients also reported pain (11%), vestibular symptoms (11%), and otorrhea (6%).

Facial nerve symptoms in FNSs have been classically described as having a slowly progressive pattern. Jackson and colleagues noted that facial paresis that progresses to complete paralysis over 6 to 12 weeks is not Bell palsy.[10] May and Hardin argued that progression of a facial paralysis beyond 3 weeks was suggestive of a neoplasm.[11] Facial twitching followed by progressive paresis is very characteristic of these tumors and should trigger suspicion for a neoplasm. Furthermore, a diagnosis of Bell palsy should not be accepted if there are no signs of recovery at 6 months.

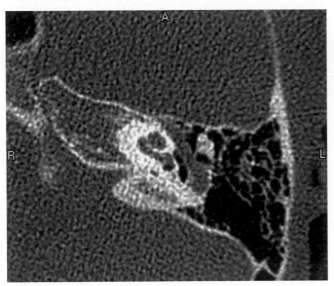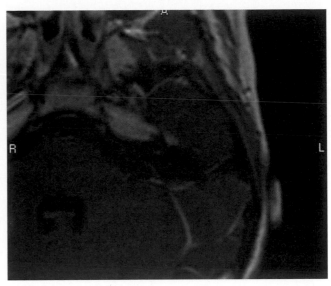

Fig. 14.2a, b Imaging characteristics of facial nerve schwannoma (FNS). (**a**) Axial computed tomography image of left-sided FNS depicts enlargement of the tympanic segment of the facial nerve. (**b**) T1-weighted postgadolinium axial magnetic resonance imaging of FNS depicts the frequently noted occurrence of skip lesions in FNSs with lesions visible in the fundus and geniculate ganglion.

However, FNSs can masquerade as Bell palsy presenting with a sudden complete paralysis with the occurrence ranging from 14–21%.[9,12,13] In addition, the presentation of recurrent facial palsy should trigger a search for neoplastic involvement of the facial nerve. One should not be lulled into the diagnosis of "recurrent Bell palsy." FNSs that arrive in the internal auditory canal and cerebellopontine angle may manifest with progressive sensorineural hearing loss similar to that caused by a vestibular schwannoma (VS). The diagnosis of FNSs in these cases may not be established until they are identified surgically. In a patient with a suspected VS, the presence of coexisting facial nerve symptoms should raise the surgeon's suspicion for an FNS. The solicitation of hyperkinesis, slowly progressive facial paralysis, recurrent ipsilateral paralysis, or asymmetric hearing loss on history or the presence of a mass in the ear canal, middle ear, or parotid should prompt radiological investigations.

Diagnostic Studies

Audiological testing should be obtained in all patients with facial paralysis. It should be mentioned that Bell palsy does not cause hearing impairment and, thus, any abnormality on the pure tone audiogram should mandate further investigation. Opinions differ on the utility of electroneurography (ENoG) and electromyography (EMG) testing in the diagnosis stage. Problems with standardization and potential sources of error as well as intertest and interdevice variability have been noted. However, the utility of these studies is optimized for those who use them frequently and are familiar with the limitations of their own test procedures. ENoG showing increased latency and/or greater amplitude reduction than expected for incomplete facial paralysis and an EMG showing fibrillations and polyphasic

potentials simultaneously can be clues for pushing one to pursue radiological evaluation. The latter is consistent with compression neuropathy.[14] These studies may help in instances where the diagnosis of an FNS is in question, with the alternative being a VS, and may help the surgeon to better prepare and counsel the patient accordingly.

Radiological imaging, meaning computed tomography (CT) and magnetic resonance imaging (MRI), are easily obtained in the modern era of medicine. Findings on CT provide a detailed look at the bony anatomy and may show dilation of the fallopian canal or intralabyrinthine segment (**Fig. 14.2a**), bone erosion around the geniculate ganglion or otic capsule, and possibly a middle ear mass. MRI with gadolinium, however, is the initial imaging study of choice and is superior in demonstrating disease in the cerebellopontine angle and extratemporally in the parotid as well as demonstrating tumor extension along the facial nerve. FNSs are isointense or slightly hypointense compared with brain on T1-weighted MRI, exhibit homogeneous enhancement with gadolinium, and demonstrate increased signal on T2-weighted images with characteristics similar to cerebrospinal fluid. Proximal tumors may imitate acoustic neuromas (**Fig. 14.2b**).

■ Facial Nerve Hemangiomas

FNHs have been considered extremely rare lesions. However, continuing advances in MRI have led to the identification of these lesions on a more frequent basis. In 1969, Pulec described a cavernous hemangioma with a diameter of 1 cm arising from the geniculate ganglion in a patient with a 3-year history of slowly progressive facial paralysis.[15]

Tumor Anatomy, Pathology, and Pathogenesis

FNHs are probably not true neoplasms but are more likely to be vascular malformations, specifically venous vascular malformations.[16] A classification for vascular lesions based on clinical, histopathological, and cytological features was introduced by Mulliken and Glowacki in 1982 and has been subsequently refined (**Table 14.1**).[17,18] The refined classification system argues that the term "hemangioma" should be reserved for benign vascular tumors that arise by cellular hyperplasia, whereas the term "malformation" should be used for errors of vascular morphogenesis that develop in utero and persist postnatally. Benoit and colleagues argue that what have been previously called FNHs exhibit clinical, histopathological, and immunohistochemical characteristics consistent with venous vascular malformations.[16]

On gross inspection, hemangiomas are rubbery red or purple masses that have the appearance of a sponge on sectioning. Histologically, FNHs appear as spaces lined by single layer of endothelial cells and filled with red blood cells. More specifically, Benoit et al provide a modern histologic description noting the presence of irregularly shaped dilated vessels with scant mural smooth muscle without an internal elastic lamina consistent with venous or lymphatic malformation.[16] Benoit and colleagues note that, in all specimens examined, lesional endothelial cells were mitotically inactive. Unlike traditional hemangiomas, facial nerve or geniculate ganglion hemangiomas do not stain positively for glucose transporter protein isoform 1 or Lewis Y antigen, and demonstrate immunoreactivity for podoplanin, a marker for lymphatic endothelial differentiation.[16]

Traditionally, it is thought that hemangiomas of the facial nerve originate from the vascular plexuses that surround the nerve. Vascularity is most intense around the geniculate ganglion and, to a lesser extent, around the internal auditory canal and midmastoid portion.[19] As a result of their origin from the vascular plexus, these tumors are typically extraneural, although infiltration of the nerve

does occur.[20] Thus, FNHs tend to occur around the geniculate ganglion. Although extension to the labyrinthine or tympanic segment can occur, extension to the internal auditory canal or beyond the cochleariform process is uncommon.[21]

Clinical Presentation

Despite being characteristically slow growing, FNHs tend to produce significant facial dysfunction at early stages out of proportion to the actual tumor size.[21] Some have suggested that this is due to a "vascular steal" phenomenon. In a review of the experience with geniculate ganglion hemangiomas at the House Clinic, which represents the largest single institution published experience in the literature, the most common presenting symptoms and signs were progressive facial paresis or paralysis and facial twitching followed by hearing loss due to either disruption of the ossicular chain or from erosion into the cochlea (**Fig. 14.3a, b**).

Table 14.2 depicts the distribution of presenting signs and symptoms. The House-Brackmann (HB) grading at presentation was I/II, III/IV, and VI in seven (38%), six (28%), and six patients (34%), respectively (**Table 14.3**).

Diagnostic Studies

While audiometry and acoustic reflex testing are important, they are nonspecific in patients with FNHs. However, the underlying hearing status is important for planning of surgical management and approach. Due to their small size and lack of unique angiographic appearance from other vascular lesions, angiography plays little role in the evaluation.

On ENoG, some lesions may demonstrate significant decrease in the response amplitude, and EMG may show a characteristic pattern of mixed regeneration and degeneration with concomitant presence of fibrillation potentials and polyphasic action potentials. This resulting dyssynchrony may explain the discrepancy seen in some patients between the severity of amplitude reduction noted on ENoG and the relatively mild facial nerve dysfunction.

High-resolution, fine-section CT and MRI are essential for the evaluation of a patient when a facial nerve hemangioma is suspected. CT may demonstrate enlargement of the geniculate ganglion and possible enlargement of distal labyrinthine or proximal tympanic segments of the facial nerve (see **Fig. 14.3a, b**). Typically, the lesion is centered on the geniculate ganglion and may exhibit adjacent nonsharp bony erosion with irregular borders, intralesional stippled calcifications, and spicules of bone. On MRI, FNHs tend to be slightly hypo- or isointense with brain on T1-weighted imaging and enhance intensely with gadolinium (**Fig. 14.3c**).

Table 14.1 Classification of the International Society for the Study of Vascular Anomalies

Vascular tumors	Vascular malformations
Hemangioma of infancy (superficial, deep, mixed)	Simple malformation
Congenital hemangioma	Capillary (Port wine stain)
Rapidly involuting versus noninvoluting	Venous
Kaposiform hemangioendothelioma	Lymphatic (microcystic versus macrocystic)
Tufted angioma	Arteriovenous malformation
Lobular capillary hemangioma	Combined malformation
Hemangiopericytoma	Capillary-lymphatic-venous
	Capillary-venous
	Capillary-venous with arteriovenous shunting

Source: Data from Benoit et al.[16]

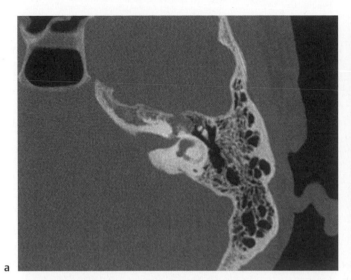

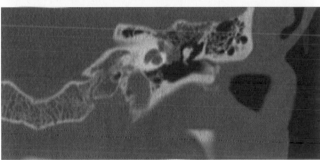

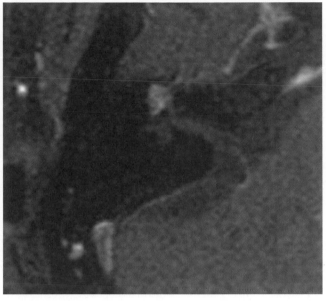

Fig. 14.3a–c Computed tomography (CT) imaging characteristics of facial nerve hemangioma. (**a**) Axial view CT image of a left-sided facial nerve hemangioma depicts adjacent nonsharp bony erosion with irregular borders and intralesional calcifications. (**b**) Coronal view CT image of a left-sided facial nerve hemangioma; cochlear fistula depicted. (**c**) T1-weighted postgadolinium axial magnetic resonance imaging of facial nerve hemangioma.

On T2-weighted imaging, FNHs tend to be hyperintense to brain, although they can be less intense than FNSs. Sometimes, intratumoral calcifications are present, and these lesions may exhibit a salt-and-pepper appearance on MRI. Lo and colleagues have shown that contrasted MRI was more sensitive in detecting hemangiomas of the internal auditory canals but missed four of six geniculate ganglion hemangiomas.[22] Thus, in patients with progressive facial palsy, a gadolinium-enhanced MRI of the internal auditory canal is the initial study of choice. If MRI is negative, then a high-resolution CT scan of the temporal bone is recommended to evaluate for geniculate ganglion hemangioma.

Table 14.2 House clinic experience: 19 patients over 20-year period, presenting symptoms and signs

Symptoms and signs	n (%)
Facial palsy (progressive onset/sudden onset)	16 (89)/1 (5)
Facial twitching	10 (56)
Synkinesis	3 (17)
Hearing loss	4 (22)
Dysequilibrium	1 (5)
Hypercusis	1 (5)
Taste disturbance	1 (5)
Retroauricular pain	1 (5)

Source: Data from Semaan et al.[21]

■ Differential Diagnosis

An estimated 5% of peripheral facial paralysis is due to tumor involvement.[23] The duration of symptoms and the infrequency of correct preoperative diagnosis speak to the inherent diagnostic difficulties. A positive response to steroids does not preclude the presence of a neoplasm. Furthermore, the presentation of a slowly progressive facial palsy, the presence of facial twitching, or the presence of ear, eye, or facial pain associated with facial weakness increases the likelihood of neoplasm. Once a neoplasm is identified along the facial nerve, the differential is limited. Schwannomas and hemangiomas are by far the most common. However, other entities exist and must be considered in the differential. With respect to the internal auditory canal and cerebellopontine angle, the differential is primarily between VS and FNS. A note of caution: enhancement of the labyrinthine segment on T1-weighted images with gadolinium

Table 14.3 House clinic experience: 19 patients over 20-year period, presenting facial function

House-Brackmann grade	n (%)
Grade I/II	1 (5)/6 (33)
Grade III/IV	3 (17)/2 (11)
Grade V/VI	3 (17)/3 (17)

Source: Data from Semaan et al.[21]

in the presence of a cerebellopontine angle mass should raise one's suspicion for an FNS, as an acoustic neuroma will not exhibit labyrinthine segment enhancement with gadolinium. Geniculate ganglion lesions with a facial nerve palsy that is out of proportion to the size of the lesion should prompt one's suspicion for a facial nerve hemangioma.

Other lesions that should be included in the differential of either FNS or FNHs include meningioma, cholesteatoma, glomus facialis, malignancy, and metastasis. Meningiomas isolated to the geniculate ganglion have been reported.[13] Larger meningiomas of the petrous apex or middle cranial fossa floor could extend to involve the facial nerve at the geniculate, but this would be a rare cause of facial paralysis. Presence of a dural tail may help to distinguish these lesions, although identification may in some cases only be possible at time of surgery.

Cholesteatoma can present as sudden complete and slowly progressive facial paralysis.[12,13] Congenital cholesteatoma can arise from the supralabyrinthine area adjacent to the geniculate ganglion and in one series accounted for 83% of congenital cholesteatomas causing facial paralysis.[13] This lesion is particularly important to differentiate from facial nerve hemangioma. CT imaging should demonstrate very sharp bone erosion versus the nonsharp erosion frequently seen in facial nerve hemangioma.

While uncommon, glomus tumors of the facial nerve have been reported.[23] A small number of glomus bodies are found in the descending segment of the facial nerve and, thus, glomus tumors of the facial nerve have been reported most commonly in the descending segment of the facial nerve.[24] These tumors typically present with facial paralysis or pulsatile tinnitus. Salient imaging features on CT include a hypervascular lesion, irregular widening of the descending portion of the facial nerve, and adjacent permeative lucency.[24]

Malignant lesions, particularly of the parotid gland, may present with facial paralysis, pain, or facial twitching. The importance here is to remember that a detailed neurotological examination for etiology must include careful palpation of the parotid and neck.

Metastasis from distant sites may be a consideration in the absence of palpable locoregional malignancy. Adenocarcinoma of the breast, lung, and prostate, as well as melanoma and rhabdomyosarcoma, may be considered. In these cases, however, it is unlikely that malignant facial nerve lesions will occur in isolation.

■ Operative Management

Facial Nerve Schwannomas

Surgical Philosophy

Traditionally, surgical resection has been the gold standard for the management of FNSs. Over the past 15 years, the management of FNSs has evolved as a result of new

Table 14.4 Proposed management algorithm for facial nerve schwannoma

- In a tumor of stable size without a bony confine, and with stable facial function of less than or equal to HB III, observe.
- In a bony-confined tumor with increasing size, worsening facial function (any grade), and/or worsening electroneurography function, consider bony decompression.
- In an enlarging tumor without a bony confine in the cerebellopontine angle or middle fossa with facial function less than or equal to HB III, consider stereotactic radiation.
- In an enlarging tumor with facial function greater or equal to HB IV or concern for adjacent structure, compressive symptoms, or stereotactic radiation failure, consider resection and grafting.

Abbreviations: HB, House-Brackmann.
Data from Wilkinson EP, Hoa M, Slattery WH III, et al. Evolution in the management of facial nerve schwannoma. Laryngoscope 2011;121(10):2065–2074.

surgical techniques and new therapeutic options including microsurgical decompression and stereotactic radiation. This evolution of treatment has resulted in longer preservation of good facial function in such patients. As a result, the authors believe that the principal goal in the management of patients with FNS should be to maximize facial function over the longest period possible in the absence of other symptoms demanding treatment. Surgical resection may be reserved for more severe declines in facial function. The experience at the House Clinic with patients with FNS has resulted in a proposed algorithm for management of these patients (**Table 14.4**).

In the absence of bony confinement in the setting of stable facial function greater than or equal to a HB III, stable tumors can be observed. However, enlarging tumors with facial function better than an HB III may consider stereotactic radiation. In the presence of bony confinement, enlarging tumors with worsening facial function and/or worsening ENoG function may be considered for bony decompression. Finally, resection and grafting may be considered for enlarging tumors with facial function HB IV or worse where concern exists for adjacent structures, in the presence of compressive symptoms, or because of stereotactic radiation failures.

Observation

Similar to the debate regarding other slow-growing tumors, there is a debate as to whether and when to intervene in patients with FNS. Some patients may be asymptomatic or may be discovered during the work-up of auditory complaints. It must be kept in mind that the best possible outcome from facial nerve excision and grafting would be a HB grade III. However, if one waits until the facial nerve degenerates, the likelihood of obtaining this outcome may be less likely. We believe that observation with serial MRI is an acceptable approach in patients with good facial function and no brainstem compressive symptoms.

Bony Decompression

As management of FNS has evolved over the past 30 years, the goal of prolonging good facial nerve function has become more prominent. The technique of bony decompression of the facial nerve from the internal auditory canal to the stylomastoid foramen has regained attention in light of this new focus in management. This technique is performed through a combined middle cranial fossa-transmastoid approach. Based on our experience, we believe that enlarging tumors with worsening facial function and/or worsening ENoG function, in the presence of bony confinement, may be considered for bony decompression.

Surgical Resection and Approach

The selection of surgical approach to FNS has not changed greatly in recent years. The surgeon must be prepared to expose the entire facial nerve from cerebellopontine angle to the stylomastoid foramen. In cases of patients without hearing, a translabyrinthine approach may be considered. However, in most cases, a middle cranial fossa approach is employed with the addition of a transmastoid approach if significant distal extension of the FNS exists (**Fig. 14.4**). Operative exposure of an FNS via middle cranial fossa approach is depicted in **Fig. 14.5**.

Access to the cerebellopontine angle and facial nerve route entry zone can be obtained by an extended middle fossa approach. Access to the horizontal segment of the facial nerve can be obtained by removal of the tegmen tympani. Tumors with extension distal to the midtympanic segment will require the addition of a transmastoid approach. This approach provides exposure from the brainstem to the stylomastoid foramen.

Radiosurgery

Stereotactic radiosurgery has become a popular treatment modality in recent years. A review of the literature regarding radiosurgical treatment of FNSs reveals that the experience with this modality is increasing (**Table 14.5**).[25–30] While preliminary results appear promising, longer-term follow-up and more definitive evaluation criteria are needed to assess the efficacy of this modality. Based on our experience, stereotactic radiosurgery may be considered for enlarging tumors with facial function less than or equal to an HB III.

Results

The management of FNSs has evolved at the House Clinic over the past 30 years.[30] In the 15 years prior to 1995, surgical resection composed the majority of treatments (85%), followed by bony decompression. Since 1995, the distribution of treatment modality has changed with bony decompression being performed most frequently (34%), followed by microsurgical resection (28%), observation

(26%), and stereotactic radiation (12%). This evolution reflects changing priorities in the management of FNS. Facial nerve grade was maintained or improved over the follow-up period (mean time = 4.6 years) in 77.8% of the decompression group and 100% of the observation and radiation groups compared with 54.8% of the resection group.

Facial Nerve Hemangiomas

Surgical Philosophy

While recent series have commented on the adherence of and intimate relationship of FNHs to the facial nerve, they still remain extraneural in location with respect to the facial nerve.[14,20,31] With this in mind, it is possible to remove these tumors while still preserving the continuity of the facial nerve. For this reason, it has been traditionally advocated that early surgery be offered for the best chance of excellent facial nerve function. In addition, complete surgical excision when possible is advocated. However, it is our experience that preservation of facial nerve continuity is important to the eventual good facial function and that the incidence of recurrence or further growth of these vascular malformations in our published experience is rare.[21] Furthermore, there is a trend toward better facial function in those patients in whom facial nerve continuity is preserved.[21] Thus, in instances where the hemangioma is particularly adherent to the facial nerve, it may be permissible to preserve the integrity of the facial nerve while leaving a small residual of tumor on the facial nerve.

Surgical Resection and Approach

If hearing is not a concern, then a transmastoid translabyrinthine approach will allow exposure of the entire course of the facial nerve and will provide the best exposure for grafting if the geniculate segment needs to be excised. In most cases, an extradural middle fossa craniotomy approach is ideal for most lesions. On rare occasions with extensive middle ear involvement, a transmastoid approach may be a helpful adjunct to the middle fossa approach. Preoperative CT may be helpful in making a final decision on surgical approach, particularly if otic capsule erosion by the tumor is seen. In such a case, the surgeon may elect a translabyrinthine approach due to the high likelihood of hearing loss due to a labyrinthine fistula.

Middle Fossa Approach

After the craniotomy window is made, the temporal lobe is supported by a retractor, and the greater superficial petrosal nerve and the skeletonized superior semicircular canal are identified. The greater superficial petrosal nerve is followed posterior to the geniculate ganglion (**Fig. 14.6**). Careful microsurgical dissection with intraoperative facial nerve monitoring is recommended especially in this region as tumor can distort the anatomy. The internal auditory

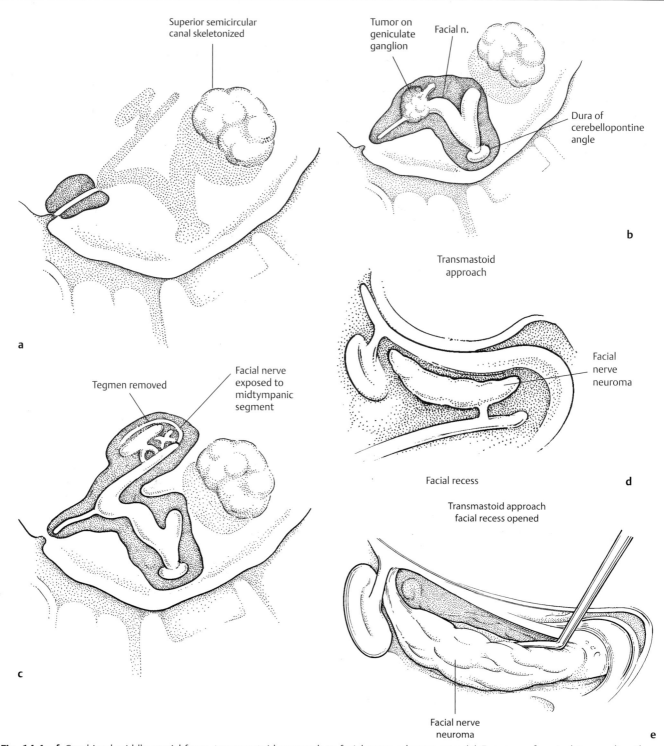

Fig. 14.4a–f Combined middle cranial fossa–transmastoid approach to facial nerve schwannoma. (**a**) Exposure of geniculate ganglion through middle fossa approach. (**b**) Greater superficial petrosal nerve and superior semicircular canal are skeletonized. The tumor is encountered at the geniculate ganglion. (**c**) Internal auditory canal and labyrinthine facial nerve are exposed medial to the geniculate ganglion. (**d**) After removal of the tegmen, the facial nerve can be exposed to approximately the midtympanic segment. (**e**) Facial nerve neuroma as seen through the transmastoid approach. Opening of the facial recess allows for exposure of the distal facial nerve.

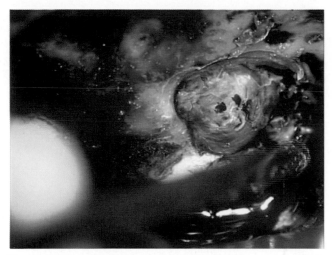

Fig. 14.5 Intraoperative view of middle cranial fossa approach to facial nerve schwannoma.

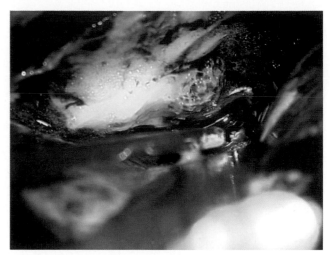

Fig. 14.6 Intraoperative view of middle cranial fossa approach to geniculate ganglion hemangioma.

canal is then dissected and the labyrinthine facial nerve is identified. The amount of internal auditory canal exposure varies with the degree of tumor extension and the need for access to place a graft.

Transmastoid Approach

When additional distal exposure is needed, a transmastoid approach to the facial nerve can be performed. The facial recess is opened and the nerve is exposed to the stylomastoid foramen. Around the facial nerve, it is best to thin the bone over it with a diamond burr with copious irrigation and to remove the overlying "eggshell" of bone with an instrument such as an annulus elevator or Rosen needle. The malleus head and incus can be removed for additional exposure with ossicular reconstruction being performed at the end of the procedure.

Tumor Removal

While most hemangiomas exhibit some degree of adherence to the facial nerve, a plane can be developed between the tumor and the nerve in some cases that will allow tumor removal and preservation of facial nerve continuity.

Graft Material and Nerve Grafting

With respect to graft material, great auricular nerve or sural nerve can be utilized to reconstruct the facial nerve should nerve continuity not be maintained. With respect to nerve grafting in the temporal bone, placement of the graft in approximation to the nerve end with or without collagen tubules usually suffices. Frozen section examination of the nerve stump is necessary not only to validate complete tumor removal, but to ensure that no tumor remains at the anastomotic site to impede axonal

Table 14.5 Review of literature for stereotactic radiation treatment of facial nerve schwannomas

Study	n	Age (yr) mean (min–max)	Sex (M/F)	Margin dose (Gy) (min–max)	HB FN grade	Tumor size
Litre et al, 2009[25]	11	45.9 (22–87)	4/7	10–16	Three improved Eight unchanged	Four decreased Six stable One increased
Kida et al, 2007[26]	14	45.4 (28–70)	6/8	11–16	Five improved Eight unchanged One worse	Eight decreased Six stable
Nishioka et al, 2009[27]	4	28.5 (20–43)	1/3	FSR: 50 Gy total	Four unchanged	Two decreased Two stable
Madhok et al, 2009[28]	6	39.5 (19–59)	3/3	12–12.5	One improved Five unchanged	Three decreased Three stable
Hillman et al, 2008[29]	2	52.0 (51–53)	2/0	12, 25 FSR	One improved One unchanged	Two stable
House Clinic experience (unpublished)	6	47.3 (21–65)	2/4	12.5–13	Six unchanged	Three decrease One stable Two increased

Abbreviations: FN, facial nerve; FSR, fractionated stereotactic radiotherapy; HB, House-Brackmann.

regrowth. (This subject is dealt with in more depth in Chapter 23 of this book.)

Results

Fifteen of the 18 patients seen at the House Clinic were managed surgically. Three patients declined surgical treatment and were observed. Of the 15 patients managed surgically, 10 patients underwent a complete excision, 4 patients underwent partial excision, and 1 patient underwent a decompression procedure. In the four cases where the facial nerve was sacrificed, a nerve reconstruction was performed with a greater auricular nerve in three cases and sural nerve in one case. Of the 11 patients who underwent surgical resection with preservation of facial nerve continuity, 8 (73%) patients exhibited a postoperative HB grade I/II. The remaining three (27%) patients recovered to a HB grade III. In the four patients who underwent facial nerve excision with grafting, one patient had a HB grade III, two patients

recovered to a HB grade IV, and one patient had a HB grade V at last follow-up.[21] With respect to tumor growth and recurrence, one patient in the observation group exhibited growth while the remaining patients in the observation group did not exhibit any tumor growth. Furthermore, all patients in the surgically managed group, regardless of complete or partial excision, did not exhibit any recurrence or growth of their tumors. The average duration of follow-up was 73 months with a range of 4 to 189 months.[21]

■ Conclusion

While facial nerve tumors are relatively uncommon, the presence of a slowly progressive facial palsy or complaints of facial spasm should heighten one's suspicion for a facial nerve tumor. Understanding the intricacies of presentation as well as the complexities of management is essential for comprehensive management of these patients.

References

1. Schmidt C. Neurinom des nervus facialis. Zentralblatt Hals-Nas-Ohrenheild 1930;16:329
2. Shirazi MA, Leonetti JP, Marzo SJ, Anderson DE. Surgical management of facial neuromas: lessons learned. Otol Neurotol 2007;28(7):958–963
3. Saito H, Baxter A. Undiagnosed intratemporal facial nerve neurilemomas. Arch Otolaryngol 1972;95(5):415–419
4. Symon L, Cheesman AD, Kawauchi M, Bordi L. Neuromas of the facial nerve: a report of 12 cases. Br J Neurosurg 1993;7(1):13–22
5. Gunther M, Danckwardt-Lilliestrom N. Gudjonsson 0, Nyberg G, Kinnefors A, Rask Andersen H, Ekvall L. Surgical treatment of patients with facial neuromas-A report of 26 consecutive operations. Otol Neurotol 2010;31(9):1493–1497
6. O'Donoghue GM, Brackmann DE, House JW, Jackler RK. Neuromas of the facial nerve. Am J Otol 1989;10(1):49–54
7. Kertesz TR, Shelton C, Wiggins RH, Salzman KL, Glastonbury CM, Harnsberger R. Intratemporal facial nerve neuroma: anatomical location and radiological features. Laryngoscope 2001;111(7):1250–1256
8. Hajjaj M, Linthicum FH Jr. Facial nerve schwannoma: nerve fibre dissemination. J Laryngol Otol 1996;110(7):632–633
9. Lipkin AF, Coker NJ, Jenkins HA, Alford BR. Intracranial and intratemporal facial neuroma. Otolaryngol Head Neck Surg 1987;96(1):71–79
10. Jackson CG, Glasscock ME III, Hughes G, Sismanis A. Facial paralysis of neoplastic origin: diagnosis and management. Laryngoscope 1980;90(10 Pt 1):1581–1595
11. May M, Hardin WB Jr. Facial palsy: interpretation of neurologic findings. Trans Sect Otolaryngol Am Acad Ophthalmol Otolaryngol 1977;84(4 Pt 1):ORL-710–ORL-722
12. Schaitkin B, May M. In: May M, Schaitkin B, eds. Tumors involving the facial nerve. New York: Thieme; 2000
13. Fisch V, Ruttner J. Pathology of intratemporal tumors involving the facial nerve. In: Fisch U, ed. Facial Nerve Surgery. Birmingham, AL: Aesculapius; 1977:448–456
14. Shelton C, Brackmann DE, Lo WW, Carberry JN. Intratemporal facial nerve hemangiomas. Otolaryngol Head Neck Surg 1991;104(1):116–121
15. Pulec JL. Facial nerve tumors. Ann Otol Rhinol Laryngol 1969;78(5):962–982
16. Benoit MM, North PE, McKenna MJ, Mihm MC, Johnson MM, Cunningham MJ. Facial nerve hemangiomas: vascular tumors or malformations? Otolaryngol Head Neck Surg 2010;142(1):108–114
17. Mulliken JB, Glowacki J. Hemangiomas and vascular malformations in infants and children: a classification based on endothelial characteristics. Plast Reconstr Surg 1982;69(3):412–422
18. Chang MW. Updated classification of hemangiomas and other vascular anomalies. Lymphat Res Biol 2003;1(4):259–265
19. Balkany T, Fradis M, Jafek BW, Rucker NC. Hemangioma of the facial nerve: role of the geniculate capillary plexus. Skull Base Surg 1991;1(1):59–63
20. Eby TL, Fisch U, Makek MS. Facial nerve management in temporal bone hemangiomas. Am J Otol 1992;13(3):223–232
21. Semaan MT, Slattery WH, Brackmann DE. Geniculate ganglion hemangiomas: clinical results and long-term follow-up. Otol Neurotol 2010;31(4):665–670
22. Lo WW, Shelton C, Waluch V, et al. Intratemporal vascular tumors: detection with CT and MR imaging. Radiology 1989;171(2):445–448
23. Petrus LV, Lo WM. Primary paraganglioma of the facial nerve canal. AJNR Am J Neuroradiol 1996;17(1):171–174
24. Connor SEJ, Gleeson MJ, Odell E. Extracranial glomus faciale tumour. J Laryngol Otol 2008;122(9):986–989
25. Litre CF, Gourg GP, Tamura M, et al. Gamma knife surgery for facial nerve schwannomas. Neurosurgery 2007;60(5):853–859, discussion 853–859
26. Kida Y, Yoshimoto M, Hasegawa T. Radiosurgery for facial schwannoma. J Neurosurg 2007;106(1):24–29
27. Nishioka K, Abo D, Aoyama H, et al. Stereotactic radiotherapy for intracranial nonacoustic schwannomas including facial nerve schwannoma. Int J Radiat Oncol Biol Phys 2009;75(5):1415–1419
28. Madhok R, Kondziolka D, Flickinger JC, Lunsford LD. Gamma knife radiosurgery for facial schwannomas. Neurosurgery 2009;64(6):1102–1105, discussion 1105
29. Hillman TA, Chen DA, Fuhrer R. An alternative treatment for facial nerve tumors: short-term results of radiotherapy. Ear Nose Throat J 2008;87(10):574–577
30. Wilkinson EP, Hoa M, Slattery WH III, et al. Evolution in the management of facial nerve schwannoma. Laryngoscope 2011;121(10):2065–2074
31. Isaacson B, Telian SA, McKeever PE, Arts HA. Hemangiomas of the geniculate ganglion. Otol Neurotol 2005;26(4):796–802

15 Extratemporal Causes of Facial Paralysis

John P. Leonetti and Sam J. Marzo

Acute facial paralysis is due to Bell palsy in ~85% of patients who present with complete, unilateral facial weakness.[1] The dangerous diagnosis of "atypical" Bell palsy has been inappropriately assigned to a variety of clinical presentations including fluctuating facial paralysis, gradual onset facial weakness, progressive facial palsy, and facial paresis involving peripheral branches of the facial nerve.[2] The etiology of facial paralysis that is anything but acute in presentation is best considered a wolf in sheep's clothing, and the appropriate investigation for a neoplastic cause must be implemented.[3] The purpose of this chapter is to discuss the diagnosis and management of extratemporal causes of facial paralysis.

■ Clinical Assessment

Patient History

The most important initial step in the evaluation of a patient with facial paralysis is taking an accurate history of the onset of the facial weakness. Extratemporal causes are usually associated with gradual-onset facial weakness, peripheral branch involvement, or fluctuating facial weakness.[4] Acute facial paralysis rarely is caused by an extratemporal neoplasm. Localized pain, referred otalgia, or trismus should alert the clinician as to the possibility of an extratemporal malignancy causing facial paralysis. Pain in this region is due to neoplastic involvement of the sensory branches of the trigeminal nerve.[5] Patients should also be questioned about any prior skin cancer treatment in the scalp or facial region as deep tumor invasion or lymphatic spread can cause ipsilateral facial paralysis.

Physical Examination

The exact extent of the presenting facial weakness must be accurately made and documented. Facial photography at rest and during animation should be made part of the patient's medical record. Dynamic facial function can also be video-recorded and stored in the patient's electronic medical record.

Neck and parotid gland palpation must be carefully performed in an effort to identify cervical lymph node metastases or a primary parotid neoplasm. The ipsilateral auricle, temporal scalp, and facial regions should be inspected for skin cancers that may directly invade the facial nerve or spread to parotid lymph nodes. The oral cavity must also be inspected and palpated as deep-lobe or parapharyngeal space tumors may not be externally visible or palpable. Any degree of trismus, due to tumor invasion of the ptygoid muscles or the temporomandibular joint, can also be assessed during the oral cavity examination.[6]

Microscopic otoscopic examination is performed as some parotid neoplasms either originate in the temporal bone or may involve the ear canal by direct cartilaginous or bony invasion.[7] Finally, a complete cranial nerve assessment is performed as occult, deep parotid tumors may invade the jugular foramen causing lower cranial nerve dysfunction, and perineural spread along the trigeminal nerve may lead to cavernous sinus extension and deficits of cranial nerves III, IV, or VI.

Diagnostic Studies

The radiological assessment of a palpable parotid mass in a patient with facial paralysis can be accomplished with either contrast-enhanced computed tomography (CT) or magnetic resonance imaging (MRI).[8] Perineural extension is better evaluated with MRI coronal views with special attention to the trigeminal nerve and the cavernous sinus (**Fig. 15.1**).[9] Temporal bone invasion, especially at

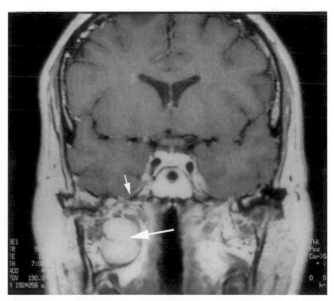

Fig. 15.1 Coronal magnetic resonance imaging view of a malignant parotid tumor (*large arrow*) causing facial paralysis with superior perineural extension along the mandibular division of the trigeminal nerve (*small arrow*).

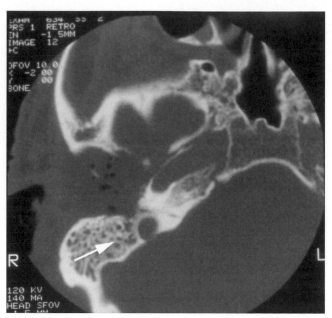

Fig. 15.2 Axial computed tomography scan view of a malignant parotid tumor causing facial paralysis with temporal bone invasion (*arrow*).

Table 15.1 Extratemporal causes for facial paralysis

Benign neoplasms

    Facial neuroma

    Hemangioma

    Ectopic paraganglioma

Malignant parotid neoplasms

    Adenoid cystic carcinoma

    Mucoepidermoid carcinoma

    Squamous cell carcinoma

    Adenocarcinoma

    Carcinoma ex-pleomorphic adenoma

Malignant cutaneous neoplasms

    Squamous cell carcinoma

    Melanoma

    Basal cell carcinoma

Temporal bone malignancies

    Squamous cell carcinoma

    Basal cell carcinoma

the stylomastoid foramen, is better evaluation with high-resolution CT imaging (**Fig. 15.2**). Nonpalpable tumor invasion of the facial nerve by primary parotid malignancies of adjacent skin cancers may only be seen on MRI selective views.[10]

The assessment of metastatic disease can be accomplished with CT or MRI views of the brain, chest, and abdomen, or whole-body positron emission tomography scanning. Peripheral bone, spine, or joint pain may suggest bone metastases, which are best evaluated with a whole-body radionucleotide bone scan.

Tissue Biopsy

Fine-needle aspiration cytology may provide a preoperative tissue diagnosis, although inaccurate results may lead to inappropriate surgical treatment. Tru-cut or core biopsy is contraindicated in the evaluation of parotid neoplasms due to the risk of tumor seeding or injury to the uninvolved portion of the facial nerve. Parotidectomy with biopsy and permanent (not frozen-section) histology is the most accurate means of making the correct diagnosis.

■ Differential Diagnosis

Infectious, inflammatory, or granulomatous disorders rarely cause extratemporal facial paralysis. Likewise, it is extremely unusual for benign parotid neoplasms to paralyze the facial nerve. Facial neuromas may originate in the parotid region or may extend into the parotid gland as a part of a temporal bone primary neoplasm. Constriction of

the nerve at the stylomastoid foramen may cause partial or complete facial weakness that is gradual in onset.

A variety of salivary gland malignancies can cause facial paralysis including, but not limited to, adenoid cystic carcinoma, mucoepidermoid carcinoma, squamous cell carcinoma, adenocarcinoma, and carcinoma ex-pleomorphic adenoma.

Scalp and facial skin cancers that can invade the facial nerve include squamous cell carcinoma, melanoma, and basal cell carcinoma. Any malignant skin lesion can penetrate deep enough to invade peripheral branches of the facial nerve.

A summary of extratemporal neoplastic lesions that may cause facial paralysis is provided in **Table 15.1**.

■ Management Options

The standard treatment for tumors confined to the parotid gland that cause facial paralysis is a parotidectomy followed by radiation therapy if the neoplasm is malignant.[11] Facial reanimation is planned according to the extent of the surgical resection, and cervical lymphadenectomy is performed in patients with high-grade malignancies or clinically palpable neck metastases. Chemotherapy is generally reserved for patients with distant metastatic spread or those who have recurrent disease despite surgical resection with or without radiotherapy.[12]

Surgical Technique

A standard preauricular incision with a slight posterior curve over the mastoid tip is extended into a cervical neck

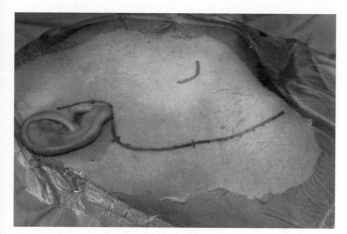

Fig. 15.3 Standard parotid incision (modified Blair) that can be utilized for transmastoid facial nerve dissection in patients presenting with facial paralysis.

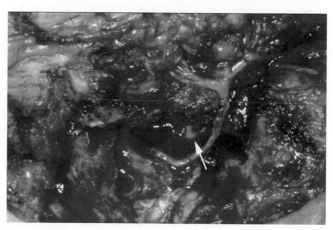

Fig. 15.4 Sural nerve interposition facial nerve grafting following malignant parotid tumor resection (*arrow*).

crease; at least two fingerwidths below the mandible is utilized for patients with tumors confined to the parotid gland (**Fig. 15.3**). A parotidectomy is performed and, if possible, the uninvolved division or branches of the facial nerve are preserved. If the facial nerve is invaded at the stylomastoid foramen, the soft tissues are back-elevated, and a simple mastoidectomy is performed. The vertical segment of the nerve is uncovered, the nerve is transsected, and a frozen section analysis is obtained to confirm a tumor-free margin. Cervical lymphadenectomy is then performed according to the tumor histology or the presence of palpable neck disease.

A postauricular incision with transsection of the external auditory meatus is employed in patients with temporal bone or temporomandibular joint involvement.[13] Following a subtotal petrosectomy, the facial nerve may be transsected as proximal as the perigeniculate region. The mandibular condylar head or the entire glenoid fossa may also be resected through this approach. The jugular bulb and petrous carotid artery are identified prior to the resection of deep lobe parotid tumors with infratemporal involvement, and the mandibular and maxillary divisions of the trigeminal nerve can be resected along the middle cranial fossa floor in patients with clinical evidence of perineural spread in this area.[14]

Facial Nerve Management

Single, peripheral branch resection requires no repair as anastamotic branches, in time, provide acceptable facial movement. Interposition cable grafting with the sural nerve is used to repair the main trunk of the facial nerve if a negative tumor margin is obtained proximally and peripherally, and if the facial musculature was not resected (**Fig. 15.4**). Cross-facial grafting may be used to reanimate the lower division on the paralyzed side in conjunction with static procedures to assist in eye closure. Likewise,

this technique is only employed in patients with preserved muscles of animation.[15]

Extensive defects following radical parotidectomy, facial musculature resection, and subtotal petrosectomy are best reconstructed with microvascular free-tissue transfer.[16] While the rectus abdominus muscle requires no intraoperative change in patient positioning and can easily fill the operative defect, the serratus muscle can serve a dual purpose of lower facial reanimation and defect reconstruction. Occuloplastic techniques are then used to provide upper facial symmetry at rest and to assist in eye closure.

Radiation Therapy

Postoperative radiotherapy has been shown to improve local control as well as long-term survival in patients with malignant parotid tumors.[17] The initial treatment plan must include the ipsilateral neck as well as the proximal skull base.

Additional stereotactic radiation may be considered for patients with perineural spread along the facial nerve at the geniculate ganglion or the trigeminal nerve divisions near the gasserian ganglion or cavernous sinus.

■ Results

Facial nerve paralysis due to extratemporal invasion by malignant parotid tumors has been considered a poor prognostic indicator.[18] In a recent review of 26 patients with lateral skull base malignancies and preoperative facial paralysis, our 1-year and 3-year overall tumor-free survival rates were 76% and 35%, respectively.[19] The goal of any cancer surgery must be to achieve a tumor-free margin, including, if necessary, the resection of the facial nerve.

■ Conclusion

Extratemporal causes for facial nerve paralysis most often are due to neoplasms of the parotid gland or the temporal bone. The clinical signs and symptoms should not be mistaken for the classic, acute presentation of Bell palsy. The appropriate radiographic assessment will guide in the treatment planning in an effort to optimize the best possible long-term results.

Acknowledgment
The authors of this chapter thank Renee Milani for her help in the preparation and critique of their manuscript.

References
1. Gantz BJ, Rubinstein JT, Gidley P, Woodworth GG. Surgical management of Bell's palsy. Laryngoscope 1999;109(8):1177–1188
2. Eneroth CM. Facial nerve paralysis. A criterion of malignancy in parotid tumors. Arch Otolaryngol 1972;95(4):300–304
3. Marzo SJ, Leonetti JP, Petruzzelli G. Facial paralysis caused by malignant skull base neoplasms. Neurosurg Focus 2002;12(5):e2
4. Woods JE. The facial nerve in parotid malignancy. Am J Surg 1983;146(4):493–496
5. Matsuba HM, Thawley SE, Simpson JR, Levine LA, Mauney M. Adenoid cystic carcinoma of major and minor salivary gland origin. Laryngoscope 1984;94(10):1316–1318
6. Magnano M, gervasio CF, Cravero L, et al. Treatment of malignant neoplasms of the parotid gland. Otolaryngol Head Neck Surg 1999;121(5):627–632
7. Leonetti JP, Smith PG, Kletzker GR, Izquierdo R. Invasion patterns of advanced temporal bone malignancies. Am J Otol 1996;17(3):438–442
8. Schwaber MK, Zealear D, Netterville JL, Seshul M, Ossoff RH. The use of magnetic resonance imaging with high-resolution CT in the evaluation of facial paralysis. Otolaryngol Head Neck Surg 1989;101(4):449–458
9. Freling NJM, Molenaar WM, Vermey A, et al; Clinical Use of MRI and Histologic Correlation. Malignant parotid tumors: clinical use of MR imaging and histologic correlation. Radiology 1992;185(3):691–696
10. Horowitz SW, Leonetti JP, Azar-Kia B, Fine M, Izquierdo RCT. CT and MR of temporal bone malignancies primary and secondary to parotid carcinoma. AJNR Am J Neuroradiol 1994;15(4):755–762
11. Pedersen D, Overgaard J, Søgaard H, Elbrønd O, Overgaard M. Malignant parotid tumors in 110 consecutive patients: treatment results and prognosis. Laryngoscope 1992;102(9):1064–1069
12. Carrillo JF, Vázquez R, Ramírez-Ortega MC, Cano A, Ochoa-Carrillo FJ, Oñate-Ocaña LF. Multivariate prediction of the probability of recurrence in patients with carcinoma of the parotid gland. Cancer 2007;109(10):2043–2051
13. Leonetti JP, Smith PG, Anand VK, Kletzker GR, Hartman JM. Subtotal petrosectomy in the management of advanced parotid neoplasms. Otolaryngol Head Neck Surg 1993;108(3):270–276
14. Fisch U, Fagan P, Valavanis A. The infratemporal fossa approach for the lateral skull base. Otolaryngol Clin North Am 1984;17(3):513–552
15. O'Brien CJ, Adams JR. Surgical Management of the Facial Nerve in the Presence of Malignancies about the Face. Curr Opin Otolaryngol Head Neck Surg 2001;9(2):90–94
16. Izquierdo R, Leonetti JP, Origitano TC, al-Mefty O, Anderson DE, Reichman OH. Refinements using free-tissue transfer for complex cranial base reconstruction. Plast Reconstr Surg 1993;92(4):567–574, discussion 575
17. Paulino AC, Marks JE, Leonetti JP. Postoperative irradiation of patients with malignant tumors of skull base. Laryngoscope 1996;106(7):880–883
18. Hocwald E, Korkmaz H, Yoo GH, et al. Prognostic factors in major salivary gland cancer. Laryngoscope 2001;111(8):1434–1439
19. Mantravadi AV, Marzo SJ, Leonetti JP, Fargo KN, Carter MS. Lateral temporal bone and parotid malignancy with facial nerve involvement. Otolaryngol Head Neck Surg 2011;144(3):395–401

16 Central Causes of Facial Paralysis

J. Gail Neely

Central facial paralysis classically presents unilaterally, contralateral to the central lesion, as (1) paresis of the lower face, with sparing of the upper face; (2) volitional paralysis, but sparing of nonvolitional spontaneous or emotional movements; and (3) usually of short duration. The basis for this classic presentation is that the majority of central facial paralyses are due to stroke in the distribution of the middle cerebral artery.[1] However, lesions in the distribution of the anterior cerebral artery or other diffuse or localized lesions may result in very different presentations of facial paralysis. Detailed knowledge of the neuroanatomy influencing facial movement is fundamental to understanding central facial paralysis.

■ Neuroanatomy

There are two distinct control mechanisms of facial motion: for voluntary movements and for involuntary and emotional movements. The older literature referred to these mechanisms as pyramidal system for voluntary movements and extrapyramidal system for involuntary movements.[2] Pyramidal pathway is a monosynaptic projection of motor neurons to the facial nucleus.[3,4] Conversely, polysynaptic "extrapyramidal" pathways via brainstem subcortical nuclei and limbic system (e.g., basal ganglia, thalamus, and limbic system amygdala) complexly interact with the cortical motor centers to influence facial movement. Newer literature focuses upon the cortical motor connections with the facial subnuclei to explain voluntary and involuntary facial expression.[1,5–9]

Cortical Motor Center Connections to Facial Subnuclei and to Facial Muscle Groups

Five cortical areas have direct connections (corticobulbar) to the four facial subnuclei in the pontine tegmentum.[7] These five cortical areas with corticobulbar fibers to the facial subnuclei are primary motor cortex (M1), supplementary motor cortex (M2), rostral cingulate motor cortex (M3), caudal cingulate motor cortex (M4), and ventral lateral premotor cortex (LPMCv). The dorsal lateral premotor cortex, originally thought to have major facial nucleus projects, has not been proven to be primarily important and has been excluded after further studies.[1] All five cortical motor regions connect bilaterally to all facial subnuclei. However, they connect in different ways. Each of the four facial subnuclei selectively innervates different groups of facial muscles (**Figs. 16.1** and **16.2**).[1,7] The strength of

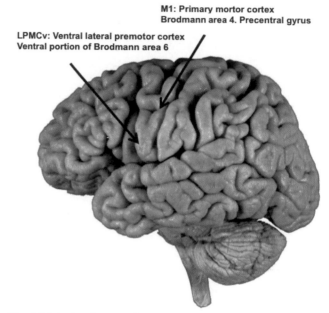

Fig. 16.1 Brain photograph of lateral cortical surface. (Used with permission from Woolsey TA, Hanaway J, Gada MH. The Brain Atlas. A Visual Guide to the Human Central Nervous System. Hoboken, NJ: John Wiley & Sons, Inc; 2008:20.)

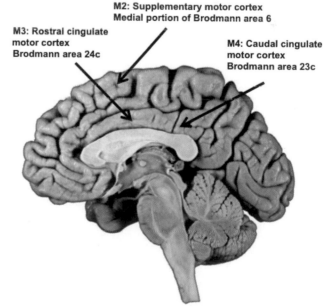

Fig. 16.2 Brain photograph of medial cortical surface. (Used with permission from Woolsey TA, Hanaway J, Gada MH The Brain Atlas. A Visual Guide to the Human Central Nervous System. Hoboken, NJ: John Wiley & Sons, Inc; 2008:24.)

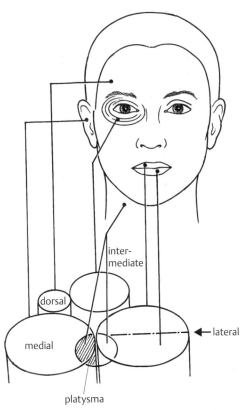

Fig. 16.3 Artist's illustration of facial subnuclei and facial muscles supplied.

corticonuclear projections are, in order, M1 and LPMCv, M2, M3, and M4.

The facial nuclei, the origin of the two facial nerves, are in the pontine tegmentum. Each facial nucleus consists of four subnuclei that are arranged in rostral-caudal columns. Two larger subnuclei are inferior (anterior), the lateral and medial subnuclei; two smaller subnuclei are located superiorly (posterior), the dorsal and intermediate subnuclei. The lateral subnucleus innervates the perioral muscles; neurons on the superior part innervate muscles of the upper lip and neurons in the inferior part muscles of the lower lip. M1, LPMCv, and M4 project predominantly to the contralateral lateral nucleus. Extremely few fibers from M1 go to the upper face. The medial subnucleus innervates auricular muscles (frontalis and platysma in humans). M2 projects bilaterally to the medial subnuclei. The dorsal and intermediate subnuclei innervate the frontalis and orbicularis oculi muscles. M3 projects bilaterally to the dorsal and intermediate subnuclei (**Fig. 16.3**).

Corona Radiata and Internal Capsule

Projection fibers to (corticopetal) and from (corticofugal) the cerebral cortex connect the cortices with subcortical structures. Corticofugal fibers converge from all directions to form a wide fan-shaped white matter structure known

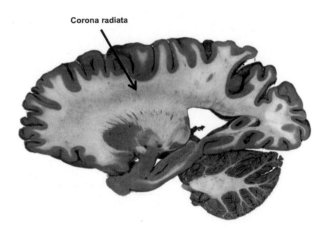

Fig. 16.4 Brain photograph of sagittal brain slice showing corona radiata. (Used with permission from Woolsey TA, Hanaway J, Gada MH. The Brain Atlas. A Visual Guide to the Human Central Nervous System. Hoboken, NJ John Wiley & Sons, Inc; 2008:96.)

as the corona radiata, which becomes the internal capsule and continues toward the brainstem in the cerebral peduncle (**Figs. 16.4** and **16.5**).[4] It is classically thought that the genu of the internal capsule contains most of the corticobulbar fibers that terminate mostly in contralateral-cranial nerve motor nuclei. However, detailed information obtained from nonhuman primates suggests facial representation in the internal capsule is more complexly organized.[6] Axons to superior levels in the brainstem, from the facial motor cortices, occupy the anterior limb, genu, and anterior portion of the posterior limb. These projections are arranged from anterior to posterior in the following order: M3, M2, LPMCv, M4, and M1. Projections from the cortex to the lower brainstem are in the posterior limb of the internal capsule in the same anterior–posterior order (**Fig. 16.6**).

Specific areas of the internal capsule receive blood supply from different striate branches of the middle cerebral artery, anterior cerebral artery, internal carotid artery, and the anterior choroidal artery.[3] Morecraft et al[6] suggested that the differential arrangement of corticofacial fibers in the internal capsule might allow small more anterior capsular lesions to affect small specific facial regions and allow more favorable recovery. However, if the lesion is more posterior in the capsule, the relatively more compact grouping of all these axons could produce greater deficits and be associated with poorer recovery.

Corticobulbar (Corticofacial) Fibers in the Brainstem

The corticobulbar tracts and the corticospinal tracts in the brainstem are easier to understand by briefly reviewing the brain segments in order from most superior (rostral) to inferior (caudal). The prosencephalon (forebrain consisting of the two cerebral hemispheres) is divided into telencephalon, which includes the cortex and basal

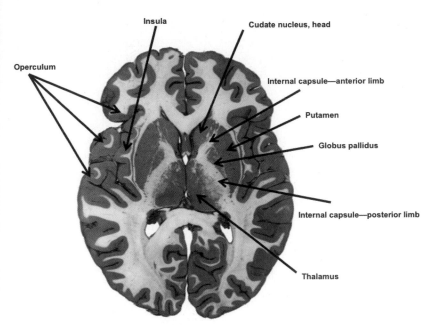

Fig. 16.5 Brain photograph of axial brain slice showing opercular cortices and internal capsule in relationship with basal ganglia. (Used with permission from Woolsey TA, Hanaway J, Gada MH. The Brain Atlas. A Visual Guide to the Human Central Nervous System. Hoboken, NJ: John Wiley & Sons, Inc; 2008:122.)

ganglia and corona radiata, and the diencephalon, which principally contains the thalamus, epithamalus, and hypothalamus, and the internal capsule. Internal capsule fibers converge to flank the midbrain as cerebral peduncles (**Fig. 16.7**). The mesencephalon (midbrain), capped by the quadrageminal plate (colliculi), the shortest segment of the brain, contains the red nucleus, substantia nigra, and connects the forebrain with the rhombencephalon (hindbrain). As the corticobulbar fibers exit the internal capsule into the cerebral peduncles, the fibers then form

two protrusions (peduncles) on the ventral surface of the midbrain that includes the crus cerebri (the mesial aspect of the peduncles) (**Fig. 16.8**). The end of the brainstem is the rhombencephalon (hindbrain), which is divided into two parts: the pons and medulla oblongata. As corticobulbar fibers exit the crus cerebri to enter the pons, they are separated into fascicles by the transverse pontocerebellar fibers.[4]

A more detailed analysis of the corticofacial fibers within the pons and medulla shows three pathways to the facial nucleus[10]:

(1) Most of the corticofacial fibers course through the ventromedial pontine base to cross midline at the

Fig. 16.6 Artist's illustration of change in location of corticobulbar fiber projections from the anterior limb to the posterior limb of the internal capsule as observed at higher and lower levels of the brainstem. GPL, globus pallidus lateral (external); GPM, globus pallidus medial (internal); LPMCv, ventral lateral premotor cortex; M1, primary motor cortex; M2, supplementary motor cortex; M3, rostral cingulate motor cortex; M4, caudal cingulate motor cortex.

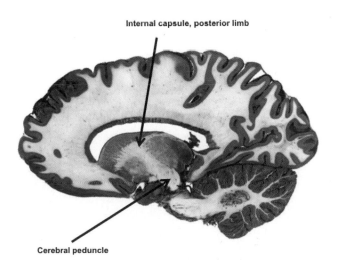

Fig. 16.7 Brain photograph of sagittal brain slice showing a cerebral peduncle. (Used with permission from Woolsey TA, Hanaway J, Gada MH. The Brain Atlas. A Visual Guide to the Human Central Nervous System. Hoboken, NJ: John Wiley & Sons, Inc; 2008:98.)

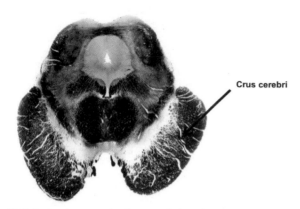

Crus cerebri

Fig. 16.8 Brain photograph of an axial slice through the midbrain showing the crus cerebri. (Used with permission from Woolsey TA, Hanaway J, Gada MH. The Brain Atlas. A Visual Guide to the Human Central Nervous System. Hoboken, NJ: John Wiley & Sons, Inc; 2008:140.)

level of the facial nucleus to innervate the contralateral facial nucleus.

(2) However, in some individuals, the corticofacial fibers course along the dorsal edge of the base of the pons in an "aberrant bundle" then cross midline at the level of the facial nucleus to innervate the contralateral facial nucleus.

(3) And in others, the corticofacial fibers loop down into the ventral part of the upper medulla, cross the midline, and ascend in the dorsolateral medullary region to reach the contralateral facial nucleus.[11]

Involuntary and Emotional Facial Expressions

Involuntary and emotional facial expressions result from a complex multisynaptic control mechanism involving the thalamus, basal ganglia, limbic system, and the motor cortices on the medial side of the cerebral hemisphere, especially the cingulate gyrus.[3,4] The thalamus has reciprocal projections to and from most of the cerebral cortex and is the major route for subcortical to cortical communication. The basal ganglia (caudate nucleus, putamen, globus pallidus, and amygdala) modulate movement and motivational aspects of behavior. The principal input to the basal ganglia from the rest of the brain is via the caudate nucleus and putamen, which projects in part to the globus pallidus and substantial nigra. The globus pallidus is the main output system to the thalamus. Disorders of this system include reduced movement with hypertonia (like Parkinson disease) or abnormal involuntary movements (dyskinesias). The amygdala is integrally associated with the basal ganglia and with the limbic (ring or border) system, which forms a ring around the thalamus and basal ganglia. The limbic system integrates external and internal sensory information, and links cortical sensory association areas and subcortical autonomic and endocrine areas

with the emotion expressive motor systems. It also has a role in memory, food intake, arousal, sexual behavior, and motivation.

These structures modulate facial expressions in the following ways.[5,8,9,12] The amygdala integrates sensory information and generates emotional responses such as rage. The emotional information is sent to higher cortical levels for memory and learning, and to subcortical levels of the hypothalamus and brainstem for autonomic, hormonal, and behavioral responses to the emotional information. This information is then sent to the rostral cigulate motor cortex (M3), which projects bilaterally to the dorsal and intermediate facial subnuclei, which innervate the upper face, especially the frontalis and orbicularis oculi. Thus, the amygdala-cingulate cortex facial nucleus system is involved in emotional expression, emotional maturation, and social adaptation.[9] Additionally, the amygdala sends emotional information to M4, which supplies the contralateral lower face. In summary, M3 and M4 are critical targets for motor expression from the limbic system in the role of emotion, attention, and cognition.[7,8] Pathology in this pathway may cause emotional paralysis of the face while maintaining normal volitional control; this is the opposite of classical central facial paralysis.

Intrapontine Course of the Facial Nerve

The pons is composed of two parts: the tegmentum and the base. The large middle cerebellar peduncles grossly demarcate the two parts: the tegmentum is the largely gray matter portion dorsally (posteriorly) and the base largely white matter protrudes ventrally (anteriorly). The ventral or base of the pons contains the multiple pontine nuclei projecting to the cerebellar cortex through which are dispersed the fascicles of the corticobulbar and corticospinal tracts. The facial nucleus lies in the lateral inferior pontine tegmentum. The facial nerve exiting the nucleus ascends to loop medially and anteriorly around the abducens nucleus close to the medial longitudinal fasciculus just lateral to the midline. As the facial nerve goes superior to the abducens nucleus, it bulges into the floor of the fourth ventricle as the facial colliculus. As it begins to pass the abducens nucleus, it curves rostrally and then descends in an inferolateral–caudal path to exit at the pontomedulary junction, superior to the pontine base (**Fig. 16.9**).[4]

Opercular Cortices and Insula

The insula is part of the deep lateral cerebral cortex, involved with taste, smell, and other somatosensory functions; portions of the frontal, frontoparietal, and temporal lobes, known as the opercula, cover it (see **Fig. 16.5**).[4] A unique syndrome involving the opercula is addressed in the following.

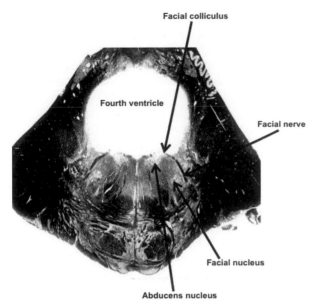

Facial colliculus

Fourth ventricle

Facial nerve

Facial nucleus

Abducens nucleus

Fig. 16.9 Brain photograph of an axial slice through the pons showing the facial and abducens nucleus in the tegmen and the descending postnuclear facial nerve transversing the base of the pons. (Used with permission from Woolsey TA, Hanaway J, Gada MH. The Brain Atlas. A Visual Guide to the Human Central Nervous System. Hoboken, NJ: John Wiley & Sons, Inc; 2008:143.)

■ Pathologic Lesions Causing Central Facial Paralysis

Symptoms and signs of neurologically associated lesions with central facial palsy help localize the lesion to the central neural axis level and side. The neuroanatomy of the central facial pathways begin broadly at the cortices and converge as they progress inferiorly. The more inferior the lesion, the closer the nuclei and tracts are arranged. Conversely, the vascular supply of the cortices cover a wide area, whereas the vascular supply of the deeper brain centers tend to be much more localized. Metastatic lesions tend to be focally limited and symptoms may range from none to extensive, dependent on the site of lesion (**Table 16.1**).

Opercular Cortex Lesions (Foix-Chavany-Marie Syndrome)

Foix, Chavany, and Marie first described a syndrome in which a sudden loss of bilateral voluntary motor control of muscles mediated by cranial nerves V, VII, IX, X, and XII occurs but nonvoluntary automatic functions of these muscles are left intact.[13] The patient cannot chew or speak, or voluntarily move either side of the face, but can laugh, cry, yawn, and swallow when food is far enough posterior in the mouth to elicit the swallowing reflex.[14] Even though this is a central origin facial paralysis, with the characteristic disassociation of voluntary and involuntary movements, it often can involve the upper face as well as the lower face like a peripheral facial paralysis. Occasionally, it can involve only one side of the face and may be confused with Bell palsy.[15]

The pathophysiology of this syndrome is the bilateral dysfunction of the opercular cortices. Five etiological categories have been described: (1) the most common and classical is that associated with bilateral strokes, (2) a subacute type from central nervous system infections, (3) a congenital developmental type,[16] (4) a reversible syndrome seen in children with epilepsy, and (5) a rare neurodegenerative type.[14]

Table 16.1 Site of lesion and associated dysfunction

Site of Lesion	Central Facial Paralysis
Lateral cerebral cortex (middle cerebral artery)[1,35]	Contralateral, lower face, volitional
Associated dysfunctions: Contralateral sensory loss and paralysis of face, arm, leg; speech and language disorder; vision and conjugate disorder	
Medial cerebral cortex (anterior cerebral artery)[1,35]	Bilateral (somewhat more contralateral), upper and lower face, emotional "blunted facial expressions"
Associated dysfunctions: Contralateral foot and leg paralysis and sensory loss; urinary incontinence; contralateral grasp and suckling reflex; mental impairment	
Midbrain and pontomesencephalic junction (central portion of cerebral peduncles)[10]	Contralateral, lower face, volitional
Base of pons (at upper and midlevel of pons, lesions are at center of pontine base; at lower level of pons, lesions are ventromedial of pontine base close to midline)[10]	Contralateral, lower face, volitional
Associated dysfunctions: Six clinical syndromes determined by degree of dysfunction and site of lesion.[36] In general: facial movement and articulation (rostral and medial basilar pons); hand coordination (rostral and mid-pons, medial and ventral); arm function (ventral and lateral to hand); leg coordination (caudal half of pons, laterally); swallowing (many regions of rostral pons); gait (medial and lateral throughout rostral to caudal); higher order dysfunctions: motor neglect, paraphasic errors, and pathological laughter (rostral and medial pons).	
Upper level medulla (medial ventral)[10,17]	Contralateral, lower face, volitional
Upper level medulla (lateral medulla)[10]	Ipsilateral, lower face, volitional
Associated dysfunctions: rotary nystagmus and vertigo with vomiting; dysphagia; unsteady gait; hoarse speech; Horner syndrome	

Brainstem Vascular Lesions Comparative Frequencies

Pontine lesions are the most frequent of the vascular ischemic infarctions of the brainstem. Only slightly more than half of these lesions present with central facial paralysis. Urban et al,[10] in studying 53 patients with local ischemic brainstem lesions, found 28 with and 25 without central facial paralysis. Site of lesion frequencies with facial paralysis were pons (17/28), medulla oblongata (5/28), pontomedullary (3/28), midbrain (2/28), and pontomesencephalic junction (1/28).[10] Facial paralysis is characteristically contralateral to the lesion, in the lower face, and affecting voluntary movement and not emotional expressions.

Midbrain Lesions

Vascular ischemic lesions in the midbrain (mesencephalon) and pontomesencephalic region are rare. When they do occur and create a central facial paralysis, they mainly occur in the central portion of the midbrain and the midbrain-pons junction and affect the cerebral peduncles.[10]

Pontine Lesions

Common vascular ischemic lesions in the pons occur in the upper and middle pons, and spread across the center of the pontine base. Lower pontine lesions shift inferomedially close to the midline.[10]

Medullar Lesions

Superior medullary lesions may result in a central facial paralysis, characterized by lower face paralysis with sparing of the upper face. Upper medullary lesions may cause the usual contralateral voluntary lower facial paralysis[10]; however, some may occur ipsilateral to the lesion, presumably by affecting the medullary loop of the corticofacial fibers after they cross the midline. If the lesion is extends slightly more rostrally into the lowest pontine tegmentum, it may affect not only the ascending loop fibers, but the lowest, most inferior (caudal) subnucleus supplying the lower face only and thus present as a confusion of upper motor and lower motor neuron lesion.[17]

Congenital Facial Paralyses

Infants with facial paralysis at birth are classified into those with birth trauma and those with congenital lesions. There is growing evidence that the congenital group, with or without syndromes known to be associated with facial paralysis, have abnormal facial nuclei.[18,19] Syndromes associated with facial paralysis are Möbius syndrome, Goldenhar syndrome, and Poland syndrome. Möbius syndrome may be classified into four categories: Group 1, small or

absent brainstem nuclei for cranial nerves VI, VII, and III, V, VIII, IX, XI, and XII at times; Group 2, degeneration of neurons in the peripheral facial nerve; Group 3, degeneration of neurons and other brain cells, and hardened tissue in brainstem nuclei; and Group 4, muscular dysfunction without lesions in cranial nerves.[20] Goldenhar syndrome encompasses a wide spectrum of abnormalities of the first and second brachial arches, including preauricular tags, microtia, unilateral maxillary and mandibular hypoplasia, epibulbar dermoids, and vertebral abnormalities. Perhaps a third of the cases are associated with facial paralysis of a peripheral type.[21] Because of the obvious cranial abnormalities, it has been tempting to ascribe the facial paralysis to the lower motor nerve per se rather than the more probable nuclear abnormality. Poland syndrome consists of unilateral absence of the pectoralis muscles, upper limb defects, and less commonly a congenital facial paralysis.[18]

Multiple Sclerosis

There are many demyelinating diseases; we consider only the most common one in this chapter. Multiple sclerosis (MS) is a central nervous system demyelinating autoimmune disease, occurring initially between 20 and 40 years of age. Initial symptoms include diplopia, red-green abnormalities or blurred vision, which may progress erratically to a variety of sensory and/or motor dysfunctions, dizziness, instability, and cognitive disorders.[22] No single symptom, sign, or laboratory test clearly confirms the diagnosis of multiple sclerosis; however, oligoclonal bands and elevated immunoglobulin G seen in cerebrospinal fluid is supportive of the diagnosis. Basic criteria required for the diagnosis are (1) two or more central nervous system areas (brain, spinal cord, and/or optic nerves) of dysfunction, (2) dysfunctions occurring at least 1 month apart, and (3) all other possible etiologies ruled out.[23] Magnetic resonance imaging of the head and/or spine is sensitive to detect and localize MS; criteria are described in the 2005 Revised McDonald Criteria.[24,25] Lesions may occur anywhere within the central nervous system; however, they are most common in the optic nerve, spinal cord, brainstem, and periventricular areas. Demyelization is the predominant pathology; however, axon loss, initially involving transport deficiencies, is also seen abundantly in lesions. Recently, it has been discovered that large areas of subpial cortical gray matter and spinal gray matter may be involved. Early lesions tend to show inflammation and demyelization and late lesions seem to be predominantly neurodegenerative, suggesting two separate pathologic mechanisms.[26]

Facial nerve involvement may occur during the clinical course of MS in as many as 52% of autopsy proven cases[27] or in ~20% of cases at some point in time during the clinical course over a little more than 4 years.[28] In the majority of cases, multiple neurological signs and symptoms occur concomitantly. However, isolated cranial nerve dysfunction may occur as the initial presenting symptom or as a symptom of relapse in ~10% of the cases; most of these cases involve the fifth or seventh cranial nerves, with very few involving the third, sixth, or eighth nerves.[29] Isolated facial nerve dysfunction of a lower motor neuron type may occur in ~5% of MS cases and precede the next MS symptom by 0.5 to 3 years, making it difficult to differentiate from Bell palsy.[28] Magnetic resonance imaging predominantly shows a lesion in the ipsilateral pontine tegmentum in the region of the facial nucleus[28]; however, occasionally a lesion may occur at the root exit zone along the intramedullary course of the facial nerve.[30,31] Interestingly, the course of facial paralysis may resolve in a few days and responds to steroids. One paper also revealed a complete normal recovery of a profound ipsilateral deafness within 1 week.[30] Another paper described a sequential bilateral hearing loss with facial paralysis on one side. The hearing loss returned spontaneously to normal on the first side within 2 months.[32] These two papers illustrate that spontaneous recovery to normal need not be a cause for celebration, but a "red flag" suggesting further study.

Guillain-Barré Syndrome

Guillain-Barré syndrome is an autoimmune peripheral nervous system disease that is rapidly progressive over hours or a few weeks, with greatest weakness within the first 2 weeks. It is not a central nervous system disease and is mentioned here only to emphasize that and to briefly review the disorder.[33] The first symptoms usually begin in the legs with paresthesias and weakness, and progress centrally, ultimately resulting in complete motor paralysis of the whole body and requiring mechanical ventilation in some. There is no known cure; however, spontaneous recovery to normal or almost normal with some residual is usual. Plasmapheresis and/or immune globulins help. Bilateral simultaneous or rapidly sequential lower motor neuron facial paralysis, like Bell palsy, may be the presenting symptom.[34]

■ Conclusion

Five cerebral motor cortices, two lateral and three medial, project somatotopically along corticobulbar tracts to converge upon all of the four facial subnuclei bilaterally. Each of the subnuclei project to specific facial muscles. Voluntary facial movements predominantly follow the major corticobulbar pathways, whereas emotional and involuntary facial expressions are mediated by the medially located cingulated motor cortices in connection with the limbic system amygdala. These anatomical arrangements explain the differential facial motor abnormalities seen in central facial paralyses.

Central facial paralyses, commonly involving the lateral cortices or their pathways, usually exhibit lower facial paralysis, with sparing of the upper face and emotional and involuntary expressions. However, lesions of the medial cortices and/or limbic connections may demonstrate the exact opposite pattern of emotional expression paralysis and normal voluntary movements. Associated signs and symptoms help localize the lesion within the central nervous system.

Acknowledgment
The author thanks Thomas A. Woolsey, MD, and Joseph T. Black, MD, for their intellectual input and review of the draft chapter.

References

1. Morecraft RJ, Stilwell-Morecraft KS, Rossing WR. The motor cortex and facial expression: new insights from neuroscience. Neurologist 2004;10(5):235–249
2. Van Gelder RS, Van Gelder L. Facial expression and speech: neuroanatomical considerations. Int J Psychol 1990;25(2):141–155
3. Afifi AK, Bergman RA. Functional neuroanatomy, 2nd ed. New York: Lange Medical Books/McGraw-Hill; 2005: 168
4. Standring S. Gray's Anatomy. The anatomical basis of clinical practice, 40th ed. London, UK: Churchill Livingstone: Elsevier; 2008: 223–394
5. Ghashghaei HT, Barbas H. Pathways for emotion: interactions of prefrontal and anterior temporal pathways in the amygdala of the rhesus monkey. Neuroscience 2002;115(4):1261–1279
6. Morecraft R, Louie J, Herrick J, et al. Organization of face representation in the internal capsule of the rhesus monkey. Neuroscience 2001;27:825–827
7. Morecraft RJ, Louie JL, Herrick JL, Stilwell-Morecraft KS. Cortical innervation of the facial nucleus in the non-human primate: a new interpretation of the effects of stroke and related subtotal brain trauma on the muscles of facial expression. Brain 2001;124(Pt 1):176–208
8. Morecraft RJ, McNeal DW, Stilwell-Morecraft KS, et al. Amygdala interconnections with the cingulate motor cortex in the rhesus monkey. J Comp Neurol 2007;500(1):134–165
9. Yuasa S. [Somatotopy in the emotional exression by the amygdala]–article in Japanese. Brain Nerve 2009;61:1395–1404
10. Urban PP, Wicht S, Vucorevic G, et al. The course of corticofacial projections in the human brainstem. Brain 2001;124(Pt 9):1 866–1876
11. Cavazos JE, Bulsara K, Caress J, Osumi A, Glass JP. Pure motor hemiplegia including the face induced by an infarct of the medullary pyramid. Clin Neurol Neurosurg 1996;98(1):21–23
12. Holstege G. Emotional innervation of facial musculature. Mov Disord 2002;17:S12–S16
13. Foix C, Chavany J, Marie J. Diplegie facio-linguo-masticatrice d'origine cortico souscorticale sans paralysie des membres. Rev Neurol (Paris) 1926;33:214–219
14. Weller M. Anterior opercular cortex lesions cause dissociated lower cranial nerve palsies and anarthria but no aphasia: Foix-Chavany-Marie syndrome and "automatic voluntary dissociation" revisited. J Neurol 1993;240(4):199–208
15. Crumley RL. The opercular syndrome—diagnostic trap in facial paralysis. Laryngoscope 1979;89(3):361–365

16. Nisipeanu P, Rieder I, Blumen S, Korczyn AD. Pure congenital Foix-Chavany-Marie syndrome. Dev Med Child Neurol 1997;39(10):696–698

17. Urban PP, Wicht S, Fitzek S, et al. Ipsilateral facial weakness in upper medullary infarction-supranuclear or infranuclear origin? J Neurol 1999;246(9):798–801

18. Jemec B, Grobbelaar AO, Harrison DH. The abnormal nucleus as a cause of congenital facial palsy. Arch Dis Child 2000;83(3):256–258

19. Verzijl HT, van der Zwaag B, Lammens M, ten Donkelaar HJ, Padberg GW. The neuropathology of hereditary congenital facial palsy vs Möbius syndrome. Neurology 2005;64(4):649–653

20. Office of Communications and Public Liaison. NINDS Moebius syndrome information page. Bethesda, MD: National Institute of Neurological Disorders and Stroke; 2008

21. Berker N, Acaroğlu G, Soykan E. Goldenhar's Syndrome (oculo-auriculo-vertebral dysplasia) with congenital facial nerve palsy. Yonsei Med J 2004;45(1):157–160

22. Office of Communications and Public Liaison. NINDS Multiple Sclerosis information page. Bethesda, MD: NIH-National Institute of Neurological Disorders and Stroke/Disorders; 2010: 1–4

23. National multiple sclerosis society. The criteria for a diagnosis of MS. 2010. Available at http://www.nationalmssociety.org/about-multiple-sclerosis/what-we-know-about-ms/diagnosing-ms/index.aspx

24. Fox RJ, Sweeney P. Multiple Sclerosis. In: Disease management project. Cleveland, OH: The Cleveland Clinic Center for Continuing Education; 2009: 1–13

25. Polman CH, Reingold SC, Edan G, et al; International Panel on MS Diagnosis. Diagnostic criteria for multiple sclerosis: 2005 revisions to the "McDonald Criteria". Ann Neurol 2005;58(6):840–846

26. Stadelmann C, Wegner C, Brück W. Inflammation, demyelination, and degeneration - recent insights from MS pathology. Biochim Biophys Acta 2011;1812(2):275–282

27. Carter S, Sciarra D, Merritt HH. The course of multiple sclerosis as determined by autopsy proven cases. Res Publ Assoc Res Nerv Ment Dis 1950;28:471–511

28. Fukazawa T, Moriwaka F, Hamada K, Hamada T, Tashiro K. Facial palsy in multiple sclerosis. J Neurol 1997;244(10):631–633

29. Zadro I, Barun B, Habek M, Brinar VV. Isolated cranial nerve palsies in multiple sclerosis. Clin Neurol Neurosurg 2008;110(9):886–888

30. Commins DJ, Chen JM. Multiple sclerosis: a consideration in acute cranial nerve palsies. Am J Otol 1997;18(5):590–595

31. Schnorpfeil F, Braune HJ. Nuclear facial palsy in multiple sclerosis: a case report. Electromyogr Clin Neurophysiol 1997;37(4):207–211

32. Oh Y-M, Oh D-H, Jeong S-H, Koo JW, Kim JS. Sequential bilateral hearing loss in multiple sclerosis. Ann Otol Rhinol Laryngol 2008;117(3):186–191

33. Office of Communications and Public Liaison. NINDS Guillain-Barre Syndrome Information Page. Bethesda, MD: National Institute of Neurological Disorders and Stroke; 2010

34. Narayanan RP, James N, Ramachandran K, Jaramillo MJ. Guillain-Barré Syndrome presenting with bilateral facial nerve paralysis: a case report. Cases J 2008;1(1):379

35. Adams RD, Victor M, Ropper AH. Principles of Neurology, 6 ed. St. Louis: McGraw Hill; 1997: 777–873

36. Schmahmann JD, Ko R, MacMore J. The human basis pontis: motor syndromes and topographic organization. Brain 2004;127(Pt 6):1269–1291

17 Hemifacial Spasm

Jacques Magnan and Claire-Lise Curto Faïs

Hemifacial spasm is characterized by the occurrence of unilateral, involuntary, sudden, and isolated spasms of one side of the face. It is rare, affecting 1 to 15 per 100,000 inhabitants depending on the series. There is no statistical difference for the side affected. Most series tend to show a female predominance. Long unrecognized, hemifacial spasm, like any face movement disorder, has a very important impact on patients' social and professional relationships that must not be overlooked during their medical care. For many years, the etiology was considered idiopathic, it is now accepted that the cause of hemifacial spasm is neurovascular compression between a vascular loop and the root exit zone of the facial nerve in the cerebellopontine angle.

■ Pathophysiology

There are two major theories regarding the pathophysiology of hemifacial spasm. "Ephaps" is the ability of two close nervous fibers to let a nerve impulse stimulating one nerve fiber to pass through both nerve fibers. In this theory, the vessel in contact with the nerve induces a chronic compression that leads to focal demyelination through which ephaptic transmissions can occur.

Ephaptic theory[1-3] is based on the following electromyographic data: in a healthy subject, the stimulation of a branch of the facial nerve only induces contractions of motor fibers innerved by this branch, whereas in patients suffering from hemifacial spasm, the same stimulation would induce contractions in the innervated expected muscles and also in other muscle territories not innervated by the particular nerve. This abnormal response is called abnormal muscle response. The spraying of contraction to other facial muscle territories is called lateral spread motor responses (**Fig. 17.1**).

In nuclear theory,[4-8] chronic stimulation of the facial nerve by a vessel induces transmission of a nerve impulse toward peripheral muscle in an orthodromic way and also in an antidromic way, toward facial nerve nucleus, which becomes hyperexcitable. This theory explains the delay that is sometimes seen when the patient becomes cured sometime after the surgical neurovascular decompression.

Nowadays, the best hypothesis involves a combination of the two theories:

- Systolic pulses of the vessel at the site of the compression create ectopic nervous stimulation. This stimulation is due to the compression itself and also to the bioelectrical changes induced by the variations of blood flow in the looped or atheromatous vessel.
- Demyelination progressively occurs and allows ephaptic transmissions.

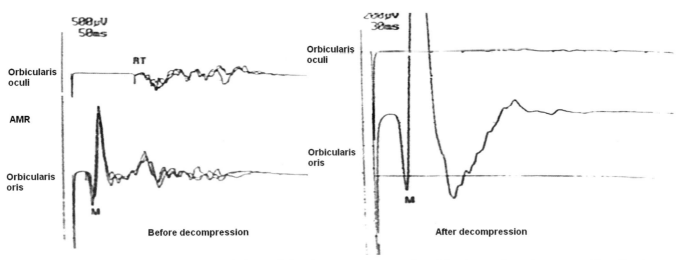

Fig. 17.1 Intraoperative facial monitoring results before and after decompression. Recording of the abnormal muscle response of hemifacial spasm from the orbicularis oculi muscle after stimulation of the inferior branch of the facial nerve. This response has a latency of 10 ms and disappears when the offending vessel is moved off the facial nerve. The intraoperative monitoring of abnormal muscle response represents a reliable test to confirm the adequate vascular decompression procedure.

- Antidromic conduction of the impulse is responsible for the facial nerve nucleus hyperexcitability, which progressively evolves on its own.
- Hyperactivity of the facial nerve explains the occurrence of hemifacial spasms after peripheral stimuli (voluntary or involuntary facial movements) or emotional stimulation via the reticulated formation.

The root entry zone or root exit zone (REZ) corresponds to the emergence of the facial nerve from the pons into the cerebellopontine angle (CPA). It is also called the Obersteiner-Redlich zone. In this zone, intraprotuberential fibers of cranial nerve VII are very superficial, and the nucleus is very close, around 1 mm. Therefore, any compression at this level could affect both the central and peripheral portion of the VII nerve, as well as its nucleus.

Moreover, this zone corresponds to a physiological transition between central nervous sheathing (oligodendrocytes) and peripheral sheathing (Schwann cells). Vascularization is very poor in this area, making the zone very fragile to any insult and representing a kind of Achilles heel along the course of the facial nerve.[9,10]

■ Diagnosis

Hemifacial spasm belongs to class of facial movement disorders. Its diagnosis is based on clinical examination. The muscle contractions observed are:

- Unilateral: The hemiface is wrinkled, the eye is half shut, the corner of the lip is pulled up on the affected side, and the tip of the nose is curved.
- Involuntary: Contractions are uncontrollable. They can occur at night, causing sleep impairment. There is no triggering factor but crisis often occurs in periods of stress, overtiredness, and/or anxiety.
- Sudden: Contractions are tonic or tonicoclonic. Initial blepharospasm is found in 90% of the cases. After a few weeks, months, or years, spasmodic contractions affect all the hemiface muscles, last for a few seconds, and disappear as quickly as it appeared. Crisis begins with clonical contractions rising from orbicularis oculi, and at its height tonical contractions of the hemiface (**Fig. 17.2**). As time progresses, the crises become more frequent and more intense.
- Isolated: There is no motor trouble or movement disorder between crises. There are never permanent contractions, and above all there is no facial weakness.

Hemifacial spasm has deep repercussion on the patient's quality of life, and most patients are anxious about the cosmetic appearance as well as the functional problems associated with uncontrolled spasms. Many patients may seek antianxiety therapies.

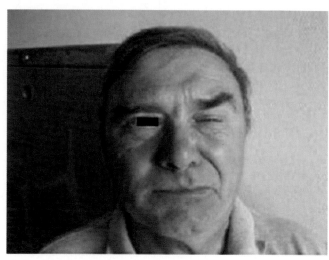

Fig. 17.2 Male, 53 years old, with left hemifacial spasm since 23 years of age.

■ Clinical Forms

- Bilateral spasm: It is rare and is a problem of differential diagnosis.
- Hemifacial spasm associated with trigeminal neuralgia: It is rare and also called painful tic convulsif.

■ Differential Diagnosis

The most common cause of hemifacial spasm is due to vascular compression at the REZ. There are other rare but important causes that can cause symptomatic spasms (1–2%) and a thorough evaluation can reveal:

- Arachnoid cysts
- Vascular lesions: Arnold-Chiari, vertebrobasilar aneurysms, ischemia of the pons
- Tumors: Brainstem or CPA tumors
- Paget disease
- Multiple sclerosis

For postparalytic spasms, a period of facial palsy is found in the patient's background or history. Spasm is then characterized by contracture at rest, clonical contractions at blinking, abnormal voluntary movements with loss of functional synergy, and, above all, facial weakness.

Neuromuscular dystonias are characterized by their central origin and affect both sides of the face. Some etiologies of this type of dystonia include the following:

- Idiopathic blepharospasm leads to complete or partial closure of the eyes.
- Oromandibular dystonia or Meige syndrome corresponds to bilateral blepharospasm associated with periodic contraction of muscles from the lower part of the face.

- Cervical dystonia or spasmodic stiff neck affects the shoulders and neck muscles.
- Convulsive tics affect mainly children and disappear when sleeping or with voluntary control.
- Partial epilepsy.
- Myokymia are most of the time very localized, especially on the orbicularis oris or orbicularis oculi, which tremble or spasm. They can be found in anxious patients, and physicians must look for an etiology such as a metabolic disorder or for multiple sclerosis.

■ Radiological Exploration[11–15,25]

Radiological evaluation of the CPA is based on magnetic resonance imaging (MRI). MRI only can provide analysis of both the nervous and vascular structures. The objectives of imaging are:

- To confirm clinical diagnosis by showing a neurovascular conflict.
- To eliminate other etiologies in the differential diagnosis.
- To identify a precise preoperative vascular lesion for surgical mapping.

Imaging usually begins with a cerebral MRI to eliminate other etiologies in the differential diagnosis and to confirm the diagnosis. The sequences commonly used are as follows:

- T2 high-resolution: This sequence gives a cisternographic view of the CPA, where cerebrospinal fluid appears hyperintense and vessels hypointense, giving an excellent contrast between cerebrospinal fluid and the neurovascular elements (**Fig. 17.3**).

- Three-dimensional T1 with gadolinium: This sequence offers good delineation of nerves and vessels and can identify venous conflicts.
- Magnetic resonance angiography sequences, such as the sequence "time of flight," highlights vascular structures where the intensity depends on the speed of intravascular blood flow. This sequence can demonstrate either arterial signals and/or venous signals.
- Fusion sequences time of flight: T2 high-resolution.

There are three radiological signs of neurovascular compression: (1) a neurovascular contact must be shown at the REZ; (2) the vessel is perpendicular to the nerve; and (3) a deformity of the nerve or the pons is observed.

MRI cannot be interpreted without any data concerning the patient's clinical background, as up to 3% of asymptomatic patients have a neurovascular contact on MRI and 0.5% of asymptomatic patients present with a neural deformity.

■ Therapeutic Care of Hemifacial Spasm

Many patients undergo various medical treatments such as antidepressants, anxiolytics, neuroleptics, etc., but none of these are effective on the spasm itself. There are only two treatments that can really treat the hemifacial spasms.

- Botulinum toxin blocks neuromuscular transmission of the nervous signal and therefore prevents the injected muscles of the face from facial contractions. Botox is commonly used to treat essential blepharospasms. Botox can also be used in selected patients to control the effects of muscle contraction associated with hemifacial spasm. The effects of Botox can be very satisfactory in some patients. However, the effect is nevertheless transitory, lasting from 2 to 4 months depending of the type and the amount of toxin injected. Botox is not a curative

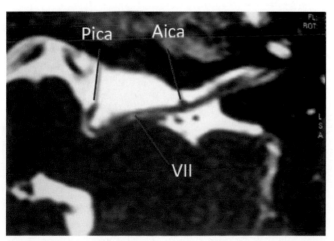
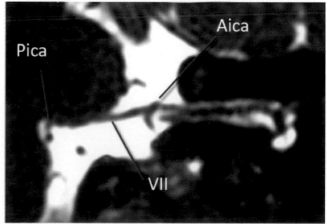

a   b

Fig. 17.3a, b T2 high-resolution magnetic resonance imaging. Conflict involving the posteroinferior cerebellar artery (*Pica*) as the offending vessel: the posteroinferior cerebellar artery is responsible for an orthogonal compression and distortion of the brainstem at the root entry zone. The anteroinferior cerebellar artery (*Aica*) is surrounding the acousticofacial bundle without distortion of the cisternal part of the cranial nerve VII (normal vascular loop).

treatment of hemifacial spasm; it only stops or slows the muscle spasms until the neuromuscular junction repairs itself and normal nerve conduction occurs and the symptoms return. For a more detailed explanation, see Chapter 26.

- Neurovascular decompression: This surgical technique was first described by W.J. Gardner to cure trigeminal neuralgia in 1959. Gardner and Sava applied the same technique to the facial nerve in 1962 to successfully cure hemifacial spasm. The widespread acceptance of this technique was due to Jannetta with the use of operative microscope; he intensively described the microvascular decompression technique.[26] Then the procedure was improved in the 1990s by Magnan with the complementary help of endoscope and the development of the minimally invasive retrosigmoid approach. Surgical decision to perform this procedure is made in cases of persistent and severe hemifacial spasm, immediately or after toxin injections that do not modify surgical prognosis and results.

■ Neurovascular Decompression for Hemifacial Spasm

Hemifacial spasm affects men and women with a discrete predominance for women. The mean age at surgery is 57.2 years (19–84) in our series, which corresponds to other authors' data. Neurovascular decompression can be approached via the retrosigmoid approach, as described by Bremond, Garcin, and Magnan in 1974.[16,17] This technique has the advantage of providing a direct and safe access to the CPA through a protected corridor to reach the acousticofacial nerve bundle and allows easy handling of all the structures crossing the CPA. The surgical access to the CPA is called "key hole surgery" as the craniotomy used is small (≈ 2 cm^2) (**Fig. 17.4**) and no mechanic cerebellar retractor is needed. Hyperventilation is used during anesthesia, lowering the postoperative side effects, particularly hearing impairment.

Under general anesthesia, the patient is installed in supine position, with monitoring of the facial nerve. The

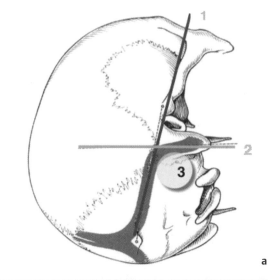

a

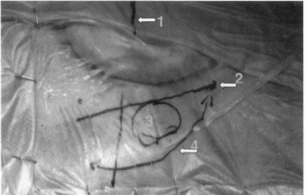

b

Fig. 17.5a, b Surgical landmarks: craniotomy is figured with the circle (3), digastric ridge (2), francfort plane (1), and the curved retroauricular incision (4).

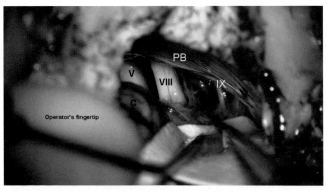

Fig. 17.4 Operative view through a right "keyhole" craniotomy. Note the size of the craniotomy compared with the operator's fingertip. C, cerebellum; PB, petrous bone; V, VIII, IX, cranial nerves.

monitoring of the cochlear nerve can be used, but this does not offer any objective advantages as any change in the auditory brainstem response is delayed from the time of injury, making this testing technique only helpful at the end of surgery to confirm hearing preservation.

The anatomic landmarks of the craniotomy are the posterior edge of the sigmoid sinus (anterior limit), the occipital line that corresponds to the posterior extension of the Frankfurt line (superior limit), and the digastric muscle groove (inferior limit) (**Fig. 17.5**).

After a curvilinear skin incision two fingers behind the pinna, an anterior skin flap and a posterior muscle-periostal flap are elevated to expose the bone of the mastoido-occipital region. The mastoid emissary vein centers the retromastoid craniotomy.

Both profound balanced anesthesia and assisted hyperventilation to reach 25 pCO$_2$ techniques are key to obtain an adequate spontaneous retraction of cerebellum when the dura mater is exposed behind the blue line of the posterior margin of the sigmoid sinus. An anteriorly based dural flap is delineated and elevated, and then the cerebellum is protected using a piece of synthetic dura mater. The surgeon can advance inferiorly into the posterior fossa through a safe corridor with the following boundaries: the posterior wall of the temporal bone anteriorly and the protected cerebellum posteriorly, until reaching and opening the posterior cisterna at the level of the lower cranial nerves. Cerebrospinal fluid escapes, and the cerebellum falls away without any pressure on it.

After opening the CPA by dissecting arachnoid wrapping around cranial nerves with the magnification of the operative microscope, a first endoscopic look of the CPA is made with a 4-mm, 30-degree angled rigid endoscope, which provides a panoramic view of all the components of the CPA and an optimal view of the REZ area without modifying the neurovascular relationships (see **Fig. 17.4**). The endoscope-assisted technique provides a clear and reliable identification of the offending vessel (or multiple offending vessels in 30%) without unnecessary retraction of cerebellum or brainstem.

Microvascular decompression begins by creating an operating field between the auditory nerve superiorly and the dissected glossopharyngeal nerve inferiorly. This starts with gentle elevation of the compressing vascular loop from the REZ of the facial nerve. This maneuver may create a

hyperstimulation of the facial nerve monitor, which should return to normal a few minutes after manipulation. This is good but inconstant data. Offending vessels can be kept away by using surgical glue. The zone of compression on the nerve is protected and isolated from any vascular contact by the use of small pieces of Teflon foam pad (Bard PTFE, Tempe, AZ). The endoscope is again used to assess and control the proper positioning of the Teflon once it has been placed at the target site.

The dura mater is sutured with local adipose tissue and fibrin glue to seal the suture. The bony defect is filled with the harvested bone paté at the drilling. Then musculoaponeurotic and skin flaps are sutured. The patient returns the day of the surgery to their room in the ward whatever the age and is usually discharged after 3 to 7 days.

Different types of vascular compromises can be observed:

- Most of the vascular compromise are observed at the REZ and are due to the posteroinferior cerebellar artery (PICA) and/or vertebral artery because of their anatomic proximity to the facial nerve (**Figs. 17.6** and **17.7**).

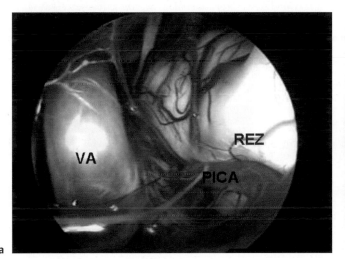

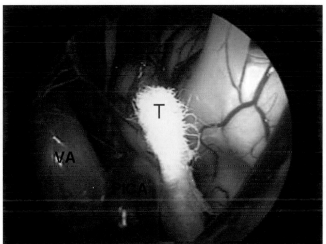

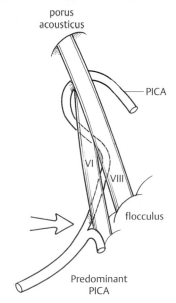

Fig. 17.6a–c The most common offending vessel: posteroinferior cerebellar artery (PICA). (**a, b**) Endoscopic views before and after decompression of a left side: note the deformity of the root exit zone (REZ) due to the PICA, which makes a print in it, and the dolichovertebral artery (VA). T, Teflon. (**c**) PICA-dominant configuration. This is the most common with PICA at the REZ. VI, VIII, cranial nerves.

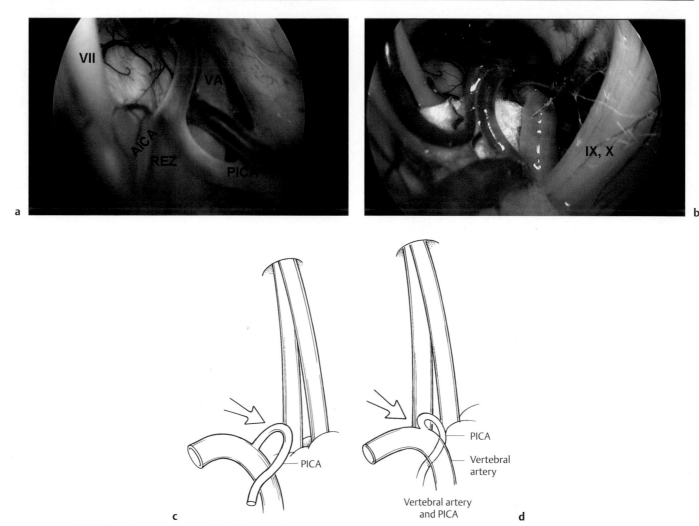

Fig. 17.7a–d (**a, b**) Endoscopic views, right side. Multiple offending vessels at the root exit zone (REZ) of the facial nerve: vertebral artery (VA), the posteroinferior cerebellar artery (PICA), and the anteroinferior cerebellar artery (AICA). VII, IX, X, cranial nerves. (**c, d**) Vertebral and/or PICA compression at REZ.

- The anteroinferior cerebellar artery (AICA) can be responsible for compressions on the cisternal portion of the nerve (**Fig. 17.8**). This type is more difficult to operate on when the AICA goes between the facial and cochleovestibular nerve because of the difficulty to mobilize the artery without risking any hearing impairment.
- Some compressions with the AICA are located within the internal auditory canal, and it is required to drill the internal auditory canal to have a good view of the facial nerve (**Fig. 17.9**). Pieces of Teflon are most of the time too large to be interposed and Neuropatch (Braun, Kronberg, Germany) can be used instead.
- In the case of a dominant form of the PICA, the AICA arises from the PICA at the REZ of the facial nerve and become the major offending vessel (**Fig. 17.10**).

Other compressions include:

- Compressions of youth: Hemifacial spasm is more common with age and increases in the elderly, in whom time, atherosclerosis, hypertension, and diabetes modify vascular walls and alter intravascular blood flow, contributing to abnormal nervous stimulation. Nevertheless, hemifacial spasm can affect young people (e.g., under the age of 30). Several causes have been suggested: thick arachnoid membrane, narrower posterior fossa, connective laxity, or anomaly of cranial nerve VII (plexiform minirootlets).
- Venous conflicts: Isolated venous conflicts are rare (0.4–4.1%). The difficulty is to identify the vein implicated and to know how to deal with it, choosing between decompression with interposing Teflon, coagulating it, or preserving it.

■ Surgical Results

Surgical care for patients suffering from hemifacial spasm has to be efficient, with a low morbidity, as always in caring for a functional disease. Efficiency varies

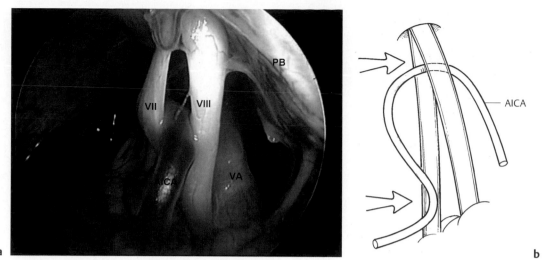

Fig. 17.8a, b (**a**) Endoscopic view, right side. Conflict by an anteroinferior cerebellar artery (AICA) in between cranial nerves VII and VIII. DV, Dandy vein; PB, petrous bone; VA, vertebral artery. (**b**) Intercochleofacial anteroinferior cerebellar artery (AICA) with two offending contacts.

from 83–97%.[18–21] In the authors' series of 553 cases, 93.6% of the patients had complete relief of their hemifacial spasm, but in 11% after revision surgery. Surgical result can be delayed (20.8% of patients in our series) an average of 6 months after first surgery. This delay corresponds to the time needed for hyperactivity of the nucleus to decrease.[18,22,24]

Surgical efficiency is highlighted in **Fig. 17.11**, which shows preoperative and postoperative quality of life evaluation in 326 patients operated on and with at least 2 years follow-up. This validated score[23] evaluates, from 0 to 4 (not affected to very affected), eight criteria of quality of life: driving, reading, television watching,

depressive mood, shunning of visual contacts, embarrassment caused by the condition, worry about others' reaction, and sleeping impairment.

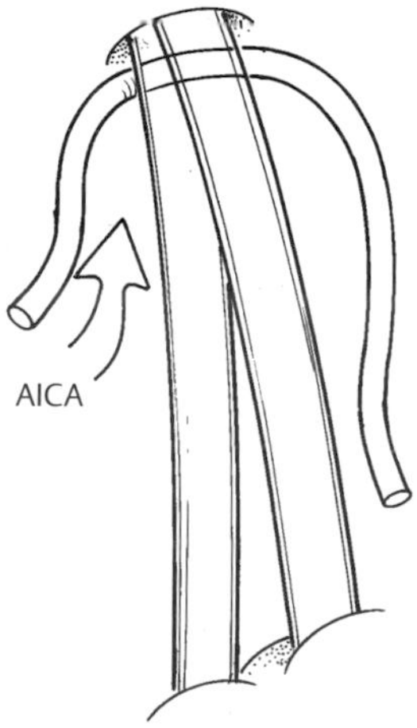

Morbidity is low, around 4%; cerebrospinal fluid leak (3%, 11 patients out of 326 analyzed), hearing impairment to deafness in 0.3%, secondary transient facial weakness occurring by viral resurgent response after 10 to 14 days, and postoperative headache or Arnold neuralgia (uncommon).

No mortality has occurred in our experience.[27–29]

■ Conclusion

Hemifacial spasm is a very disabling disease with an impact on one's self-image and on the patient's quality of life. Its pathophysiology remains unclear, probably involving peripheral vascular compression responsible for nervous deformity, focal demyelination, intrinsic modifications of vascular walls contributing to ectopic stimulation of facial nerve, and a nuclear hyperactivity.

If the diagnosis is clinical, radiological examination by MRI allows eliminating differential diagnosis and gives surgeons a precise vascular mapping of the CPA, thanks to the use of high-resolution sequences T2 and magnetic resonance angiography. Most of conflicts occur between the vertebral artery or the posteroinferior cerebellar artery and the facial nerve at its REZ in the pons.

Surgical treatment based on neurovascular decompression combining the use of both microscope and preoperative endoscope is the only curative treatment. It is efficient and has a very low morbidity rate. The good results obtained are long-lasting, and patients rapidly go back to the socio-professional lives they expected.

Fig. 17.9 The anteroinferior cerebellar artery (AICA) at porus. Some compressions with the AICA are located within the internal auditory canal, and it is required to drill the internal auditory canal to have a good view of the facial nerve.

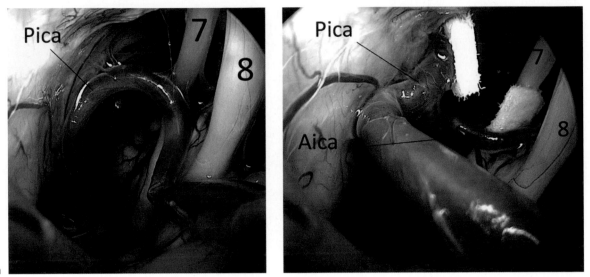

Fig. 17.10a, b Endoscopic views, right side, before and after decompression. Dominant form of posteroinferior cerebellar artery (*Pica*). Note the offending effect of the anteroinferior cerebellar artery (*Aica*) at its origin. (7) Facial nerve, (8) auditory nerve.

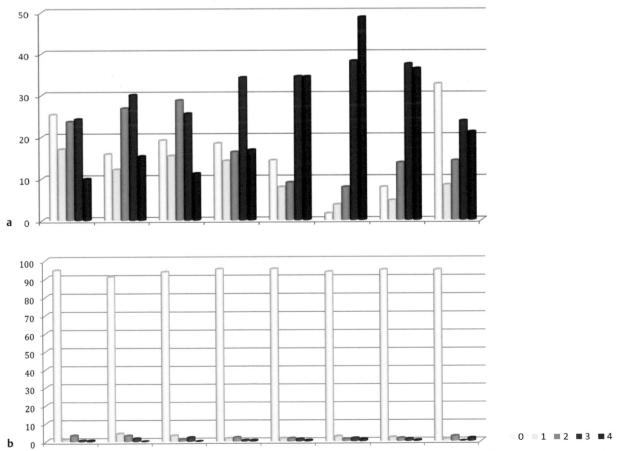

Fig. 17.11a, b The patient reported scores from 0 to 4 (not affected to very affected). (**a**) Preoperative quality of life. (**b**) Postoperative quality of life.

References

1. Nielsen VK, Jannetta PJ. Pathophysiology of hemifacial spasm: III. Effects of facial nerve decompression. Neurology 1984;34(7): 891–897
2. Krishnan AV, Hayes M, Kiernan MC. Axonal excitability properties in hemifacial spasm. Mov Disord 2007;22(9):1293–1298
3. Montero J, Junyent J, Calopa M, Povedano M, Valls-Sole J. Electrophysiological study of ephaptic axono-axonal responses in hemifacial spasm. Muscle Nerve 2007;35(2):184–188
4. Møller AR, Jannetta PJ. Hemifacial spasm: results of electrophysiologic recording during microvascular decompression operations. Neurology 1985;35(7):969–974
5. Møller AR, Sen CN. Recordings from the facial nucleus in the rat: signs of abnormal facial muscle response. Exp Brain Res 1990;81(1):18–24
6. Møller AR. Interaction between the blink reflex and the abnormal muscle response in patients with hemifacial spasm: results of intraoperative recordings. J Neurol Sci 1991;101(1):114–123
7. Wilkinson MF, Kaufmann AM. Monitoring of facial muscle motor evoked potentials during microvascular decompression for hemifacial spasm: evidence of changes in motor neuron excitability. J Neurosurg 2005;103(1):64–69
8. Yamakami I, Oka N, Higuchi Y. Hyperactivity of the facial nucleus produced by chronic electrical stimulation in rats. J Clin Neurosci 2007;14(5):459–463
9. De Ridder D, Møller A, Verlooy J, Cornelissen M, De Ridder L. Is the root entry/exit zone important in microvascular compression syndromes? Neurosurgery 2002;51(2):427–433, discussion 433–434
10. Campos-Benitez M, Kaufmann AM. Neurovascular compression findings in hemifacial spasm. J Neurosurg 2008;109(3):416–420
11. Girard N, Poncet M, Caces F, et al. Three-dimensional MRI of hemifacial spasm with surgical correlation. Neuroradiology 1997;39(1):46–51
12. Sarrazin JL, Marsot-Dupuch K, Chaÿas A. [Pathology of the cerebellopontine angle]. J Radiol 2006;87(11 Pt 2):1765–1782
13. Naraghi R, Tanrikulu L, Troescher-Weber R, et al. Classification of neurovascular compression in typical hemifacial spasm: three-dimensional visualization of the facial and the vestibulocochlear nerves. J Neurosurg 2007;107(6):1154–1163
14. Sindou M, Keravel Y. [Neurosurgical treatment of primary hemifacial spasm with microvascular decompression]. Neurochirurgie 2009;55(2):236–247
15. Girard N, Magnan J, Caces F, Chays A, Raybaud C. Imagerie de l'angle pontocérébelleux et du-conduit auditif interne normal et pathologique. EMC Oto-Rhino-Laryngologie 1998;20-047-A-80: 25p
16. Bremond GA, Garcin M, Magnan J, Bonnaud G. L'abord a minima de l'espace ponto-cerebelleux. Cah ORL 1974;19:443–460
17. Bremond GA, Garcin M. Microsurgical approach to the cerebellopontine angle. J Laryngol Otol 1975;89(3):237–248
18. Goto Y, Matsushima T, Natori Y, Inamura T, Tobimatsu S. Delayed effects of the microvascular decompression on hemifacial spasm: a retrospective study of 131 consecutive operated cases. Neurol Res 2002;24(3):296–300
19. Samii M, Günther T, Iaconetta G, Muehling M, Vorkapic P, Samii A. Microvascular decompression to treat hemifacial spasm: long-term results for a consecutive series of 143 patients. Neurosurgery 2002;50(4):712–718, discussion 718–719
20. Moffat DA, Durvasula VS, Stevens King A, De R, Hardy DG. Outcome following retrosigmoid microvascular decompression of the facial nerve for hemifacial spasm. J Laryngol Otol 2005;119(10):779–783
21. Cheng WY, Chao SC, Shen CC. Endoscopic microvascular decompression of the hemifacial spasm. Surg Neurol 2008;70 (Suppl 1):S1, 40–46
22. Sindou MP. Microvascular decompression for primary hemifacial spasm. Importance of intraoperative neurophysiological monitoring. Acta Neurochir (Wien) 2005;147(10):1019–1026, discussion 1026
23. Tan EK, Fook-Chong S, Lum SY, Thumboo J. Validation of a short disease specific quality of life scale for hemifacial spasm: correlation with SF-36. J Neurol Neurosurg Psychiatry 2005;76(12): 1707–1710
24. Badr-El-Dine M, El-Garem HF, Talaat AM, Magnan J. Endoscopically assisted minimally invasive microvascular decompression of hemifacial spasm. Otol Neurotol 2002;23(2):122–128
25. Elaini S, Miyazaki H, et al. Correlation between Magnetic Resonance Imaging and surgical findings in vasculoneural compression syndrome. Int Adv Otol 2009;5(3):1
26. Jannetta PJ. The cause of hemifacial spasm: definitive microsurgical treatment at the brainstem in 31 patients. Trans Sect Otolaryngol Am Acad Ophthalmol Otolaryngol 1975;80(3 Pt 1):319–322
27. Magnan J, Caces F, Locatelli P, Chays A. Hemifacial spasm: endoscopic vascular decompression. Otolaryngol Head Neck Surg 1997;117(4):308–314
28. Magnan J, Sanna M. Endoscopy in Neuro-otology. New York: Thieme; 1999
29. Miyazaki H, Deveze A, Magnan J. Neuro-otologic surgery through minimally invasive retrosigmoid approach: endoscope assisted microvascular decompression, vestibular neurotomy, and tumor removal. Laryngoscope 2005;115(9):1612–1617

18 Facial Nerve Monitoring

Emily Z. Stucken, Kevin D. Brown, and Samuel H. Selesnick

Injury to the facial nerve is one of the most feared and potentially devastating complications of otologic and neurotologic surgery. The facial nerve is at risk in otologic and neurotologic surgeries as a result of its tortuous course in the temporal bone and the cerebellopontine angle. To reduce risk of damage to the facial nerve, intraoperative nerve monitoring systems have been developed.

■ Indications for Facial Nerve Monitoring

Cerebellopontine Angle Tumors

The decision to use facial nerve monitoring is surgeon and case specific; its use has been described in nearly all otologic and neurotologic procedures.[1,2] Facial nerve monitoring has been consistently recommended in resection of cerobellopontine angle tumors and tumors of the internal auditory canal.[3] Here, it has achieved widespread use due to the limited anatomic exposure, the altered anatomy of the facial nerve caused by tumor compression and displacement, and increased vulnerability associated with the absence of epineurium in this region. Not uncommonly, the appearance of the facial nerve may also be transformed; the nerve's fibers may become splayed into a thin ribbon of tissue rather than its normal cylindrical shape. Dissection can become dangerous in these situations, especially as tumor size increases. In these instances, electrophysiologic facial nerve identification can occur before visual identification.

Middle Ear Surgery

The decision to use facial nerve monitoring when operating in the middle ear is surgeon dependent. Some have advocated the use of facial nerve monitoring in routine as well as complex middle ear cases.[1] Routine use was shown to be more cost-effective than the cost associated with selective use of facial monitoring combined with the management of complications of facial nerve injury in cases of nonuse.[4] Other surgeons elect to use facial nerve monitoring only in situations of chronic or recurrent middle ear disease. Patients with chronic ear disease, cholesteatoma, and patients with prior surgery may have obscured/absent anatomic landmarks. In these cases, facial nerve monitoring may allow the surgeon to dissect with greater safety in the midst of cholesteatoma, granulation tissue, and fibrosis.[1,5] Facial nerve monitoring may also be useful to detect a dehiscent facial nerve before it can be visualized in the surgical field. [1,6–8]

Pediatric Otology

The facial nerve continues to develop through age 4.[9] The mastoid tip also continues to develop and enlarge during this time, and as it does the facial nerve moves from a relatively lateral position to a more medial, adult position. Pediatric patients that require otologic surgery may have congenital abnormalities of their inner, middle, or external ear, predisposing them to have aberrant facial nerve anatomy.[10] In cases of congenital aural atresia, the facial nerve has been shown to have greater anatomic variability. Specifically, it tends to lie more anterior and superior in position in its vertical segment.[11] Facial nerve monitoring in these cases may help confirm the location of the facial nerve and prevent injury.

■ Types of Facial Nerve Monitoring

History

The first example in the literature of facial nerve monitoring was published by Krause in 1898, at which time electrical stimulation was described. During a cochlear nerve section, Dr. Krause noted that "unipolar faradic irritation of the nerve trunk . . . resulted in contractions of the right facial region, especially of the orbicularis oculi, as well as the branches supplying the nose and mouth."[12] The receptive portion of facial nerve monitoring still consisted of an assistant observing the face under the drapes. Facial nerve monitoring has progressed since this original description, evolving into a highly technological science that often employs auxiliary personnel to execute. In the past, devices that sensed facial muscle contraction were employed. The most commonly employed facial nerve monitoring systems at present are electromyography (EMG) systems; however, other systems such as video monitoring and direct monitoring of nerve impulses are available.

Electromyography

EMG uses facial muscle response as an indicator of facial nerve continuity and activity.[13] EMG can be used intraoperatively to alert a surgeon when the facial nerve is nearby. It can also be used to survey the operative field before dissecting in an area. A nerve stimulator can identify the nerve and map the location of the nerve in the surgical field. At the conclusion of dissection, the nerve stimulator can be used to confirm nerve continuity and give prognostic information regarding the functional status of the nerve. In addition, important information can be captured without nerve stimulation. For example, neurotonic discharges arising during a dissection can serve as warnings of impending facial nerve injury.

It is important to note that what is being measured is compound muscle action potentials, or the electrical activity being generated in a muscle, which reflects the health of the nerve innervating the muscle being monitored. EMG electrodes do not measure the compound nerve action potential (CNAP), which is the electrical activity generated by the nerve itself.

Setup

There are many systems commercially available. Once the patient has been properly positioned, nerve electrodes are inserted into the facial muscles in the authors' typical setup (**Fig. 18.1**). The authors use two electrodes each in the orbicularis oculi, orbicularis oris, and frontalis muscles. Guo et al performed a prospective study examining placement of electrodes to give optimal compound muscle action potential output. They recommend that the orbicularis oculi electrodes be placed at the orbital rim and the upper eyelid with needles separated by 1.5 cm, and that the orbicularis oris electrodes be placed 5 mm lateral to the oral commisure and 2 cm away at the lower lip.[14] Ground electrodes for the intramuscular electrodes and for the nerve stimulator are placed into the trapezius muscle. The electrodes are secured with clear adhesive strips, and care is taken to not run wires over the eyes. All wires should be draped over the patient such that they exit the table away from the operative site. The electrode wires are connected to a circuit box that directly interfaces with a monitor. A sterile stimulation probe is included in the instrument setup and is connected to the circuit box once the surgical field is set up. At this point, the patient is sterilely prepped and draped. Electrodes are prepped if the face is to be included in the surgical field. The authors prefer to employ a neurophysiologist to monitor EMG tracings, although some surgeons use a loudspeaker system that emits audible responses to electrical or mechanical stimulation of the facial nerve.

Anesthesia

Both nondepolarizing and depolarizing long-acting neuromuscular blockers commonly used to induce and maintain paralysis during anesthesia will impair the proper functioning of EMG nerve monitoring. Therefore, it is important to avoid use of muscle relaxants during cases in which EMG nerve monitoring is to be used, with the exception of succinylcholine at induction. Succinylcholine is short-acting with a half-life of 3.5 minutes, allowing for complete emergence from neuromuscular blockade within 15 minutes.[15] This 15-minute period after induction is generally inconsequential. Some have described the use of partial neuromuscular blockade monitored by twitches.[16,17] The authors, however, do not find partial paralysis to be necessary or assistive in otologic and neurotologic cases, and some researchers have even found that partial paralysis decreases spontaneous and mechanically evoked EMG activity.[18] Of note, EMG nerve monitoring is unaffected by inhalational or intravenous anesthetic agents, so adequate anesthesia may be obtained without the use of neuromuscular blockers.[18] Local anesthetic is commonly used at the incision site and within the ear canal; however, care must be taken to avoid overinjection near the stylomastoid foramen or into the middle ear to prevent infiltration of local anesthetic along the facial nerve.

Operative Use

At the start of the operation, it is prudent to test the integrity of the EMG circuit. Baseline EMG data should be recorded before commencement of the procedure. If the surgical procedure is amenable, the function of the circuit should be verified before dissection near the facial nerve by stimulating another motor nerve. In the case of skull base approaches to a cerebellopontine angle tumor, this can be achieved by stimulating cranial nerve XI at the jugular foramen. Any dysfunction in the EMG system should be addressed before proceeding to tumor dissection. In middle ear cases, a control motor nerve is not available within the field.

A stimulation probe may be used to confirm the location of the facial nerve in the operative field. Probes may be either monopolar or bipolar. Bipolar probes offer a theoretical advantage of having the ability to stimulate a smaller area of the nerve; however, their use requires a precise

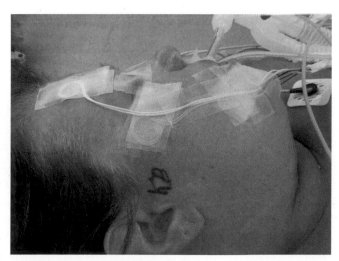

Fig. 18.1 Placement of electrode leads.

orientation between the probe and the nerve. This may be precluded by anatomic constraints. Monopolar probes are more commonly used.[15] Such probes can be used to map the path of the nerve and to distinguish the facial nerve from surrounding tissue such as arachnoid, tumor, cholesteatoma, granulation tissue, or fibrosis. When confirming the location of the nerve, the probe should be set to the lowest intensity to identify a threshold and allow for a neuromuscular response without delivering a potentially damaging amount of energy. Two stimulation probe systems are available: those that deliver a constant current and those that deliver a constant voltage. Despite the theoretical differences between the two systems, neither has achieved clinical advantage[19]; both systems are currently used.

Electromyography Tracings

The EMG system will provide data that reflects the status of the facial nerve in the surgical field. It is important to remember that there are many sources of interference introduced by objects in the operative field. Four distinct EMG tracings (**Fig. 18.2; Table 18.1**) can be seen, which reflect the activity of the facial nerve and its dependent musculature.[20] Random muscle activity provides a background of electromyographic deflections on which pulsed responses, repetitive (train) activity, and nonrepetitive (burst) activity may be seen. A uniform increase in random muscle activity generally heralds a diminution of the effects of anesthesia. Pulsed responses are seen with electrical stimulation of the nerve using a stimulation probe. Pulsed responses are used to confirm the presence of the nerve in the surgical field. Neurotonic trains of EMG activity may occur as a result of traction, pressure, or caloric irritation of the nerve. Prolonged train activity may signal impending injury to the facial nerve. Burst activity

Table 18.1 Types of electromyography activity in facial nerve monitoring

Electromyography Tracing	Neuromuscular Correlate
Background electromyographic deflections	Random muscle activity
Pulsed responses	Use of stimulation probe
Train activity	Traction, pressure, or caloric irritation
Burst activity	Surgical manipulation

is generally seen with surgical manipulation of the nerve and serves as a warning that the site of dissection or the technique employed by the surgeon should be modified. It is important to note that the absence of EMG burst activity does not confirm that the nerve is safe; this could also result from a nonconducting nerve.

When localizing the facial nerve in the field of dissection, the lowest intensity should be used to stimulate the nerve: this is the nerve threshold. A nerve that has been stretched or otherwise traumatized may require increasing levels of stimulation to achieve a neuromuscular response. Numerous studies have examined the correlation between stimulation level, neuromuscular response, and postoperative facial nerve functional outcomes.[21-26] Morton et al examined postoperative outcomes of immediate facial palsy, delayed facial palsy, or no facial palsy, and found an inverse relationship between stimulation levels and facial nerve outcomes such that lower stimulation levels were associated with better outcomes.[27] Isaacson et al also found intraoperative monitoring parameters (proximal stimulation threshold and proximal-to-distal response amplitude ratio) to be reliable in predicting facial nerve outcomes.[28] In a prospective study, however, Axon et al did not find intraoperative stimulation thresholds to accurately predict postoperative function in patients with poor postoperative facial function.[29]

Pitfalls of Electromyography

EMG is a technological aid to otologic and neurotologic surgery, but it should never replace a thorough surgical fund of knowledge. Intraoperatively, information suggested by the monitor may be in contradiction to clinical findings. The surgeon must use sound anatomic knowledge as an overriding guide. A concern has been raised that facial nerve monitoring systems may give an inexperienced surgeon a level of false confidence and may result in an inappropriately aggressive dissection.[2] Furthermore, there are areas of intrinsic fallibility within the EMG system that can lead to equivocal results. Electrical interference from operating room equipment and electrocautery can interfere with EMG monitoring and preclude accurate monitoring.

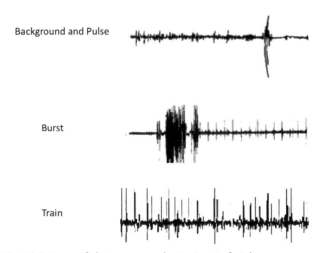

Fig. 18.2 Types of electromyography tracings in facial nerve monitoring.

Other Types of Facial Nerve Monitoring

Although EMG is the most commonly used facial monitoring platform, other types of monitoring have been used and are currently being studied. CNAP monitoring is a technique that involves attachment of electrodes directly to nerves such that readings reflect conduction properties of the nerve being monitored.[30–33] CNAP monitoring has the potential to offer continuous monitoring of the nerve status. CNAP monitoring is also unaffected by neuromuscular blockade. CNAP does, however, require manipulation of the nerve for electrode placement, which places the nerve at added danger. Nerve monitoring systems using videoanalysis of facial movements have been developed and are currently being studied.[34,35] These systems have the potential to be unaffected by interference such as that from electrocautery.

■ Outcomes with Facial Nerve Monitoring

Since the advent of facial nerve monitoring, numerous comparative studies have been published that have cemented the role of facial nerve monitoring in neurotologic surgery.[36–43] Hammerschlag and Cohen found a significant reduction of facial paralysis in cerebellopontine angle surgery with the use of facial nerve monitoring; they noted a 3.6% incidence of facial paralysis with intraoperative monitoring compared with a 14.5% incidence with previously unmonitored cases.[36] Several studies describe an increase in facial function when using facial nerve monitoring for acoustic neuroma resection and a decrease in patients with poor outcomes.[38,39]

Kwartler et al describe a significant improvement in facial nerve results with nerve monitoring in the postoperative period and at time of discharge, though this association lost statistical significance by 1 year postoperatively. Of note, when subgroups were analyzed with respect to size of tumor, those tumors smaller than 2.5 cm did not show a difference in outcomes with use of the facial nerve monitoring system.[40]

Nissen et al found a nonsignificant trend toward improved facial nerve function results with use of intraoperative facial nerve monitoring; this effect was more pronounced with large size tumors.[41] Morikawa et al found that intraoperative nerve monitoring not only resulted in improved facial nerve functionality, but also significantly increased the number of tumors that were able to be completely resected.[42] In a study published by Kartush et al, it was noted that preservation of facial nerve function with nerve monitoring could be extrapolated to the cochlear nerve, which benefitted indirectly from careful dissection within the internal auditory canal.[43]

■ Conclusion

The use of facial nerve monitoring systems has become well established in otologic and neurotologic surgery. Intraoperative monitoring has improved outcomes in cerebellopontine angle surgery, most prominently with large tumors. Many have found it useful in middle ear and mastoid surgeries, and in pediatric otology. Facial nerve monitoring systems continue to evolve, and we will likely see refinement of EMG as well as other types of monitoring systems in the future. Armed with sound anatomic knowledge and meticulous surgical planning, the surgeon will continue to find that intraoperative facial nerve monitoring will positively impact outcomes in otologic and neurotologic surgeries.

References

1. Silverstein H, Smouha EE, Jones R. Routine intraoperative facial nerve monitoring during otologic surgery. Am J Otol 1988;9(4):269–275
2. Jackler RK, Selesnick SH. Indications for cranial nerve monitoring during otologic and neurotologic surgery. Am J Otol 1994;15(5):611–613
3. The Consensus Development Panel. National Institutes of Health Consensus Development Conference Statement on Acoustic Neuroma, December 11-13, 1991. Arch Neurol 1994;51(2):201–207
4. Wilson L, Lin E, Lalwani A. Cost-effectiveness of intraoperative facial nerve monitoring in middle ear or mastoid surgery. Laryngoscope 2003;113(10):1736–1745
5. Leonetti JP, Matz GJ, Smith PG, Beck DL. Facial nerve monitoring in otologic surgery: clinical indications and intraoperative technique. Ann Otol Rhinol Laryngol 1990;99(11):911–918
6. Noss RS, Lalwani AK, Yingling CD. Facial nerve monitoring in middle ear and mastoid surgery. Laryngoscope 2001;111(5):831–836
7. Pensak ML, Willging JP, Keith RW. Intraoperative facial nerve monitoring in chronic ear surgery: a resident training experience. Am J Otol 1994;15(1):108–110
8. Choung YH, Park K, Cho MJ, Choung PH, Shin YR, Kahng H. Systematic facial nerve monitoring in middle ear and mastoid surgeries: "surgical dehiscence" and "electrical dehiscence". Otolaryngol Head Neck Surg 2006;135(6):872–876
9. Schaitkin BM, Shapiro A, May M. Disorders of the facial nerve. In: Lalwani AK., Grundfast KM., eds. Pediatric otology and neurotology. Philadelphia, PA:Lippincott-Raven;1998:457–475
10. Jahrsdoerfer RA. The facial nerve in congenital middle ear malformations. Laryngoscope 1981;91(8):1217–1225
11. Schuknecht HF. Congenital aural atresia. Laryngoscope 1989;99(9):908–917
12. Krause F. Surgery of the brain and spinal cord, Vol. II. New York, NY: Rebman; 1912
13. May M, Wiet RJ. Iatrogenic injury: Prevention and management. In: May M, ed. The facial nerve. New York, NY: Thieme; 1986:549–560
14. Guo L, Jasiukaitis P, Pitts LH, Cheung SW. Optimal placement of recording electrodes for quantifying facial nerve compound muscle action potential. Otol Neurotol 2008;29(5):710–713
15. O'Malley MR, Moore BA, Haynes DS. Neurophysiologic intraoperative monitoring. In: Bailey BJ, Johnson JT, Newlands SD. Head and neck surgery-Otolaryngology 4th Ed. Vol II. Philadelphia, PA: Lippincott Williams & Wilkins;2006:1943–1960

16. Ho LC, Crosby G, Sundaram P, Ronner SF, Ojemann RG. Ulnar train-of-four stimulation in predicting face movement during intracranial facial nerve stimulation. Anesth Analg 1989;69(2): 242–244

17. Lennon RL, Hosking MP, Daube JR, Welna JO. Effect of partial neuromuscular blockade on intraoperative electromyography in patients undergoing resection of acoustic neuromas. Anesth Analg 1992;75(5):729–733

18. Yingling CD, Ashram YA. Intraoperative monitoring of cranial nerves in neurotologic surgery. In: Cummings CW. Otolaryngology head and neck surgery, 4th Ed. Philadelphia, PA: Elsevier Mosby; 2005:3877–3911

19. Prass R, Lüders H. Constant-current versus constant-voltage stimulation. J Neurosurg 1985;62(4):622–623

20. Prass RL, Kinney SE, Hardy RW Jr, Hahn JF, Lüders H. Acoustic (loudspeaker) facial EMG monitoring: II. Use of evoked EMG activity during acoustic neuroma resection. Otolaryngol Head Neck Surg 1987;97(6):541–551

21. Magliulo G, Zardo F. Facial nerve function after cerebello-pontine angle surgery and prognostic value of intraoperative facial nerve monitoring: a critical evaluation. Am J Otolaryngol 1998;19(2):102–106

22. Berges C, Fraysse B, Yardeni E, Rugiu G. Intraoperative facial nerve monitoring in posterior fossa surgery: prognostic value. Skull Base Surg 1993;3(4):214–216

23. Zeitouni AG, Hammerschlag PE, Cohen NL. Prognostic significance of intraoperative facial nerve stimulus thresholds. Am J Otol 1997;18(4):494–497

24. Beck DL, Atkins JS Jr, Benecke JE Jr, Brackmann DE. Intraoperative facial nerve monitoring: prognostic aspects during acoustic tumor removal. Otolaryngol Head Neck Surg 1991;104(6): 780–782

25. Silverstein H, Willcox TO Jr, Rosenberg SI, Seidman MD. Prediction of facial nerve function following acoustic neuroma resection using intraoperative facial nerve stimulation. Laryngoscope 1994;104(5 Pt 1):539–544

26. Goldbrunner RH, Schlake HP, Milewski C, Tonn JC, Helms J, Roosen K. Quantitative parameters of intraoperative electromyography predict facial nerve outcomes for vestibular schwannoma surgery. Neurosurgery 2000;46(5):1140–1146, discussion 1146–1148

27. Morton RP, Ackerman PD, Pisansky MT, et al. Prognostic factors for the incidence and recovery of delayed facial nerve palsy after vestibular schwannoma resection. J Neurosurg 2011;114(2): 375–380

28. Isaacson B, Kileny PR, El-Kashlan HK. Prediction of long-term facial nerve outcomes with intraoperative nerve monitoring. Otol Neurotol 2005;26(2):270–273

29. Axon PR, Ramsden RT. Intraoperative electromyography for predicting facial function in vestibular schwannoma surgery. Laryngoscope 1999;109(6):922–926

30. Colletti V, Fiorino FG, Policante Z, Bruni L. New perspectives in intraoperative facial nerve monitoring with antidromic potentials. Am J Otol 1996;17(5):755–762

31. Colletti V, Fiorino FG. Advances in monitoring of seventh and eighth cranial nerve function during posterior fossa surgery. Am J Otol 1998;19(4):503–512

32. Richmond IL, Mahla M. Use of antidromic recording to monitor facial nerve function intraoperatively. Neurosurgery 1985; 16(4):458–462

33. Schmid UD, Sturzenegger M, Ludin HP, Seiler RW, Reulen HJ. Orthodromic (intra/extracranial) neurography to monitor facial nerve function intraoperatively. Neurosurgery 1988;22(5): 945–950

34. Filipo R, Pichi B, Bertoli GA, De Seta E. Video-based system for intraoperative facial nerve monitoring: comparison with electromyography. Otol Neurotol 2002;23(4):594–597

35. De Seta E, Bertoli GA, De Seta D, Covelli E, Filipo R. New development in intraoperative video monitoring of facial nerve: a pilot study. Otol Neurotol 2010;31(9):1498–1502

36. Hammerschlag PE, Cohen NL. Intraoperative monitoring of facial nerve function in cerebellopontine angle surgery. Otolaryngol Head Neck Surg 1990;103(5 (Pt 1):681–684

37. Harner SG, Daube JR, Ebersold MJ, Beatty CW. Improved preservation of facial nerve function with use of electrical monitoring during removal of acoustic neuromas. Mayo Clin Proc 1987;62(2):92–102

38. Leonetti JP, Brackmann DE, Prass RL. Improved preservation of facial nerve function in the infratemporal approach to the skull base. Otolaryngol Head Neck Surg 1989;101(1):74–78

39. Silverstein H, Rosenberg SI, Flanzer J, Seidman MD. Intraoperative facial nerve monitoring in acoustic neuroma surgery. Am J Otol 1993;14(6):524–532

40. Kwartler JA, Luxford WM, Atkins J, Shelton C. Facial nerve monitoring in acoustic tumor surgery. Otolaryngol Head Neck Surg 1991;104(6):814–817

41. Nissen AJ, Sikand A, Welsh JE, Curto FS, Gardi J. A multifactorial analysis of facial nerve results in surgery for cerebellopontine angle tumors. Ear Nose Throat J 1997;76(1):37–40

42. Morikawa M, Tamaki N, Nagashima T, Motooka Y. Long-term results of facial nerve function after acoustic neuroma surgery—clinical benefit of intraoperative facial nerve monitoring. Kobe J Med Sci 2000;46(3):113–124

43. Kartush JM, Larouere MJ, Graham MD, Bouchard KR, Audet BV. Intraoperative cranial nerve monitoring during posterior skull base surgery. Skull Base Surg 1991;1(2):85–92

19 Acute Management of the Effects of Facial Paralysis

Michael B. Gluth and Marcus D. Atlas

Clinical management issues related to acute facial paralysis can be divided into three categories. The first involves management directed at underlying conditions causing facial paralysis (i.e., infection, tumor). The second is concerned with treating the dysfunctional facial nerve itself (i.e., neuritis, trauma) and its branches.[1,2] The final category, and often the one associated with the greatest potential for positive intervention, includes management and prevention of the *negative effects* of acute facial paralysis. Examples of these include ophthalmic pathology such as corneal exposure injury,[3,4] psychiatric effects such as anxiety or depression, and manifestations of oral sphincter incompetence. The focus of this chapter is on the practical clinical management of this latter category: the negative sequelae of facial paralysis in the acute and subacute settings. The first of these two categories as well as definitive management of the effects of facial paralysis in the chronic setting are dealt with in Chapters 21 through 26 of this book.

■ Management of the Eye

Orbicularis oculi palsy negatively impacts the eye in several ways. First, lagophthalmos (inability to close the eye) results in an increased duration of time during which the cornea is exposed to drying and irritating influences. Second, the loss of lower eyelid muscle tone in combination with other factors such as gravity, frequent wiping, and excess stretching often result in paralytic ectropion. This, too, results in increased corneal exposure as well as a disturbance of the normal tear flow mechanism via outward deflection of the lower eyelid and lacrimal punctum relative to the globe. It also results in impaired cosmesis and bothersome tearing to a degree that can be socially disruptive.

If orbicularis oculi palsy is encountered in the setting of concomitant trigeminal nerve loss, the absence of the usual protective influence of corneal sensation (i.e., loss of Bell phenomenon, absent blink reflex) also increases the risk of corneal exposure. Furthermore, it is possible that the site of lesion may have an impact on risk of corneal injury so far as it is possible for pregeniculate lesions to negatively affect lacrimal output via derangement in function of the greater superficial petrosal nerve.

The problems of increased corneal exposure and decreased lacrimation, especially with corneal anesthesia, may lead to the most dreaded ocular complication associated with facial palsy—namely, exposure-related corneal pathology causing decreased vision. Specifically, this includes a spectrum of scattered corneal punctate epithelial loss, epithelial erosions, and ulceration involving deeper layers. These may result in corneal vascularization or stromal scarring with associated visual deficits. If secondary infection occurs as well, corneal ulceration and scarring can be more severe.

The management of the eye in facial paralysis will be influenced by the expected prognosis and cause. Temporary facial paralysis (weeks or a few months) may be treated nonsurgically, but long-term facial paralysis requires more definitive, usually surgical, treatment of the eye. These include gold weight implantation,[5,6] lower eyelid procedures, and all forms of facial reanimation.

Most patients in the early stages can be managed with the nonsurgical measures described here, but if corneal exposure persists, surgical measures such as gold weight implantation may be used in the early stages of facial paralysis. Gold weight implantation is aesthetically superior, reversible (if required), and preferred to tarsorrhaphy.

Drops/Ointment

Sterile artificial tears (ideally preservative-free) are recommended at a frequency of two drops every 1 to 2 hours while awake to combat corneal desiccation (**Table 19.1**). The most commonly encountered artificial tear preparations contain a form of methylcellulose; however, numerous varieties exist. Bland ophthalmic ointment is applied just inside the lower eyelid prior to sleep for protection at night. Furthermore, it is recommended that the patient additionally apply ointment once every 4 hours during the waking hours if redness persists despite application of drops. Unfortunately, ointment can be somewhat messy and necessarily causes blurred vision for a moderate duration of time following application.

Eye Taping

If performed properly, eye taping can be useful in combination with ocular lubricants to treat lagophthalmos and paralytic ectropion. Variations in technique exist for waking hours and for bedtime. While awake, patients are recommended to place a crescent-shaped piece of tape (preferably a paper variety that is conducive to adhesion with the thin sensitive eyelid skin) over the upper eyelid and rectangular piece horizontally over the lower eyelid to

Table 19.1   Various selected sterile ophthalmic lubricants

U.S. trade name	Manufacturer	Ingredients
Artificial tears		
Bion Tears	Alcon Laboratories (Fort Worth, TX)	Hydroxypropyl methylcellulose 0.3%, dextran 0.1%
Genteal	Novartis (Basel, Switzerland)	Hydroxypropyl methylcellulose 0.3%
Genteal Gel	Novartis	Hydroxypropyl methylcellulose 0.3%, carboxymethylcellulose 0.25%
Isopto Tears	Alcon Laboratories	Hydroxypropyl methylcellulose 0.5%
Hypotears PF	Novartis	Polyvinyl alcohol 1%
Refresh Plus	Allergan (Irvine, CA)	Carboxymethylcellulose 0.5%
Refresh Celluvisc	Allergan	Carboxymethylcellulose 1%
Refresh Classic	Allergan	Polyvinyl alcohol (1.4%), povidone 0.6%
Systane Ultra	Alcon Laboratories	Polyethylene glycol 0.4%
Tears Naturale	Alcon Laboratories	Hydroxypropyl methylcellulose free 0.3%, dextran 0.1%
Theratears Preservative Free	Advanced Vision Research (Ann Arbor, MI)	Sodium carboxymethylcellulose 0.25%
Ointments		
Duolube	Bausch & Lomb (Rochester, NY)	Mineral oil, white petrolatum
Lacrilube	Allergan	Mineral oil, white petrolatum, nonionic lanolin derivatives (*has preservatives*)
Refresh PM	Allergan	Mineral oil, white petrolatum
Systane Ointment	Alcon Laboratories	Mineral oil, white petrolatum, anhydrous lanolin
Tears Naturale PM	Alcon Laboratories	Mineral oil, white petrolatum, anhydrous lanolin

lift the lower lid. While sleeping, the eyelids can be carefully taped in a closed position with a piece that spans vertically over the lateral aspect of the eye from the forehead, over both closed eyelids, and then onto the cheek (**Fig. 19.1**).

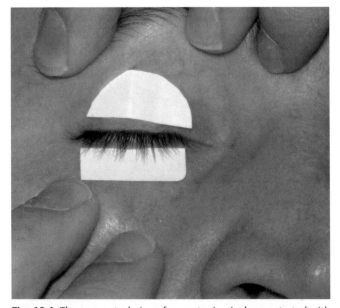

Fig. 19.1 The proper technique for eye taping is demonstrated with a crescent piece on the upper eyelid and smaller rectangular piece on the lower eyelid.

Although a helpful adjuvant, eye taping has some potential associated pitfalls. Caution should be made to ensure that the tape is not in contact with the globe as this can cause contact abrasion, especially in cases where corneal sensation is impaired. Taping can be particularly difficult at night when concomitant application of ointment may render tape relatively nonadhesive; nighttime taping is often abandoned for this reason. Furthermore, placement of tape should not involve excessive stretching or shearing forces on the lower eyelid as this can exacerbate ectropion.

Moisture Chamber/Humidification

For promotion of a moist ocular environment, several tools and techniques are available. The most simple involves the use of mechanical air humidifying devices within the home and workplace as well as the avoidance of fans. To provide a barrier to wind and air current exposure, large-lens eyeglasses or low-tint sunglasses can be worn while awake. Specialized plastic side shields can also be attached to eyewear for this same purpose.

For sleep, several options are available. When specialized tools are unavailable, simple loose application of plastic wrap, which will adhere to the forehead and cheek when set with a thin layer of ointment, can be helpful, although this has a tendency to displace with sleep motion. Loose-fitting swim goggles form an acceptable moisture chamber but tend to be poorly tolerated overnight.

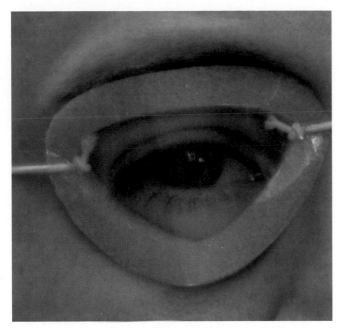

Fig. 19.2 An eye bubble is helpful in promoting humidification and protection during sleep.

Commercially manufactured eye bubble moisture chambers are also available specifically for this purpose. These are variably held in place either by a thin elastic band or surrounding adhesive tape. A pressure patch at night is not recommended due to the risk of abrasion (**Fig. 19.2**).

Soft Lenses

Soft contact lenses have been advocated by some clinicians for their ability to protect and humidify the eye. However, there may be some tendency for these to easily displace in the setting of lower eyelid ectropion and lagophthalmos. Soft lenses can also be expensive; thus, their use is perhaps best limited to patients that already had them in possession for vision correction prior to the onset of facial paralysis.

Punctal Plugs

When paralytic ectropion of the lower eyelid is severe, conjunctival irritation and epidermidalization may lead to punctual stenosis and blocked lacrimal outflow. In such cases, simple punctual dilation and placement of stenting plugs can be helpful but are infrequently used.

Eyelid Suture

Simple temporary eyelid suture techniques have been advocated, but most patients with corneal exposure are best treated with the measures described or more definitive surgery if exposure is still a problem. This includes cases that are expected to recover.

Simple temporary eyelid suture techniques or "temporary tarsorrhaphy" involve placement of a small non-resorbing suture *without* the removal of lid margin soft tissues or other intentional means of inducing permanent adhesions between opposing eyelid margins. These sutures can be removed several weeks after placement, usually without negative effects. Generally a size 5.0 suture is passed horizontally with 5 mm between needle entry/exit puncture sites in the gray line or just outside the eyelid margins. Although medial, para-median, and lateral suture techniques have been described, the latter seems most common. As an alternative, some clinicians prefer to pass suture only through the upper eyelid to be used in combo with taping to the cheek. If partial recovery in eyelid motor function is encountered, it is generally best to remove temporary sutures so as to avoid excessive stretching or discomfort.

■ Psychiatric Support

The negative psychosocial effects of facial paralysis are profound.[7-10] And yet somehow medical practitioners may overlook these at times. Unlike many other maladies, it is essentially impossible for patients to prevent facial paralysis from being evident in most of their social interactions. Unfortunately, there tends to be high degree of rejection and social discomfort from society at large when confronted with facial disfigurement. As a result, affected individuals often become quite self-conscious and withdrawn.

The psychiatric consequences of this scenario are important to consider even (if not especially) in the acute clinical setting. Patients with facial paralysis tend to suffer high levels of anxiety in the immediate period following onset, especially when prognosis is uncertain. This has some particular clinical implications. First, the importance of the clinician to possess a working knowledge of the natural history of various conditions that cause facial paralysis and the ability to properly interpret electrodiagnostic testing cannot be understated. These afford the ability to clearly outline what is known from a prognostic standpoint, thereby providing the patient with insight and in some cases with reassurance. Second, medical treatment of anxiety may be appropriate in the acute setting, especially when a patient suffers from a preexisting anxiety disorder or when his/her personality profile or professional demands makes coping a particular challenge.

Most patients who are affected for more than a few weeks by facial disfigurement are almost certain to experience some degree of depression. Both the management of anxiety and depression should be coordinated with the patient's primary care provider. It is also highly recommended to pursue psychiatry consultation in the acute setting for patients with a poor prognosis for complete or early recovery as indicated by mechanism of injury and electrodiagnostic testing.

Perhaps most important is the need for compassion, empathy, and individualized care on behalf of the medical provider. For example, organizing professional counseling sessions with a cosmetic make-up specialist has been advocated for female patients to soften the severity of the appearance of facial paralysis.[11] Such a referral demonstrates care on the part of the clinician and allows the patient to gain a small measure of control in what can feel like a very helpless situation.

■ Management of Oral Incompetence

Palsy of the perioral musculature, particularly the orbicularis oris and buccinator, will result in dysfunction of the oral sphincter mechanism. Although dysfunction related to the eye tends to be the greatest source of psychosocial distress acutely following onset of facial paralysis, oral incompetence will often become a greater source of patient concern in the subacute and chronic settings. Oral incompetence is manifested by drooling, leakage when eating, cheek biting, inability to whistle, inability to blow, defective speech articulation, and impaired cosmesis.

Patients with an uncertain prognosis that are struggling with oral incompetence in the subacute setting will often benefit from speech therapy consultation,[12]

especially those with preexisting swallowing difficulties or related risk factors. The goals of such a consultation are to promote acquisition of adaptive maneuvers for speech and swallowing as well as construction of an optimized dietary plan.

In the case of patients that, by virtue of the mechanism of facial injury, are judged to have a poor prognosis for recovery, early physical therapy consultation is especially important. The development of specialized facial paralysis physical therapy rehabilitation programs that may include electromyography biofeedback can greatly assist in retraining the development of functional facial movements and minimizing oral incompetence.[13,14] Such retraining efforts are probably optimized if started as early as possible, even while motor reinnervation is still in the infant stages. Details regarding specific physical therapy rehabilitation protocols are covered in Chapter 25.

If drooling is a major problem, anticholinergic medications can be useful; however, the benefits of usage must be counterbalanced by consideration of the potential side effect of decreased lacrimal output. Elevation of the corner of the mouth with taping techniques may be attempted, but these generally are not as useful as is the case with the eye. In cases where a slow or poor recovery is expected, early surgical static facial reanimation may be the best course of action to deal with oral incompetence.[15]

References

1. Adour KK. Medical management of idiopathic (Bell's) palsy. Otolaryngol Clin North Am 1991;24(3):663–673
2. Salinas RA, Alvarez G, Daly F, Ferreira J. Corticosteroids for Bell's palsy (idiopathic facial paralysis). Cochrane Database Syst Rev 2010;3(3):CD001942
3. Lee V, Currie Z, Collin JRO. Ophthalmic management of facial nerve palsy. Eye (Lond) 2004;18(12):1225–1234
4. Jelks GW, Smith B, Bosniak S. The evaluation and management of the eye in facial palsy. Clin Plast Surg 1979;6(3):397–419
5. Atlas MD, Talbot A, Delaney M, Chang A. Gold weight Implants in Facial Paralysis. Aust J Otolaryngol 1995;2:193–195
6. Catalano PJ, Bergstein MJ, Biller HF. Comprehensive management of the eye in facial paralysis. Arch Otolaryngol Head Neck Surg 1995;121(1):81–86
7. Brach JS, VanSwearingen JM, Delitto A, Johnson PC. Impairment and disability in patients with facial neuromuscular dysfunction. Otolaryngol Head Neck Surg 1997;117(4):315–321
8. Coulson SE, O'dwyer NJ, Adams RD, Croxson GR. Expression of emotion and quality of life after facial nerve paralysis. Otol Neurotol 2004;25(6):1014–1019
9. Hirschenfang S, Goldberg MJ, Benton JG. Psychological aspects of patients with facial paralysis. Dis Nerv Syst 1969;30(4):257–261
10. Neely JG, Neufeld PS. Defining functional limitation, disability, and societal limitations in patients with facial paresis: initial pilot questionnaire. Am J Otol 1996;17(2):340–342
11. Kanzaki J, Ohshiro K, Abe T. Effect of corrective make-up training on patients with facial nerve paralysis. Ear Nose Throat J 1998;77(4):270–274
12. Brach JS, VanSwearingen JM. Physical therapy for facial paralysis: a tailored treatment approach. Phys Ther 1999;79(4):397–404
13. Cronin GW, Steenerson RL. The effectiveness of neuromuscular facial retraining combined with electromyography in facial paralysis rehabilitation. Otolaryngol Head Neck Surg 2003;128(4):534–538
14. Ross B, Nedzelski JM, McLean JA. Efficacy of feedback training in long-standing facial nerve paresis. Laryngoscope 1991;101(7 Pt 1):744–750
15. Hadlock TA, Greenfield LJ, Wernick-Robinson M, Cheney ML. Multimodality approach to management of the paralyzed face. Laryngoscope 2006;116(8):1385–1389

Due to its proximity, lesions of the eighth cranial nerve have significant impact upon the integrity and function of the facial nerve. Because of this, treatment decisions for acoustic neuromas (more correctly named "vestibular schwannomas") are guided by a desire to reduce patient symptoms, while sparing residual facial nerve function and minimizing complications from treatment. These decisions have become complex as radiological advances have increased our ability to detect small, minimally symptomatic lesions.

Only 5% of facial nerve weakness is related to the presence of a tumor, and facial paralysis rarely presents as an initial symptom of an acoustic neuroma. In fact, facial paralysis is typically only a manifestation of a large, compressive lesion that is situated in a narrow region of the internal auditory canal (IAC). These tumors can cause nerve dysfunction by inducing nerve ischemia, obstructing cerebrospinal fluid (CSF), or direct compression. In fact, the finding of facial nerve dysfunction should alert the clinician that the lesion may not be an acoustic neuroma, but may instead represent a facial nerve neuroma or other cerebellopontine angle (CPA) neoplasm. Still, progressive facial paralysis can be a late symptom of an acoustic neuroma. In a 1992 study, most patients with acoustic neuromas had nearly 4 years of hearing loss, tinnitus, or vertigo prior to their diagnosis. If facial nerve paralysis developed, the diagnosis was made in the same year.[1]

Classically, slowly progressive or recurrent facial paralysis heralds the presence of either a facial nerve tumor or an extrinsic lesion compressing the facial nerve. Facial twitching should suggest to the examiner that the facial nerve is in a state of irritation and heighten suspicion regarding the presence of a tumor. In general, motor fibers of the facial nerve are tolerant to gradual external pressure secondary to its rich blood supply and dense fibrous covering, but the nerve may be splayed on the surface of the tumor and have little resilience.

Hearing loss, tinnitus, imbalance, headache, and facial numbness are many times more common than facial nerve weakness at the time of diagnosis. Facial pain, while frequently seen in disorders such as Ramsay Hunt syndrome or malignant neoplasms involving the facial nerve, is uncommonly associated with acoustic neuromas. Numbness of the ear canal and conchal bowl, however, can be a clinical finding associated with an acoustic neuroma. This was first described by Hitselberger and House in 1966 as hypesthesia to pin prick testing and, in the context of limited imaging capability, was used as an early clinical sign of the presence of a tumor.[2] Additional studies have confirmed that somatic sensory afferents carried by the facial nerve, via the sensory auricular branch, are found in posterior external auditory canal and inferior conchal bowl.[3] As imaging capabilities have advanced, the utility of "Hitselberger sign" has diminished, but it still helps confirm radiological findings.

Facial schwannomas are relatively rare, slow-growing tumors that may present with facial weakness and should be in the differential for a CPA or IAC neoplasm. Typically, these tumors are mistaken for acoustic neuromas when they are primarily confined to the IAC and do not enter the meatal foramen or fallopian canal. A series by McMenomey et al described 32 primary facial nerve tumors, of which 38% were believed to be acoustic neuromas preoperatively.[4] Unfortunately, there are no tests at the clinician's disposal (other than preoperative imaging) to differentiate intracanalicular acoustic neuromas from facial schwannomas. The most important imaging sign is presence of tumor in the labyrinthine segment of the facial nerve, which differentiates a facial nerve tumor from an acoustic neuroma.

Electroneuronography involves active stimulation of the extratemporal facial nerve and has not proven a reliable diagnostic test for these lesions. The intratemporal facial nerve is particularly susceptible to dysfunction secondary to the growth of these tumors due to the narrowness of the meatal foramen. Facial twitching and spasm should heighten the clinician's suspicion of a facial nerve neuroma, and patients should be counseled about intraoperative findings that may warrant decompression procedures versus resection.

■ Limiting Risk of Facial Paralysis

There is considerable controversy and variable practice patterns for the management of acoustic neuromas. Treatment decisions must consider a constellation of factors, such as the age of the patient, the overall health of the patient, the symptoms caused by the tumor, and the progression of symptoms attributable to the tumor.[5] If a patient and surgeon elect microsurgical management, treatment-specific considerations must be made regarding the position of the tumor, preoperative hearing, and anatomic features. The patient must be well informed regarding the risks of surgery, which may be substantial in view of these factors. As with all benign tumors, management decisions must be made with emphasis toward minimizing complication and morbidity, while achieving favorable outcome.

For many patients, observation is appropriate for acoustic tumors. Multiple meta-analyses have demonstrated that, particularly in the IAC, a large proportion of acoustic neuromas are quiescent, and symptoms are not related to size or patient age.[6] Recent studies cite that over long-term follow-up, approximately less than one-third of intracanalicular tumors demonstrate radiological evidence of growth, although hearing deterioration occurs regardless of growth.[7–10] From a series of 70 patients older than 65 with acoustic neuroma followed for a mean duration of 4.8 years, 42% of tumors did not grow or regressed.[11] In patients who are asymptomatic from an audiologic, vestibular, and facial nerve standpoint, the main impetus toward intervention may be a patient's desire to address the anxiety associated with an intracranial mass. It is important to be knowledgeable about the natural history of these tumors, and the patient must be informed that if symptoms develop, or radiographic characteristics change, intervention may become warranted.

Observation is not always innocuous, however, and may lead to sudden and complete hearing loss, imbalance, or facial nerve weakness. Facial weakness is an ominous sign that a patient may suffer the sudden onset of facial paralysis from tumor growth, and it should be treated aggressively. Still, the rate of facial nerve weakness as a presenting symptom of an acoustic neuroma is ~5%, and although this rate is low, subsequent facial nerve paralysis can have devastating and permanent effects. Despite multivariate analyses on the natural history of acoustic neuromas, no clinical or radiological factors have been identified as predictive of tumor behavior.

Radiosurgical management of acoustic neuromas can be a favorable option for many reasons. The treatment is brief, does not require general anesthesia, and sidesteps multiple complications that are nearly exclusively associated with surgical resection. Initially, it was described as an adjunct for incompletely resected acoustic neuromas, but more recently, it is offered as a primary modality for treatment. Treatment goals with radiosurgical techniques are inherently very different from surgical aims. There is an expanding body of literature suggesting that radiation may arrest vestibular schwannoma tumor growth, possibly through radiation-induced fibrosis and damage to tumor vasculature. The patient must be made aware that the tumor will remain after treatment, and that those symptoms such as hearing loss, imbalance, and tinnitus may progress.[12]

The effectiveness of radiation for management of these tumors is a particularly difficult subject of research secondary to the slow-growing nature of these tumors and heterogeneity in outcomes measures (i.e., radiographic criteria for growth, audiometry, vestibular symptoms, and tinnitus handicap). There is considerable variability in the description of the natural history of these tumors, and the application of radiation is transitioning to those tumors that have radiographic evidence suggesting growth. There is a 6- to 12-month period of transient tumor expansion after radiation in ~16% of treated patients, suggested to be a result of the edema associated with central tumor necrosis, which further confounds reported measures.[13] Radiosurgery methods vary from center to center, based on available equipment and personnel. Investigations are ongoing comparing the long-term advantages and effects of different administration techniques such as Gamma Knife (Elekta, Stockholm, Sweden), Cyberknife (Accuray, Sunnyvale, California), LINAC (linear accelerator radiotherapy), and fractionated radiotherapy. Published results are promising and suggest a high (> 95%) 10-year tumor control rate, with a limited immediate side-effect profile.

The marginal dose of radiation administered is a critical predictive factor for facial paresis with radiotherapy. Earlier studies described a rate of facial nerve paresis of ~21% when the average marginal tumor dose was 16 Gy using a Gamma Knife system.[14] Currently, most centers use a marginal tumor dose between 12 and 14 Gy; facial nerve outcomes have improved considerably. The rate of facial nerve weakness after radiotherapy is now cited at < 1% for both Gamma Knife and LINAC systems.[14,15] Likewise, the rate of trigeminal neuropathy has fallen from 16% to 4.4% as the marginal doses were decreased, and the trigeminal nerve is rarely affected by radiation for intracanalicular tumors.[16] Vertigo, tinnitus, hydrocephalus, xerophthalmia, sudden hearing loss, risk of radiation-induced malignancy, and accelerated vertebrobasilar atherosclerosis are described complications of radiotherapy, although their incidence in the setting of low-dose radiotherapy is unclear.

If the tumor continues to grow despite radiotherapy, literature suggests that surgical resection becomes more difficult and is associated with poorer facial nerve outcome. In a recent review by Friedman and colleagues, 46% of patients treated with salvage microsurgery had complete facial weakness at their first postoperative visit.[17] Histologically, this is supported by studies that have demonstrated significant tumor fibrosis and facial nerve adherence after radiotherapy.[18,19] It is possible that as the technology for radiotherapy administration changes, its effect on the facial nerve and surrounding structures will be further reduced.

◼ Microsurgery

There are three commonly used approaches for acoustic neuroma resections: the translabyrinthine craniotomy, the middle fossa craniotomy, and the retrosigmoid craniotomy. Each affords a different view of the CPA and has advantages and disadvantages that will be reviewed. Facial nerve outcomes have improved as imaging and monitoring have made advances. Magnetic resonance imaging has improved the clinician's ability to detect small, minimally symptomatic acoustic neuromas. Intraoperative facial nerve monitoring has had dramatic effects on dissection technique.

Since its introduction, intraoperative facial nerve monitoring has played a vital role in improving facial nerve integrity from 67%, to current studies that cite facial nerve anatomic integrity of > 98%.[20] Multiple studies have suggested intraoperative parameters that aid with prediction of both immediate and long-term facial nerve outcomes.[21,22] These can further inform intraoperative decision making and guide rehabilitative procedures that may be done to prevent exposure keratitis. If facial nerve stimulation, proximal to the site of tumor resection, remains 0.04 mA or less, than there is a 77% probability that the patient will have House-Brackmann (HB) grade I/II facial nerve function at 8 days postoperatively.[23] Electrophysical facial nerve monitoring has proven more sensitive that observation or video capture technology, and remains a useful tool for minimizing morbidity in acoustic neuroma surgery.[24]

Translabyrinthine Craniotomy

Since the development of the translabyrinthine approach for CPA tumors by Dr. William F. House in the early 1970s, there have been relatively few modifications to this approach, and it remains a workhorse in the surgical management of acoustic neuromas. Facial nerve monitoring and auditory brainstem response monitoring have made tumor dissection safer for the patient and have improved clinical outcomes. An advantage of this approach is its wide exposure of the IAC and brainstem with very limited cerebellar retraction. It affords excellent hand position at a relatively shallow depth of field, making it a comfortable

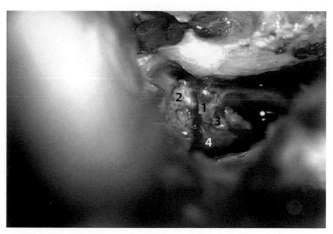

Fig. 20.2 Translabyrinthinc craniotomy, right ear. A high-magnification view of the internal auditory canal. (*1*) Transverse crest. (*2*) Superior vestibular nerve. (*3*) Inferior vestibular nerve. (*4*) Tumor.

procedure for the surgeon. The facial nerve can be visualized throughout its entire intratemporal course, affording perspective during tumor dissection.

Early studies suggested that the translabyrinthine craniotomy was the gold standard in facial nerve preservation microsurgery of the IAC, although more recent studies suggest that the experienced surgeon can achieve similar outcomes through the middle fossa craniotomy.[25,26] Studies performed at the House Clinic indicated that 98.5% of patients treated with this approach between 1984 and 1989 had an anatomically intact facial nerves postoperatively.[27] This approach permits identification of the proximal and distal facial nerve during tumor dissection, has consistent intraoperative landmarks, and provides a panoramic view suitable for removal of large tumors (**Figs. 20.1, 20.2, 20.3, 20.4, 20.5, and 20.6**).

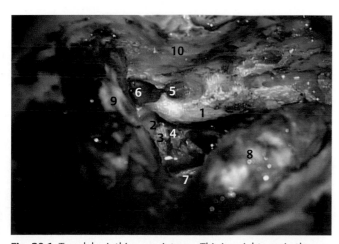

Fig. 20.1 Translabyrinthine craniotomy. This is a right ear, in the surgical position, approached for a small (1.5 cm) acoustic neuroma. (*1*) Descending segment, facial nerve. (*2*) Vertical crest (Bill bar). (*3*) Superior vestibular nerve. (*4*) Transverse crest. (*5*) The incus has been removed, and the Eustachian tube has been packed with temporalis muscle. (*6*) Epitympanum. (*7*) Posterior fossa dura. (*8*) Sigmoid sinus, with a thin layer of bone on its surface (Bill island). (*9*) Middle fossa dura. (*10*) External auditory canal.

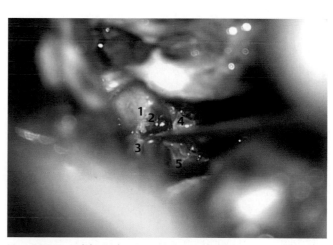

Fig. 20.3 Translabyrinthine craniotomy, right ear. The dissection begins with proximal identification of the facial nerve. (*1*) Vertical crest (Bill bar). (*2*) Facial nerve, labyrinthine segment. (*3*) Superior vestibular nerve, reflected posteriorly. (*4*) Transverse crest. (*5*) Tumor reflected posteriorly.

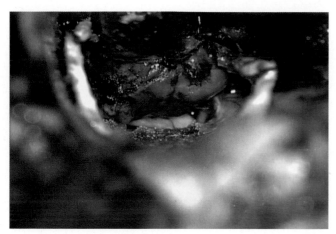

Fig. 20.4 Translabyrinthine craniotomy, right ear. The proximal seventh and eighth nerve complexes are identified. Intracapsular debulking of the tumor may aid with visualization.

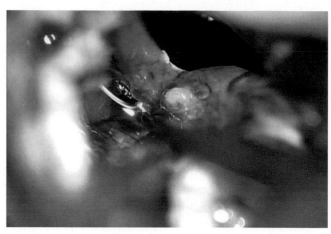

Fig. 20.6 Translabyrinthine craniotomy, right ear. Note the nodularity on the tumor surface. In this case, the tumor was densely adherent to the facial nerve in this location, and the plane was sharply dissected.

While facial nerve transection is extremely rare in this approach, injuries to the sensory contribution of the facial nerve are common (**Fig. 20.7**). A review of 224 patients who underwent acoustic neuroma resection revealed that few (2–6%) patients noted tearing while eating, xerophthalmia, or taste abnormalities preoperatively. When questioned postoperatively, 44% of those patients described tearing while eating. Reduction in tearing was noted in 72%, and taste alterations were noted in 48%. Recovery was variable in this study, and the authors suggested nervus intermedius dysfunction should be included in reporting criteria.[28]

A high-riding jugular bulb or an anteriorly positioned, dominant sigmoid sinus are not contraindications to translabyrinthine approach. The presence of active chronic otitis media is, however, considered a contraindication and may require a staged procedure with ear canal overclosure.

The most noteworthy disadvantage exclusive to the translabyrinthine craniotomy is the passage through inner ear structures and subsequent sacrifice of hearing. While there are reports of hearing preservation through a partial labyrinthectomy, with meticulous waxing and resurfacing of the semicircular canals intraoperatively, this practice is not commonplace.[29] Also, with cochlea and cochlear nerve preservation, descriptions of cochlear implantation have been published, although circumstances warranting this approach are rare.[30] Frequently, placement of an osseointegrated bone conduction hearing device can be performed at the time of tumor resection, although considerations must be made toward avoiding communication with the mastoid cavity and subsequent development of a CSF leak. This permits hearing perception bilaterally, but patients must be counseled that this ability does not afford sound localization, as sound is simply rerouted to the contralateral, functional cochlea.

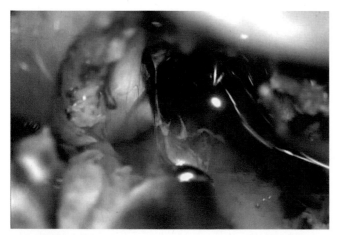

Fig. 20.5 Translabyrinthine craniotomy, right ear. A plane between the facial nerve and the tumor is identified and followed, using a combination of blunt and sharp dissection. A suction irrigator helps with visualization by washing away minor bleeding.

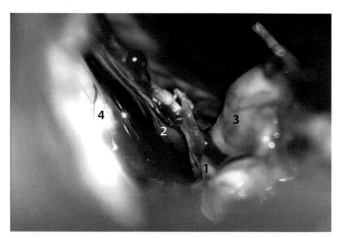

Fig. 20.7 Translabyrinthine craniotomy, right ear. Tumor resection is nearly complete. Note the tumor is adherent to the nervus intermedius. (*1*) Nervus intermedius. (*2*) Facial nerve. (*3*) Tumor. (*4*) Trigeminal nerve.

Early after introduction of the translabyrinthine craniotomy, the medical community expressed concerns regarding the risk of meningeal and intracranial contamination with otogenic bacteria. Instead, meningitis is described as extremely rare in most series, at ~1%. A CSF leak, however, increases the risk of meningitis to roughly 14%.[31] A large review of 600 cases cited the rate of CSF leak after translabyrinthine approach, either through the incision or the eustachian tube and presenting as rhinorrhea, as 1.8%.[32] Abducens paralysis, lower cranial nerve injury, major intracranial vessel injury, or parenchymal injuries are extremely rare. The mortality rate from complications of this approach is extremely low (< 1%), although medical comorbidities, as with any major surgery, must be fully addressed preoperatively. Special consideration must be made toward the period of vestibular rehabilitation postoperatively, which may involve several days of nausea, visual tracking difficulty, and bed rest.

At the authors' institution, patients are observed in the intensive care unit for one evening postoperatively, and early ambulation is encouraged. Facial nerve monitoring is prerequisite; perioperative antibiotics are continued for 24 hours postoperatively; abdominal fat grafting and Eustachian tube plugging are routine. Lumbar drains are reserved for patients at high risk for CSF leak, such as preoperative hydrocephalus or intracranial hypertension.

Middle Fossa Craniotomy

The middle fossa craniotomy approach to the IAC was likewise first described by Dr. William F. House, although it was initially described as a technique for management of cochlear otosclerosis. Its usage for management of acoustic neuroma grew as imaging capabilities have changed, and clinicians are able to detect small tumors with serviceable hearing. Its primary advantage over the translabyrinthine approach is its ability to preserve auditory function, and it is ideally suited for resection of the small, intracanalicular acoustic neuroma (**Figs. 20.8** and **20.9**).

The procedure begins with a 5 × 5-cm temporal craniotomy above the zygoma, with the patient in the supine position, preferably with the zygoma parallel to the operating bed. Mannitol and furosemide are administered to permit dural relaxation. As the floor of the middle fossa is identified, the surgeon must be aware that the geniculate ganglion is dehiscent in ~15% of patients and may be injured during dural elevation. The dura should be elevated from a posterior to anterior direction when exposing the roof of the temporal bone to minimize these traction injuries to the geniculate ganglion. The greater superficial petrosal nerve can typically be identified after dural elevation and traced posteriorly to the geniculate ganglion. The greater superficial petrosal nerve can be stimulated, via antidromic conduction, to confirm its identity.[33]

Drilling to provide exposure of the IAC should be performed on the posterior surface of the petrosal bone to

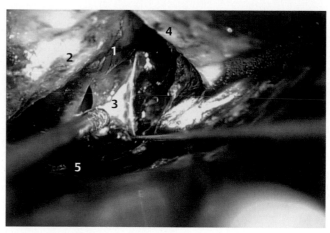

Fig. 20.8 Middle fossa craniotomy, left ear. The dura is reflected from the internal auditory canal (IAC). An acoustic neuroma can be seen situated laterally in the IAC. A House-Urban retractor has been placed under the lip of the porus acousticus. The patient received diuretics and was hyperventilated to facilitate retraction. (1) Tumor. (2) Arcuate eminence. (3) Dura of the IAC. (4) Cochlea. (5) Middle fossa dura.

avoid direct or thermal injury to the facial nerve. The IAC can then be skeletonized from the porus medially to the labyrinth and cochlea laterally. The dura of the IAC is then opened on its posterior surface and reflected anteriorly. Given its superior position in the IAC, the facial nerve may be in an unfavorable position for tumor resection. Unfortunately, this determination cannot be made preoperatively, and tumor dissection requires patience, meticulous technique, and careful understanding of anatomic relationships.

Despite the anatomic considerations that can position the facial nerve between the surgeon and the tumor, multiple series have demonstrated favorable facial nerve outcomes that compare well with the translabyrinthine approach, with HB scores of I to II in > 96%.[34,35] Still, anatomic and technical challenges, as identified through

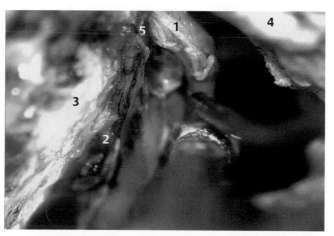

Fig. 20.9 Middle fossa craniotomy, left ear. The dura has been reflected from the internal auditory canal, and the facial nerve has been identified. The cochlear nerve is not visible at this point of the dissection. (1) Facial nerve. (2) Tumor. (3) Arcuate eminence. (4) Cochlea. (5) Vertical crest (Bill bar).

radiography and electrophysical testing, must be fairly presented to the patient prior to selection of approach. The largest series describing this approach in acoustic neuroma microsurgery indicate a hearing preservation rate of 60–73%.[34-36] Although the cochlear nerve is typically preserved during this approach, the cochlear artery, which runs on the superior surface of the nerve, may be injured during tumor dissection. Also, the cochlea and labyrinth mark the anterior limit of the IAC bony dissection, and if these landmarks prove difficult to visualize, they may be easily violated.

The middle fossa craniotomy has the disadvantages of a greater area of dural exposure, the need for temporal lobe retraction, and challenging surgical anatomy. While brain retraction can be mitigated by patient positioning to avoid jugular vein compression, administration of mannitol, and quick, decisive tumor exposure, complications such as venous infarct and stroke are extremely rare. The rate of CSF leak is still rare, although slightly higher than the translabyrinthine approach, secondary to challenges created by a pneumatized petrous apex, tegmen mastoideum, or tympani dehiscence.[36] Meningitis rates, fortunately, are still very rare, and the risk of epidural hematoma can be mitigated by placement of a Penrose drain beneath the craniotomy flap, to be removed on the first postoperative day.

At the authors' institution, we routinely employ caloric testing to aid with decision making, as inferior vestibular nerve tumors present additional challenge during hearing preservation surgery. The presence of a well-pronounced auditory brainstem response, and visualization of CSF in the fundus of the IAC on T2-weighted magnetic resonance imaging, influences decision making in determining suitable cases for hearing preservation surgery. CSF in the fundus of the IAC portends a higher rate of hearing preservation (77%) in middle fossa surgery compared with those cases in which the distal IAC is obstructed by tumor (52%).[37] Similar to the translabyrinthine approach, patients spend one evening in the intensive care unit for neurological checks, and early ambulation and vestibular rehabilitation are encouraged. Lumbar drains are not typically placed perioperatively, except in special circumstances.

■ Retrosigmoid Craniotomy

The restrosigmoid craniotomy can be utilized for resection of almost any ear acoustic neuroma, although small, laterally positioned tumors may not be accessible via this approach without injuring the labyrinth (**Fig. 20.10**). It is most suitable for patients with medially situated tumors and serviceable hearing. The entire posterior surface of the temporal bone can be visualized, and as the labyrinth is not violated, it can be used in hearing preservation techniques. Likewise, the jugular foramen can be visualized, which makes it a versatile approach for CPA management for patients with neurofibromatosis type 2, who

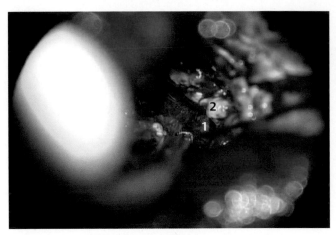

Fig. 20.10 Retrosigmoid craniotomy, left ear. The facial nerve is not visualized until the tumor has nearly been removed. The cochlear nerve is obscured by pledgets placed for hemostasis. (*1*) Facial nerve. (*2*) Tumor.

may have concurrent jugular foramen lesions. The greatest disadvantages of this approach are its poor anterior visualization during dissection, the violation of dura and cerebellar retraction, and the rate of postoperative headache. Postoperative headaches may be prolonged over many months, and even years, and is theoretically a manifestation of aseptic meningitis related to intradural bone dust or excessively taught dural closure. While bone dust may be reduced by careful irrigation prior to opening the dura, the rate of headache still remains higher than the other approaches (10%), and patients must be informed of this risk preoperatively.[38]

For the retrosigmoid approach, facial nerve outcomes can approach the outcomes seen in the translabyrinthine and middle fossa approaches, when subtotal and partial resections are performed.[39] The rate of hearing preservation has been cited as high as 73.2%, although a recent meta-analysis suggested a rate of 47%.[40,41] The cochlear nerve is frequently obscured by the tumor, and its blood supply runs on its superomedial surface, next to the facial nerve. Because the facial nerve and cochlear nerve are not identified until the end of the surgery, most centers report slightly poorer functional outcomes. Endoscopes can be used to visualize the lateral IAC, and reduced recurrence rates have been reported. Unfortunately, if the patient's hearing is poor immediately postoperatively (as evaluated by a Weber test), the prognosis for hearing recovery is poor.

■ Long-Term Facial Nerve Outcomes

In all microsurgical cases, identification of the facial nerve proximal and distal to the tumor helps with determination of dissection depth and provides a baseline stimulation threshold prior to tumor removal. The majority of facial nerve weakness after microsurgery for acoustic neuromas represents neuropraxia in the setting of a structurally intact facial nerve. Ninety percent of facial nerves that stimulate well intraoperatively are HB grade I/II at 1 year postoperative.[42] Several papers have described a fixed point in time at which the prognosis for facial nerve recovery can be determined. Arriaga et al[27] suggested that if postoperative facial nerve function is extremely poor (HB grade V/VI), then the possibility of an acceptable facial nerve outcome at 1 year postoperative (HB I–IV) still remains 69.8%. This was supported by work from Fenton et al, who evaluated the immediate postoperative facial nerve function and found that if it was greater than HB grade III, there remained a 77% chance of the patient having a HB II or III at a 2-year postoperative visit.[43] While immediate postoperative facial weakness is more common in middle fossa and retrosigmoid approaches, outcomes appear similar at 1 year postoperatively.[44]

Tumor size and patient age, but not the approach, appear to most strongly influence long-term facial nerve function.[45,46] At 1 year postoperatively, Wiet et al demonstrated that small tumors (< 1.5 cm) have a > 90% chance of HB grade I/II, intermediate tumors (1.5 to 3.0 cm) have a 75% chance of HB grade I/II, and large tumors (> 3.0 cm) had a 30% chance of HB grade I/II.[46] The authors of this chapter affirm that facial nerve outcomes improved as they gained experience. Not surprisingly, larger tumors tend to splay the facial nerve and render dissection more challenging. If the tumor is densely adherent to the nerve, then it has become common practice to leave a small rind of tumor on the surface of the facial nerve, in lieu of causing permanent facial nerve dysfunction. These cases are followed with repeat gadolinium-enhanced magnetic resonance imaging in 6 months to evaluate residual tumor, and a repeat scan is performed in 1 year to evaluate for tumor growth. Tumor residual smaller than 2–3 mm rarely grows to the point of requiring re-resection, partly because of the extensive IAC decompression performed as part of the approach. Reduced tumor growth is likely related to tumor devascularization during the initial dissection, and only 11% of subtotal resections require revision procedures.[47] In the small percentage of cases in which tumor re-resection is required, typically a revision of the same approach may be performed, as the planes of dissection are usually still maintained, despite the presence of scar tissue. Advanced patient age has also been found to be a risk factor for long-term postoperative facial weakness, which may represent a diminished vascular supply to the nerve.

Surgeon experience and hospital volume have been strongly linked to favorable postoperative overall outcomes, with high-volume facilities being 15 times more likely to achieve routine, favorable postoperative outcomes.[48] The effect this has upon facial nerve outcome is only anecdotal at this point, but as demonstrated in other surgical fields, surgeon experience likely improves outcomes.[49–52]

If a patient demonstrates facial weakness postoperatively, but the proximal nerve had stimulated vigorously prior to conclusion of the surgery, the patient is managed with postoperative glucocorticoids and supportive care. Dexamethasone is routinely initiated at 4 mg intravenously every 6 hours and tapered at 48 hours postoperatively. In the immediate postoperative period, steroids have the added benefit of decreasing perioperative nausea, facial edema, and headache. Steroids are occasionally continued as an outpatient, if there are no major medical contraindications. It is very rare to see delayed wound healing or CSF leak as a complication of short-term perioperative steroids, although many patients experience transient mood disturbances, insomnia, hyperglycemia, or blood pressure effects at these dosages. Occasionally, facial nerve weakness may develop several days postoperatively (delayed facial nerve paralysis); this is still treated with high-dose steroids. Fortunately, the vast majority of delayed facial nerve weakness seen in the perioperative period will recover. Still, immediate facial paralysis has been identified as a risk factor in long-term facial paralysis.[53] More severe paralyses, HB grades IV/VI, are associated with a higher risk of long-term weakness and potential development of synkinesis.

Rarely, in large tumors, the facial nerve may be transected as a result of tumor removal. If the facial nerve is transected intraoperatively, reanastamosis of the nerve ends should be attempted at the same setting. Blood, inflammation, and edema make staging a second procedure more challenging, and all reasonable efforts should be made toward primary reanastamosis. It is highly unlikely that the proximal end of the facial nerve will be identified in a staged procedure, making the likelihood of success very small. Early reanastamosis helps avoid the deleterious effects of Wallerian degeneration and muscle atrophy that occur after a prolonged delay prior to repair. If a segment of nerve is surgically absent, considerations may be made toward cable grafting, with the most common donor sites being the greater auricular nerve, the medial antebrachial cutaneous nerve, or the sural nerve. Synthetic nerve conduits and scaffolds make intuitive sense in proximal facial nerve repair (i.e., anastamosis is particularly challenging in the labyrinthine segment secondary to the narrow caliber of the nerve). Nerve tubules make anastomosis of the intracranial facial nerve easier. The intracranial facial nerve lacks an epineurium, so suturing of the nerve can be very difficult. The tubules have given excellent results without the need for suturing. This is an exciting, quickly developing area of research in facial nerve repair.

■ Delayed Facial Paralysis

Occasionally, patients may demonstrate a well-functioning facial nerve immediately after surgery, whose function may deteriorate at some point in the postoperative period, usually within the first 72 hours. This phenomenon has been attributed to viral reactivation and occurs in ~10–30% of patients, regardless of surgical approach and tumor dimensions.[54] Other theories are that it represents a process related to postoperative fat packing, a vascular phenomenon, or postoperative edema.

In 2004, a series of 348 patients with acoustic neuroma managed with microsurgery was reviewed in which 8 patients developed delayed facial paralysis occurring more than 72 hours postoperatively.[55] Antibodies specific for antiherpes viruses 1 and 2, as well as varicella zoster viruses, were markedly elevated, suggesting that the patients developed a viral reactivation associated with their facial weakness. From this research, it became customary for us to treat patients with famciclovir (500 mg twice a day × 3 days preoperatively, and 500 mg twice a day × 5 days postoperatively) to reduce the risk of delayed facial paralysis. In a comparison study, we found that the rate of delayed facial paralysis was significantly diminished by usage of perioperative antivirals, particularly in patients who underwent a translabyrinthine approach.[56]

■ Conclusion

Regardless of treatment approach, permanent facial nerve injury is a relatively rare occurrence for the management of the small and intermediate-sized acoustic neuroma. Large (> 3 cm) tumors are associated with a higher incidence of postoperative facial nerve paralysis, regardless of surgical approach. Treatment algorithms should be directed by the patient's wishes, and a careful risk-benefit analysis should be performed prior to surgical approach selection.

References

1. Selesnick SH, Jackler RK. Clinical manifestations and audiologic diagnosis of acoustic neuromas. Otolaryngol Clin North Am 1992;25(3):521–551
2. Hitselberger WE, House WF. Acoustic neuroma diagnosis. External auditory canal hypesthesia as an early sign. Arch Otolaryngol 1966;83(3):218–221
3. Eshraghi AA, Buchman CA, Telischi FF. Sensory auricular branch of the facial nerve. Otol Neurotol 2002;23(3):393–396
4. McMenomey SO, Glasscock ME III, Minor LB, Jackson CG, Strasnick B. Facial nerve neuromas presenting as acoustic tumors. Am J Otol 1994;15(3):307–312
5. Doherty JK, Friedman RA. Controversies in building a management algorithm for vestibular schwannomas. Curr Opin Otolaryngol Head Neck Surg 2006;14(5):305–313
6. van Leeuwen JP, Cremers CW, Thewissen NP, Harhangi BS, Meijer E. Acoustic neuroma: correlation among tumor size, symptoms, and patient age. Laryngoscope 1995;105(7 Pt 1):701–707
7. Al Sanosi A, Fagan PA, Biggs ND. Conservative management of acoustic neuroma. Skull Base 2006;16(2):95–100
8. Yoshimoto Y. Systematic review of the natural history of vestibular schwannoma. J Neurosurg 2005;103(1):59–63
9. Charabi S, Tos M, Thomsen J, Charabi B, Mantoni M. Vestibular schwannoma growth—long-term results. Acta Otolaryngol Suppl 2000;543:7–10
10. Raut VV, Walsh RM, Bath AP, et al. Conservative management of vestibular schwannomas - second review of a prospective longitudinal study. Clin Otolaryngol Allied Sci 2004;29(5):505–514
11. Rosenberg SI. Natural history of acoustic neuromas. Laryngoscope 2000;110(4):497–508
12. Hempel JM, Hempel E, Wowra B, Schichor Ch, Muacevic A, Riederer A. Functional outcome after gamma knife treatment in vestibular schwannoma. Eur Arch Otorhinolaryngol 2006;263(8):714–718
13. Roos DE, Brophy BP, Bhat MK, Katsilis ES. Update of radiosurgery at the Royal Adelaide Hospital. Australas Radiol 2006;50(2):158–167
14. Kondziolka D, Lunsford LD, McLaughlin MR, Flickinger JC. Long-term outcomes after radiosurgery for acoustic neuromas. N Engl J Med 1998;339(20):1426–1433
15. Mendenhall WM, Friedman WA, Buatti JM, Bova FJ. Preliminary results of linear accelerator radiosurgery for acoustic schwannomas. J Neurosurg 1996;85(6):1013–1019
16. Chopra R, Kondziolka D, Niranjan A, Lunsford LD, Flickinger JC. Long-term follow-up of acoustic schwannoma radiosurgery with marginal tumor doses of 12 to 13 Gy. Int J Radiat Oncol Biol Phys 2007;68(3):845–851
17. Friedman RA, Brackmann DE, Hitselberger WE, Schwartz MS, Iqbal Z, Berliner KI. Surgical salvage after failed irradiation for vestibular schwannoma. Laryngoscope 2005;115(10):1827–1832
18. Lee F, Linthicum F Jr, Hung G. Proliferation potential in recurrent acoustic schwannoma following gamma knife radiosurgery versus microsurgery. Laryngoscope 2002;112(6):948–950
19. Lee DJ, Westra WH, Staecker H, Long D, Niparko JK, Slattery WH III. Clinical and histopathologic features of recurrent vestibular schwannoma (acoustic neuroma) after stereotactic radiosurgery. Otol Neurotol 2003;24(4):650–660, discussion 660
20. Esses BA, LaRouere MJ, Graham MD. Facial nerve outcome in acoustic tumor surgery. Am J Otol 1994;15(6):810–812
21. Grayeli AB, Guindi S, Kalamarides M, et al. Four-channel electromyography of the facial nerve in vestibular schwannoma surgery: sensitivity and prognostic value for short-term facial function outcome. Otol Neurotol 2005;26(1):114–120
22. Neff BA, Ting J, Dickinson SL, Welling DB. Facial nerve monitoring parameters as a predictor of postoperative facial nerve outcomes after vestibular schwannoma resection. Otol Neurotol 2005;26(4):728–732
23. Bernat I, Grayeli AB, Esquia G, Zhang Z, Kalamarides M, Sterkers O. Intraoperative electromyography and surgical observations as predictive factors of facial nerve outcome in vestibular schwannoma surgery. Otol Neurotol 2010;31(2):306–312
24. De Seta E, Bertoli G, De Seta D, Covelli E, Filipo R. New development in intraoperative video monitoring of facial nerve: a pilot study. Otol Neurotol 2010;31(9):1498–1502 10.1097/MAO.0b013e3181f20822
25. Arriaga MA, Luxford WM, Berliner KI. Facial nerve function following middle fossa and translabyrinthine acoustic tumor surgery: a comparison. Am J Otol 1994;15(5):620–624
26. Hillman T, Chen DA, Arriaga MA, Quigley M. Facial nerve function and hearing preservation acoustic tumor surgery: does the approach matter? Otolaryngol Head Neck Surg 2010;142(1):115–119 10.1016/j.otohns.2009.10.015
27. Arriaga MA, Luxford WM, Atkins JS Jr, Kwartler JA. Predicting long-term facial nerve outcome after acoustic neuroma surgery. Otolaryngol Head Neck Surg 1993;108(3):220–224

28. Irving RM, Viani L, Hardy DG, Baguley DM, Moffat DA. Nervus intermedius function after vestibular schwannoma removal: clinical features and pathophysiological mechanisms. Laryngoscope 1995;105(8 Pt 1):809–813

29. Hirsch BE, Cass SP, Sekhar LN, Wright DC. Translabyrinthine approach to skull base tumors with hearing preservation. Am J Otol 1993;14(6):533–543

30. Arístegui M, Denia A. Simultaneous cochlear implantation and translabyrinthine removal of vestibular schwannoma in an only hearing ear: report of two cases (neurofibromatosis type 2 and unilateral vestibular schwannoma). Otol Neurotol 2005;26(2):205–210

31. Selesnick SH, Liu JC, Jen A, Newman J. The incidence of cerebrospinal fluid leak after vestibular schwannoma surgery. Otol Neurotol 2004;25(3):387–393

32. Sanna M, Taibah A, Russo A, Falcioni M, Agarwal M. Perioperative complications in acoustic neuroma (vestibular schwannoma) surgery. Otol Neurotol 2004;25(3):379–386

33. Arriaga MA, Haid RT, Masel DA. Antidromic stimulation of the greater superficial petrosal nerve in middle fossa surgery. Laryngoscope 1995;105(1):102–105

34. Arts HA, Telian SA, El-Kashlan H, Thompson BG. Hearing preservation and facial nerve outcomes in vestibular schwannoma surgery: results using the middle cranial fossa approach. Otol Neurotol 2006;27(2):234–241

35. Meyer TA, Canty PA, Wilkinson EP, Hansen MR, Rubinstein JT, Gantz BJ. Small acoustic neuromas: surgical outcomes versus observation or radiation. Otol Neurotol 2006;27(3):380–392

36. Brackmann DE, House JR III, Hitselberger WE. Technical modifications to the middle fossa craniotomy approach in removal of acoustic neuromas. Am J Otol 1994;15(5):614–619

37. Goddard JC, Schwartz MS, Friedman RA. Fundal fluid as a predictor of hearing preservation in the middle cranial fossa approach for vestibular schwannoma. Otol Neurotol 2010;31(7):1128–1134

38. Silverstein H, Norrell H, Wanamaker H, Flanzer J. Microsurgical posterior fossa vestibular neurectomy: an evolution in technique. Skull Base Surg 1991;1(1):16–25

39. Hillman T, Chen DA, Arriaga MA, Quigley M. Facial nerve function and hearing preservation acoustic tumor surgery: does the approach matter? Otolaryngol Head Neck Surg 2010;142(1):115–119

40. Sameshima T, Fukushima T, McElveen JT Jr, Friedman AH. Critical assessment of operative approaches for hearing preservation in small acoustic neuroma surgery: retrosigmoid vs middle fossa approach. Neurosurgery 2010;67(3):640–644, discussion 644–645

41. Sughrue ME, Yang I, Aranda D, Kane AJ, Parsa AT. Hearing preservation rates after microsurgical resection of vestibular schwannoma. J Clin Neurosci 2010;17(9):1126–1129

42. Lalwani AK, Butt FY, Jackler RK, Pitts LH, Yingling CD. Facial nerve outcome after acoustic neuroma surgery: a study from the era of cranial nerve monitoring. Otolaryngol Head Neck Surg 1994;111(5):561–570

43. Fenton JE, Chin RY, Fagan PA, Sterkers O, Sterkers JM. Predictive factors of long-term facial nerve function after vestibular schwannoma surgery. Otol Neurotol 2002;23(3):388–392

44. Isaacson B, Telian SA, El-Kashlan HK. Facial nerve outcomes in middle cranial fossa vs translabyrinthine approaches. Otolaryngol Head Neck Surg 2005;133(6):906–910

45. Mass SC, Wiet RJ, Dinces E. Complications of the translabyrinthine approach for the removal of acoustic neuromas. Arch Otolaryngol Head Neck Surg 1999;125(7):801–804

46. Wiet RJ, Mamikoglu B, Odom L, Hoistad DL. Long-term results of the first 500 cases of acoustic neuroma surgery. Otolaryngol Head Neck Surg 2001;124(6):645–651

47. Freeman SR, Ramsden RT, Saeed SR, et al. Revision surgery for residual or recurrent vestibular schwannoma. Otol Neurotol 2007;28(8):1076–1082

48. Slattery WH, Schwartz MS, Fisher LM, Oppenheimer M. Acoustic neuroma surgical cost and outcome by hospital volume in California. Otolaryngol Head Neck Surg 2004;130(6):726–735

49. Bach PB, Cramer LD, Schrag D, Downey RJ, Gelfand SE, Begg CB. The influence of hospital volume on survival after resection for lung cancer. N Engl J Med 2001;345(3):181–188

50. Birkmeyer JD, Siewers AE, Finlayson EV, et al. Hospital volume and surgical mortality in the United States. N Engl J Med 2002;346(15):1128–1137

51. Rosemurgy AS, Bloomston M, Serafini FM, Coon B, Murr MM, Carey LC. Frequency with which surgeons undertake pancreaticoduodenectomy determines length of stay, hospital charges, and in-hospital mortality. J Gastrointest Surg 2001;5(1):21–26

52. Dimick JB, Cattaneo SM, Lipsett PA, Pronovost PJ, Heitmiller RF. Hospital volume is related to clinical and economic outcomes of esophageal resection in Maryland. Ann Thorac Surg 2001;72(2):334–339, discussion 339–341

53. Isaacson B, Kileny PR, El-Kashlan HK. Prediction of long-term facial nerve outcomes with intraoperative nerve monitoring. Otol Neurotol 2005;26(2):270–273

54. Megerian CA, McKenna MJ, Ojemann RG. Delayed facial paralysis after acoustic neuroma surgery: factors influencing recovery. Am J Otol 1996;17(4):630–633

55. Franco-Vidal V, Nguyen DQ, Guerin J, Darrouzet V. Delayed facial paralysis after vestibular schwannoma surgery: role of herpes viruses reactivation—our experience in eight cases. Otol Neurotol 2004;25(5):805–810

56. Brackmann DE, Fisher LM, Hansen M, Halim A, Slattery WH. The effect of famciclovir on delayed facial paralysis after acoustic tumor resection. Laryngoscope 2008;118(9):1617–1620

21 Surgical Management of the Eye

Guy G. Massry

Facial nerve paresis has potentially significant ophthalmic and oculoplastic implications. Distal branches of the nerve innervate the orbicularis oculi muscle, which functions as the protractor of the eyelids. With muscle weakness comes variable degrees of reduced eyelid closure, eyelid malposition, ocular exposure, epiphora, and potentially significant corneal disease.[1,2] Some patients manifest symptoms that are mostly inconvenient and a nuisance. Others are severely bothered and may exhibit irritation, frank pain, and potentially visual loss.[3]

It is incumbent on all physicians who manage patients with facial paresis to evaluate and treat the ocular manifestations of the disease or work directly with someone who can. Most of the consequences of the facial paresis are visual and embarrassing (facial asymmetry), cause loss of function (facial movement), and psychological. Ocular manifestations, on the other hand, can lead to severe and permanent visual disability.

This chapter reviews the evaluation and management of patients with facial paresis as it relates to the eyes. Both conservative and surgical interventions are reviewed. The procedures described are those that the author has found to be reliably and reproducibly successful over time.

■ Anatomy

The frontal or temporal branch of the facial nerve innervates the upper division of the orbicualris oculi muscle, whose function is to close the upper eyelid and secondarily to depress the brow.[4] This branch also innervates the frontalis muscle, the primary elevator of the forehead and brow, and the corrugator and depressor supercilli muscles, which act as medial brow depressors. The zygomatic and some branches of the buccal division of the nerve innervate the lower lid portion of the orbiculars oculi muscle, which acts as the protractor of the lower lids.[4] Besides closing the eyelids and depressing the brows, specific potions of the orbicularis oculi are involved in the active process of tear drainage.[5] With this in mind, the characteristic ophthalmic manifestations of facial nerve damage become obvious and include (**Fig. 21.1**):

1. Brow ptosis (from frontalis weakening)
2. Upper lid retraction, lagophthalmos, and incomplete closure (from orbicularis weakness)
3. Lower lid laxity, weakness, or frank ectropion (from orbicularis weakness)

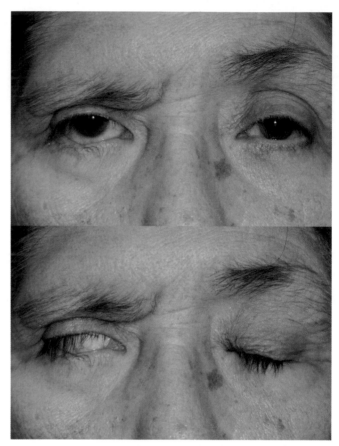

Fig. 21.1 Elderly woman with facial paresis on the right. Note (*top*) brow ptosis, relative upper lid retraction, with (*below*) lagophthalmos, poor lid closure, ocular exposure, and incipient lower lid ectropion.

4. Epiphora from lower lid weakness, reduced tear pump, and punctual malposition if ectropion present
5. Ocular exposure, corneal dryness, and corneal abrasion or ulcer (from poor corneal coverage)

■ Ophthalmic Evaluation

The range of ocular and periocular complications related to facial nerve dysfunction is varied and ranges from a mild inconvenience to potential threats to vision. For this reason, a thorough ophthalmic evaluation is needed in every case, and an individualized plan should be created to protect the eye, restore function, and re-create appearance.[6] Ocular protection and restoration of function are necessary steps in the process, and doing so in the most aesthetically acceptable way is desired.

Visual acuity is assessed and if reduced the cause sought out. In these patients, vision is usually reduced related to ocular surface irregularities (corneal dryness, abrasion, or infection) or welling up of tears from poor drainage. An examination of the pupils, motility, visual fields, and fundus is performed. Obviously, special time and attention is given to the slit-lamp and external evaluations. There are a number or corneal protective mechanisms that are assessed. These include tear production, eyelid closure, corneal sensation, and the Bell phenomenon. Reflex tear production is controlled in part by a distal autonomic branch of the facial nerve (the greater superficial petrosal nerve).[7] As such, tear production may decrease in facial paresis. As already mentioned, lid closure can be reduced if the orbicularis muscle is sufficiently damaged.

The cornea receives sensory innervations from the first division of cranial nerve V (ophthalmic nerve). If the pathology causing facial nerve disease also involves cranial nerve V, then corneal sensation may be affected. Corneal innervation is an integral part of maintaining epithelial integrity of the cornea. If sensation is reduced (neurotrophic cornea), corneal exposure is more difficult to treat. In addition, if sensation is reduced, the patient may not complain

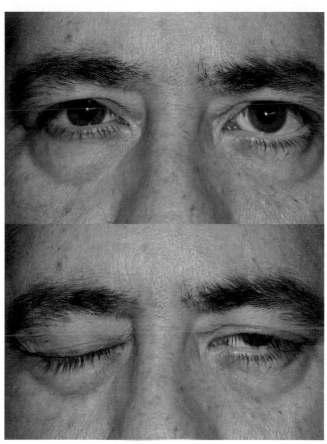

Fig. 21.3 Similar patient as in Fig. 21.2. In this instance, the Bell reflex is not intact. In these cases, corneal symptoms are observed even in more mild cases of nerve paresis.

of pain, which is a primary warning sign to seek medical attention. Finally, the Bell phenomenon is a reflex supraduction of the globe (elevation) when the lids close (Fig. 21.2). It protects the corneal surface when lid closure is reduced as the globe elevates under the upper lid. When reduced, the cornea is exposed during times of poor lid closure (Fig. 21.3). When all these mechanisms are intact, the cornea can typically withstand some degree of dryness and exposure. In the setting of facial nerve weakness, if one or all of these mechanisms fails, the cornea can decompensate.

■ Conservative Therapy

The most important steps in managing the ocular issues in facial paresis are to restore corneal protection. In cases that are milder where the cornea is generally stable, several noninvasive steps can be taken. The patient can manually lower the upper eyelid various times throughout the day and even tape (or patch) it closed for periods if necessary. This reduces exposure and may improve symptoms. Ocular lubrication with various over-the-counter lubricants can be applied on a frequent basis. Lubricant ointments

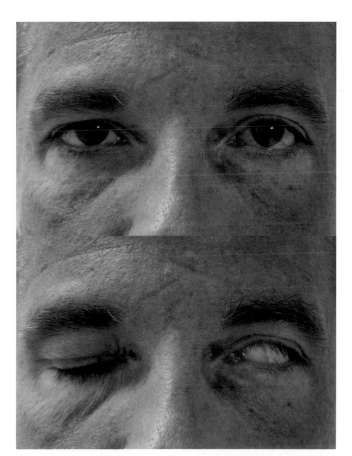

Fig. 21.2 Facial paresis patient with left-sided eyelid involvement. Note (top) open eyes and (below) forced eyelid closure. With the eyes closed (below), there is an intact Bell phenomenon. This typically conveys greater corneal protection even when paresis is more severe.

provide more protection of the cornea but blur vision. The author typically suggests such ointments at bedtime as vision is not an issue then, and they provide greater protection than tears for nocturnal lagophthalmos. At night, the lids can be taped closed, swimmer goggles can be used (acting as a humidifier), a humidifier can be placed in the bedroom, air conditioning can be turned off, and lubricants can be applied. If patients can be kept comfortable and out of harm's way with any of these measures and they tolerate their implementation, then surgery can be avoided. If not, surgical intervention should be considered.

■ Surgery

Brow Lift

Lifting a paretic brow can be a challenging endeavor. If paresis is mild and the concerns are primarily aesthetic, an endoscopic procedure, temporal lift, or even transeyelid browpexy may suffice. In more significant brow paresis, frontalis weakness limits the final result. In these cases, especially in patients who are older with preexisting forehead rhytids,[8] a direct brow lift is preferred. In the most severe cases, a perisoteal suspension is added for support. With meticulous three-layered closure, the scars heal well and are barely noticeable. The most difficult area to camouflage an incision is in the medial eyebrow where the thicker sebaceous skin tends to scar more significantly.

An ellipse is drawn above the brow in the area that is ptotic. After infiltration with anesthesia, an incision beveled in the direction of the brow hairs is made. The skin and subcutaneous tissue is excised, and hemostasis is assured. The wound is closed in layers. First deep tissue (muscle/subcutaneous fat) is secured with interrupted absorbable suture (5–0 Vicryl [Ethicon, Inc., Somerville, NJ] recommended). If periosteal fixation is performed, the deep sub-brow tissue at the inferior edge of the wound is engaged with a 4–0 Prolene suture (Ethicon, Inc.). This tissue is secured to the periosteum at the desired level by passing the suture through the deep brow tissue at the upper edge of the wound and tying the knot. This gives more brow support and creatures a more fixed brow position. Subcutaneous interrupted bites of the same 5–0 Vicryl suture are used to oppose the wound edges. The bites should be taken very close to the skin edge as to reduce tension on the wound. Finally, the skin is closed with a running 6–0 nylon suture. A running vertical mattress technique is preferred, but as long as the skin edges are intact and everted, any closure is appropriate (**Fig. 21.4**).

A direct brow lift is a very effective technique in the appropriate patient. When periosteal fixation is employed, brow animation is reduced. However, the author typically uses this technique only in the most severe cases where the paretic brow has little or no animation to start with.

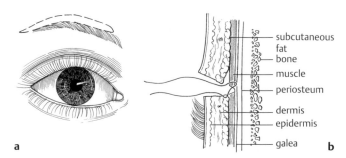

Fig. 21.4a, b Illustration demonstrating (**a**) demarcated ellipse of supra-brow tissue to be excised, and (**b**) deep sub-brow tissue being secured to periosteum (if performed).

Lower Eyelid Suspension

A variety of lower lid suspension techniques have been described to reinforce a lax eyelid with reduced tone. In cases of facial paresis, an appropriate outcome is harder to attain as the lower lid loses one of its primary support mechanisms: orbicularis tone. The orbicularis muscle is the primary eyelid protractor, and its tonic activity is needed to lend constant support to a structure whose tendency is to normally descend with age.[9] The other major influences on lower lid position are canthal tendon integrity, soft (skin, muscle, fat) and hard (bone) tissue support, and various ligaments that secure the lower lid and cheek to bone (orbitomalar ligament, etc.).[9] In younger patients who have not developed canthal tendon laxity and whose facial soft tissue and skeleton have not undergone involutional changes (atrophy), the main indicator of lid position in patients with facial paresis will be the orbicularis tone. If weakness is mild, eyelid lubrication may be all that is needed. However, if weakness is more severe, a lid suspension is warranted. Often, only a small permanent lateral tarsorrhaphy is adequate. In patients with more significant loss of eyelid support, greater canthal tendon laxity, and more severe orbicularis paresis, a more comprehensive support is needed. A traditional canthoplasty ("lateral tarsal strip procedure")[10] with or without the addition of a tarsorrhaphy is performed.

Tarsorrhaphy

A lateral tarsorrhaphy functions to enhance support for the paretic lower lid, to reduce ocular exposure by reducing the size of the palpebral aperture (horizontally and vertically), and to transfer the elevating effect of the upper lid to the lower lid. It can be performed on its own or in addition to a true canthal suspension (canthoplasty). In cases where immediate corneal coverage is needed on a temporary basis (a few weeks), a temporary tarsorrhaphy can be performed. The terminal upper and lower lid margins are anesthetized. A 4–0 silk suture is passed in a horizontal mattress fashion from upper to lower lid through skin/muscle and lid margin. The suture is tied over a foam bolster and secured. Rarely, the suture is left for longer than 2 weeks, so as to avoid skin erosion.

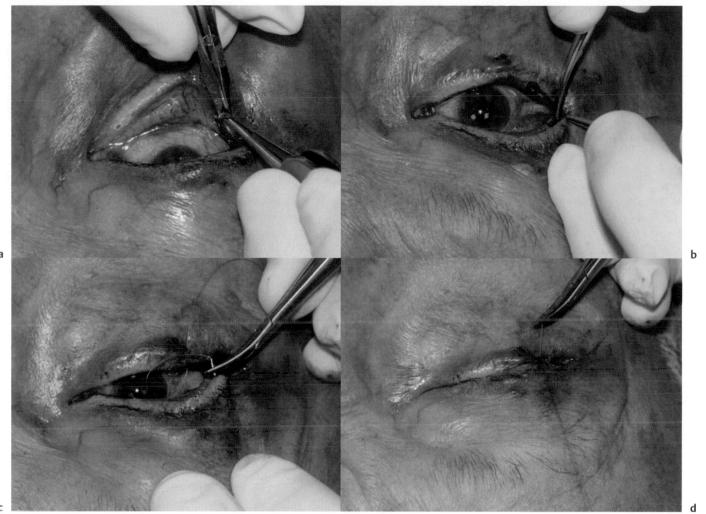

Fig. 21.5a, b Surgical series demonstrating permanent tarsorrhaphy procedure. (a) The muco-cutaneous junction of the lower lid is trimmed to the commisure posterior to the cilia. The same will be performed to the upper lid. (b) The anterior and posterior lamella are split to allow edges to evert when secured. (c) A 5-0 Chromic suture is passed between the anterior and posterior lamella of corresponding parts of the upper and lower lid. (d) The wound is closed.

If longer support is needed, a permanent intermarginal adhesion is created.[11] The terminal mucocutaneous junction of the upper and lower lids is trimmed and made continuous at the lateral commisure. The anterior and posterior lamella are split (this allows eversion of the lid margin edges when secured for adhesion), and a permanent or longer-acting absorbable suture is passed between anterior and posterior lamella of the upper to lower lid and secured. The author recommends to use a 5–0 chromic suture, which typically dissolves at 2 weeks (**Fig. 21.5**).

The tarsorrhaphy may shorten the horizontal palpebral fissure somewhat (**Fig. 21.6**), but this is typically not noticed as the loss of sphincter action of the paretic eye widens this distance as a consequence of muscle paresis. If the adhesion needs to be modified (made larger or smaller), it can be adjusted in the office under local anesthesia. When performing a permanent tarsorrhaphy, it is important to trim the mucocutaneous junction

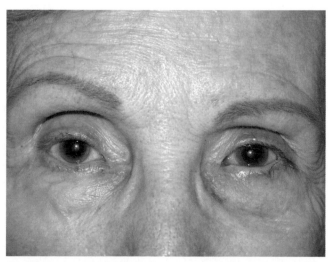

Fig. 21.6 A patient who had a 6 mm permanent tarsorrhaphy on the left. Note the small difference seen in the horizontal palpebral aperture.

posterior to the cilia so that if it is severed in the future, the incidence of trichiasis and lid margin irregularities is reduced.

Canthoplasty

The canthoplasty technique recommended is similar to that initially described by Anderson and Gordy in 1979.[10] The lateral canthus and temporal lower lid are anesthetized. A 7- to 8-mm canthotomy is performed. A tarsal tongue is fashioned in the standard way. This consists of a cantholysis (releasing the inferior crus of the lateral canthal tendon), separating the anterior and posterior lamella, trimming the mucocutaneous junction, and releasing the conjunctiva subtarsally (**Fig. 21.7**). The tarsal tongue is de-epithelialized, shortened appropriately, engaged with a 4–0 Vicryl suture on a half circle needle (P-2), sutured to the inner orbital rim periosteum (Whitnall tubercle), and secured. The canthus is then closed (**Fig. 21.8**). A lateral

tarsorrhaphy is added as needed to provide additional support and reduce the dimensions of the palpebral fissure for better corneal coverage.

In cases when lower lid support is severely lacking, a hammock-type sling can be added to support the lower lid.[12] This is most useful when midface strength has been sufficiently reduced that the weight of the cheek drags the lower lid down. The author prefers midface suspension techniques,[13] with or without spacer grafts,[14] in this scenario, as they are performed transconjunctivally as this techniques does not further manipulate the weakened orbicularis muscle. When a sling is performed, the material used can be a homologous or autologous (fascia lata) or alloplastic material. It is threaded through the lower lid posterior to the orbicularis muscle and anterior to the tarsus just under the eyelid margin. It is secured to the medial and lateral canthal tendon attachments (**Fig. 21.9**). The author has performed this procedure on only selected cases as the suspensions techniques mentioned have proven reliably successful.

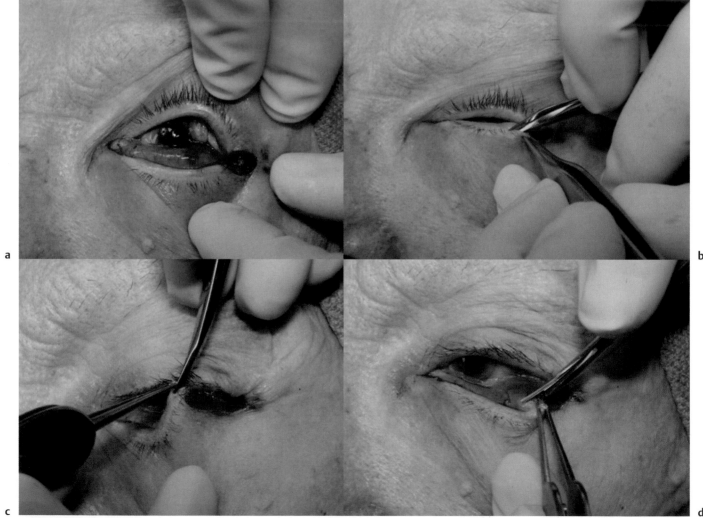

Fig. 21.7a–d Surgical series of a canthoplasty procedure. (**a**) a canthotomy is performed. (**b**) The anterior and posterior lamella is separated. (**c**) The muco-cutaneous junction is removed. (**d**) A sub-tarsal incision is made.

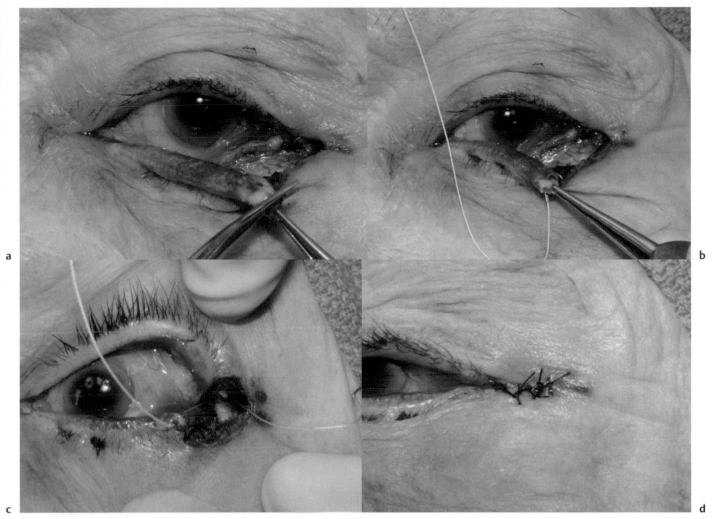

Fig. 21.8a–d Continuation of **Fig. 21.7**. (**a**) The tarsus is shortened. (**b**) A 4-0 Vicryl suture engages the de-epithelialized tarsal tongue. (**c**) The tarsus is sutured to the inner orbital rim periosteum at Whitnall's tubercle. (**d**) The canthus is closed.

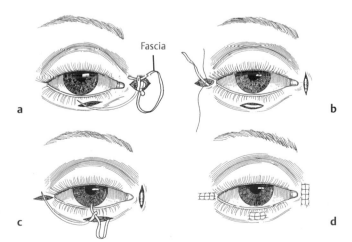

Fig. 21.9a–d Illustration of lower lid "hammock" suspension with fascial graft. (**a**) A vertical medial canthal incision is made and the fascial graft is sutured to the medial canthal tendon. (**b**) The graft is fed through the lower lid between tarsus and orbicularis just below the lid margin. (**c**) The graft is brought out a lateral canthal incision and secured with proper tension to the lateral orbital rim periosteum. (**d**) The incisions are closed.

Gold Weight Implant

Gold weights are very successfully used as a lid-loading material in upper lid recession for paralytic lagophthalmos.[15–19] They vary in size from 0.6 to 1.8 g. The 1.4-g weight is preferred as the author has found these provide the best results with fewest complications. In the upright position, the weight aids in lid closure when the levator relaxes (a normal consequence of attempted lid closure). Platinum weights are also now available[20] and may be of benefit in those patients who are allergic to gold.

The author's technique for gold weight placement is similar to traditional procedures with few modifications. The weight is placed slightly higher in the lid to prevent unsightly appearance and reduce the incidence of extrusion (**Fig. 21.10**). This requires a slightly heavier weight as the load effect of the weight is reduced with higher placement.

The eyelid crease is marked and anesthetized. The skin and orbicularis muscle are cut and the orbital septum divided. The levator aponeurosis (which the author slightly recesses) and the tarsus are identified. The gold

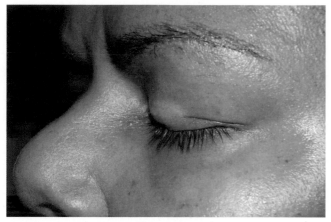

Fig. 21.10 A patient had gold weight implant placed over tarsus of left upper lid. The weight is very noticeable (and palpable) with lid closure

weight is placed between the superior tarsal boarder and the recessed levator aponeurosis (2 mm recession), and then secured to these structures with 6–0 Vicryl suture (**Fig. 21.11**). The orbicularis is then closed with numerous interrupted bites for adequate coverage of the implant. The skin is closed with a running 6–0 nylon suture.

Palpebral Spring

Palpebral springs are a wire material implanted into the eyelids whose tension allows tighter closure of the lids. While the spring may be a good resource for some patients and surgeons, their complication rates can be high even with experienced surgeons (extrusion, contour issue, etc.), and the procedures mentioned have been successful in the author's experience. For a detailed discussion on the use of springs, please refer to Chapter 22 and to various published reports of their use.[21–24]

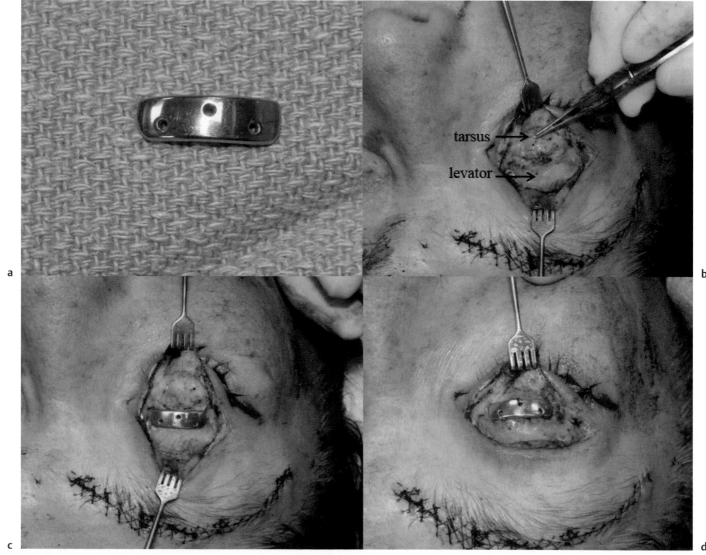

Fig. 21.11 Gold weight implantation surgical series. (**a**) 1.4 gram gold weight. (**b**) Exposure of the tarsus and levator aponeurosis. (**c**) Gold weight placed in surgical site above tarsus and below recessed levator. (**d**) Gold weight sutured to tarsus below and levator above.

■ Conclusion

Periorbital rejuvenation of the patient with facial paresis requires a thorough ophthalmic evaluation and familiarization with both invasive and noninvasive techniques of corneal protection. This chapter has outlined therapeutic modalities that have shown to be reliable in attaining this goal. It is important to emphasize that restoration of function and ocular protection are the primary objectives of these procedures. In doing so, every attempt should be made to maintain patient aesthetics whenever possible.

References

1. Seiff SR. Surgical management of seventh nerve paralysis and floppy eyelid syndrome. Curr Opin Ophthalmol 1999;10(4): 242–246
2. Collin JR, Leatherbarrow B. Ophthalmic management of seventh nerve palsy. Aust N Z J Ophthalmol 1990;18(3):267–272
3. Demirci H, Frueh BR. Palpebral spring in the management of lagophthalmos and exposure keratopathy secondary to facial nerve palsy. Ophthal Plast Reconstr Surg 2009;25(4):270–275
4. Shovlin JP, Lemke B. Clinical Eyelid Anatomy. In: Bosniak S, ed. Principals and Practice of Ophthalmic Plastic and Reconstructive Surgery. Philadelphia, PA: WB Saunders Co; 1996:261–280
5. McCord CD, Codner MA. Classic Surgical Anatomy. In: McCord CD, Codner MA, eds. Eyelid and Periorbital Surgery. St. Louis, MO: Quality Medical Publishing, Inc.: 2008:3–47
6. Jelks GW, Smith B, Bosniak S. The evaluation and management of the eye in facial palsy. Clin Plast Surg 1979;6(3):397–419
7. Ginsberg LE, De Monte F, Gillenwater AM. Greater superficial petrosal nerve: anatomy and MR findings in perineural tumor spread. AJNR Am J Neuroradiol 1996;17(2):389–393
8. Booth AJ, Murray A, Tyers AG. The direct brow lift: efficacy, complications, and patient satisfaction. Br J Ophthalmol 2004; 88(5):688–691
9. Massry GG. Comprehensive Lower Eyelid Rejuvenation. Facial Plast Surg. Scalfani AP, Seigert R, eds. Keller GS ed. 2010;(3): 209–221
10. Anderson RL, Gordy DD. The tarsal strip procedure. Arch Ophthalmol 1979;97(11):2192–2196
11. Gilbard SM. Involutional and Paralytic Ectropion. In: Bosniak S, ed. Principals and Practice of Ophthalmic Plastic and Reconstructive Surgery. Philadelphia, PA: WB Saunders Co;1996:222–237
12. Lee V, Currie Z, Collin JRO. Ophthalmic management of facial nerve palsy. Eye (Lond) 2004;18(12):1225–1234
13. Shorr N, Fallor MK. "Madame Butterfly" procedure: combined cheek and lateral canthal suspension procedure for post-blepharoplasty, "round eye," and lower eyelid retraction. Ophthal Plast Reconstr Surg 1985;1(4):229–235
14. Cohen MS, Shorr N. Eyelid reconstruction with hard palate mucosa grafts. Ophthal Plast Reconstr Surg 1992;8(3):183–195
15. Seiff SR, Boerner M, Carter SR. Treatment of facial palsies with external eyelid weights. Am J Ophthalmol 1995;120(5): 652–657
16. De Min G, Babighian S, Babighian G, Van Hellemont V. Early management of the paralyzed upper eyelid using a gold implant. Acta Otorhinolaryngol Belg 1995;49(3):269–274
17. Abell KM, Baker RS, Cowen DE, Porter JD. Efficacy of gold weight implants in facial nerve palsy: quantitative alterations in blinking. Vision Res 1998;38(19):3019–3023
18. Harrisberg BP, Singh RP, Croxson GR, Taylor RF, McCluskey PJ. Long-term outcome of gold eyelid weights in patients with facial nerve palsy. Otol Neurotol 2001;22(3):397–400
19. Rofagha S, Seiff SR. Long-term results for the use of gold eyelid load weights in the management of facial paralysis. Plast Reconstr Surg 2010;125(1):142–149
20. Silver AL, Lindsay RW, Cheney ML, Hadlock TA. Thin-profile platinum eyelid weighting: a superior option in the paralyzed eye. Plast Reconstr Surg 2009;123(6):1697–1703
21. McNeill JI, Oh YH. An improved palpebral spring for the management of paralytic lagophthalmos. Ophthalmology 1991;98(5): 715–719
22. May M. Gold weight and wire spring implants as alternatives to tarsorrhaphy. Arch Otolaryngol Head Neck Surg 1987;113(6): 656–660
23. Levine RE, Shapiro JP. Reanimation of the paralyzed eyelid with the enhanced palpebral spring or the gold weight: modern replacements for tarsorrhaphy. Facial Plast Surg 2000;16(4): 325–336
24. Terzis JK, Kyere SA. Experience with the gold weight and palpebral spring in the management of paralytic lagophthalmos. Plast Reconstr Surg 2008;121(3):806–815

22 Rehabilitation with the Enhanced Palpebral Spring

Robert E. Levine

The ocular manifestations of facial paralysis are a major source of both local and systemic disability. Locally, the inability to blink and close the upper eyelid, coupled with the malposition of the lower lid, results in corneal drying and roughness, which in turn causes severe discomfort and transient visual loss (which can elevate to permanent loss due to scarring). If the visual loss is severe, or becomes severe because of the necessity of filling the eye with lubricants, the patient is left with only the uninvolved eye available for use. Now monocular, stereo-acuity is lost. On a systemic level, being chronically uncomfortable, with the need to constantly be instilling lubricants, taping the eye, and functioning monocularly, without depth perception, is truly disabling. The patient's entire day (and, in some cases, entire life) becomes focused around caring for the eye and keeping it comfortable.

In short-term paralysis cases, a bandage contact lens, lubricants, moisture chamber, support of the lower lid with tape, and taping the eye shut at bedtime often provide adequate management. However, the patients with long-term (6 months or more) facial paralysis generally require a surgical solution. For repositioning the lower lid, a suitable combination of canthoplasties, stents or slings, and/or malar suspension is effective.

Reanimating the upper lid is a formidable challenge. As a result, many clinicians have settled for tarsorrhaphy. Tarsorrhaphy does not reanimate the eye, but it does often protect it. It is, however, disfiguring and may add to the psychological load the patient with facial paralysis is already facing. In some instances, the tarsorrhaphy becomes a fixed tarsal window and fails to protect the eye. Except for a small lateral tarsorrhaphy, it precludes the adjunctive use of a bandage contact lens, which is often a great help in dry eyes and eyes with neurotrophic keratitis. It also limits the patient's field of vision.

A popular approach to improving upper lid closure is implantation of a gold or platinum weight in the eyelid. In very mild cases of facial paralysis, this little boost may be enough to solve the problem. In more severe cases, however, a heavy weight is required, which is unsightly. More importantly, because eye closure with the weight is gravity dependent, it fails to close the eye at night, when the patient is supine. Patients are then left with still having to tape the eye each night or sleep with their head elevated with multiple pillows. Additionally, weights do not significantly increase blink speed.

Because of the limitations of tarsorrhaphies and weights, the author prefers the use of the enhanced palpebral spring procedure to reanimate the paralyzed upper eyelid. In the author's experience with over 2,000 such procedures over the past 40 years, this procedure has been a major contributor not only to the immediate problem of eye closure, but to the patient's rehabilitation. The primary focus of this chapter is to explain the rehabilitative aspects of this enhanced palpebral spring procedure.

◼ Patient Preparation

The patient is prepared and draped in the normal manner for lid surgery. The eye is protected with a scleral shell. Bupivacaine 0.5% mixed with an equal amount of lidocaine 2% with epinephrine is infiltrated along the lateral two-thirds of the upper lid fold. This mixture of anesthetic is also infiltrated along the tarsus at the center of the upper lid and along the lateral orbital rim. Care is taken when injecting to avoid distortion of lid anatomy or levator function. Basal sedation, given preoperatively, should be limited to short-acting agents that will not interfere with the patient's state of consciousness during the procedure, as cooperation is needed to open and close the eyes and to sit up on the operating table.

◼ Implanting the Spring

With a protective scleral shell in place, an incision is made along the lateral two-thirds of the lid crease and carried across the orbital rim laterally (**Fig. 22.1**). Dissection is

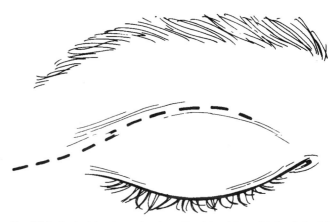

Fig. 22.1 An incision is made along the lateral two-thirds of the lid crease and carried across the orbital rim laterally. (Used with permission from Levine RE. Lid reanimation with the palpebral spring. In Tse DT, ed. Color Atlas of Oculoplastic Surgery. 2nd ed. Philadelphia, PA: Lippincott Williams & Wilkins, 2011:190–196.)

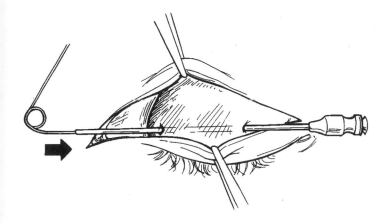

Fig. 22.2 A 22-gauge blunted spinal needle with the stylette in place is passed from the medial end of the dissection to emerge laterally in the plane between orbicularis and tarsus. (Used with permission from Levine RE. Lid reanimation with the palpebral spring. In Tse DT, ed. Color Atlas of Oculoplastic Surgery. 2nd ed. Philadelphia, PA: Lippincott Williams & Wilkins, 2011:190–196.)

carried downward at the medial end of the incision to expose the tarsal plate. Dissection is also carried upward and laterally to expose the orbital rim.

A 22-gauge blunted spinal needle with the stylette in place is passed from the medial end of the dissection to emerge laterally in the plane between orbicularis and tarsus (**Fig. 22.2**). The passage should be performed overlying midtarsus. The needle is angulated slightly downward at its lateral extent. The exit of the needle tract should be close to lateral orbital rim periosteum. The lid is everted to confirm that the needle has not inadvertently perforated the tarsus. The previously prepared wire spring (fashioned pre-operatively using 0.01 inch 35NLT wire from Ft. Wayne Metals, Ft. Wayne, IN) that has been sterilized, either by gas or low-temperature sterilization, is passed through the needle and the needle is withdrawn.

A cross-section of the lid illustrates placement of the needle over the midtarsus in the plane between the tarsus and orbicularis (**Fig. 22.3**). The wire spring should be resting on the epitarsal surface but not pressing on it.

The scleral shell is removed and the fulcrum of the spring is brought into the desired position along the orbital rim (**Fig. 22.4**). The spring should be placed in a position where its curves conform perfectly to the eyelid contour. The fulcrum of the spring is secured to the lateral orbital rim periosteum with three 4–0 Mersilene sutures (Ethicon, Inc., Somerville, NJ), taking an extra bite of the periosteum with each stitch. The lower limb of the spring should terminate at the point corresponding to the pupillary line in primary distance gaze. Loops are fashioned at each end and the spring is cut to size. The loops should be flat and tightly closed to leave no sharp edges. The medial loop is enveloped in 0.2-mm-thick Dacron patch material (Bard DeBakey, Tempe, AZ), to which it is secured by means of three 7–0 nylon sutures tied internally. The Dacron patch material is creased in a Gelfoam press (JEDMED, St. Louis, MO) before surgery and autoclaved with the other instruments. The folded Dacron envelope is cut to size at surgery. The crease in the patch material should be directed downward so that the spring and patch together provide a

smooth inferior surface. The loop at the end of the inferior arm is directed upward for the same reason. Suturing of the loop to the Dacron is facilitated by resting the Dacron on a retractor.

The end of the spring with its Dacron envelope is secured to the tarsus with 7–0 nylon sutures (**Fig. 22.5**). In time, the end of the spring will be reinforced to the tarsus by granulation tissue integrating into the Dacron patch.

The upper loop should be perpendicular to the fulcrum so that it can press against the superior orbital rim. The upper loop of the spring is secured to the undersurface of the superior orbital rim periosteum with three 4–0 Mersilene

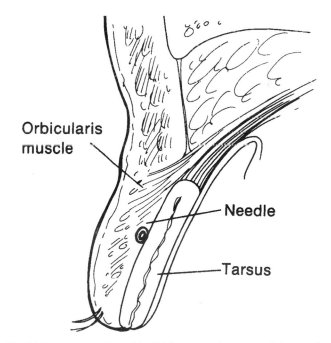

Orbicularis muscle

Needle

Tarsus

Fig. 22.3 A cross-section of the lid illustrates placement of the needle over the midtarsus in the plane between the tarsus and orbicularis. (Used with permission from Levine RE. Lid reanimation with the palpebral spring. In Tse DT, ed. Color Atlas of Oculoplastic Surgery. 2nd ed. Philadelphia, PA: Lippincott Williams & Wilkins, 2011:190–196.)

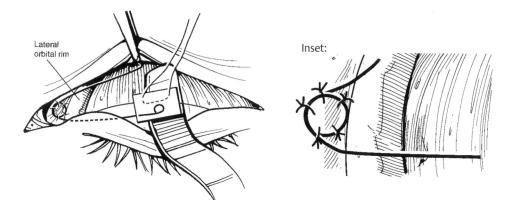

Lateral orbital rim

Inset:

Fig. 22.4 The scleral shell is removed and the fulcrum of the spring is brought into the desired position along the orbital rim. **Inset:** The spring should be placed in a position where its curves conform perfectly to the eyelid contour. (Used with permission from Levine RE. Lid reanimation with the palpebral spring. In Tse DT, ed. Color Atlas of Oculoplastic Surgery. 2nd ed. Philadelphia, PA: Lippincott Williams & Wilkins, 2011:190–196.)

sutures. An extra bite of the periosteum may be taken in each stitch before tying. When placing sutures to secure either the fulcrum or the upper loop of the spring to the orbital rim periosteum, it is safer to sew in the direction away from the globe.

■ Enhanced Palpebral Spring Implantation: Surgical Procedure

Currently, levator tightening is usually combined with the spring implantation. This procedure is referred to as "enhanced palpebral spring implantation." Three double-armed 5–0 Mersilene levator sutures are placed from tarsus through levator. The medial two of these sutures are placed through the Dacron patch as well (which helps fixate it) prior to being continued into levator. Adding the levator tuck increases the blink speed and decreases the pseudoptosis. It also allows for more exact tension on the spring, by adjusting the tension on the levator sutures.

With the patient seated, after the upper loop of the spring has been fixated, the levator sutures are tightened

to the maximum point short of becoming a tether for the lid. This is generally the best point of balance of forces. If the eye is overly open in primary gaze or if the blink speed is slowed, the levator sutures can be loosened.

Enhanced palpebral spring implantation is shown in **Fig. 22.6**. Deeper tissues overlying the spring are closed with 5–0 plain gut suture to ensure that the spring and the Mersilene sutures are well covered. Skin and muscle are closed with running 6–0 plain gut fast-absorbing suture or 6–0 Prolene suture.

■ Postoperative Care

Intravenous antibiotics are used intraoperatively, and oral prophylactic antibiotics are continued for 10 days. Intravenous steroids are also given intraoperatively, and a methylprednisone dose pack is used postoperatively. Antibiotic ointment is applied onto the wound twice daily until the wound is healed and skin sutures have been absorbed or removed. Ice packs are applied to the lid during the first 48 hours after surgery. Warm tap water compresses (or some other form of moist heat) are then substituted and continued until lid swelling subsides.

■ Rehabilitative Aspects of the Spring

Ocular Protection

The ability to blink provides the windshield wiper function required to spread tears across the cornea. This prevents the cornea from drying out during the day. In addition, being able to close the eye protects it at night without having to tape it shut. Because the spring works in any position, no extra pillows are required (**Fig. 22.7**).

Avoidance of Blurred Vision

As a result of increased ocular protection, less viscous lubricants can be used. Especially in the cases of patients

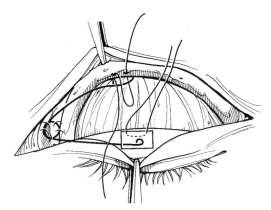

Fig. 22.5 The end of the spring with its Dacron (Bard Debakey, Tempe, AZ) envelope is secured to the tarsus with 7–0 nylon sutures. (Used with permission from Levine RE. Lid reanimation with the palpebral spring. In Tse DT, ed. Color Atlas of Oculoplastic Surgery. 2nd ed. Philadelphia, PA: Lippincott Williams & Wilkins, 2011:190–196.)

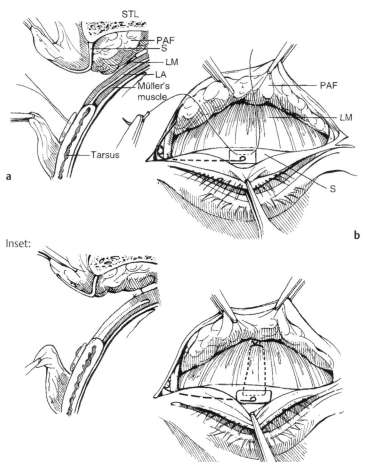

a

Inset:

b

c

Fig. 22.6a–c Enhanced palpebral spring implantation. (**a**) Levator aponeurosis and inferior aspect of the muscular portion of the levator are exposed. Centrally, the superior portion of the tarsus is also exposed. A double-armed 5–0 Mersilene suture (Ethicon, Inc., Somerville, NJ) is placed through midtarsus. (**b**) Each arm of the suture is brought through the Dacron (polyester; DuPont, Wilmington, DE) covering the spring. (**c**) It is then passed back through the Dacron and continues superiorly through the levator to emerge just above the point at which the aponeurosis meets the levator muscle. Temporary knots are tied. If necessary, an additional lateral suture and possibly an additional medial suture are placed in a similar manner through tarsus and levator. **Inset:** The course of suture is illustrated in cross-section. The surgeon should check to ensure that the suture has not perforated tarsus or conjunctiva. (Used with permission from Levine RE. Lid reanimation with the palpebral spring. In Tse DT, ed. Color Atlas of Oculoplastic Surgery. 2nd ed. Philadelphia, PA: Lippincott Williams & Wilkins, 2011:190–196.)

who required ointment around the clock previously, their vision is significantly improved by being able to substitute moderate viscosity drops for ointment, or if tear function is normal, to no longer require supplemental lubricants.

Improved Cosmesis

It is not always possible to eliminate all the pseudoptosis that accompanies palpebral spring surgery. Whereas in the normal eye, closure is turned off when the eye opens, in this instance the downward force vector created by the spring is overcome by the upward force vector provided by the levator. In patients with weak levators, the levator cannot be strengthened (tightened) enough to fully overcome the spring, and pseudoptosis results. Nevertheless, even the patient with pseudoptosis looks better than one with a significant tarsorrhaphy or a large weight (which also causes pseudoptosis, for the same reasons that the spring causes pseudoptosis).

Another aspect of the cosmetic improvement is the visibility of movement in an otherwise nonmoving half of the face. An active natural blink softens the impression of abnormality of that side of the face.

Improved Visual Field

Even a moderate lateral tarsorrhaphy can create a significant visual field defect in the direction of the lid adhesion. The author recalls an automobile mechanic whose major reason for wanting to get rid of his tarsorrhaphy and replace it with a spring was because he constantly bumping into equipment in his garage.

Allowing for Additional Eye Surgery

Patients whose facial nerve deficit resulted from an intracranial tumor frequently have associated fifth and sixth nerve deficits. In the author's experience with ~5,000 patients with facial paralysis, patients with a profound fifth nerve deficit have neurotrophic keratitis and require complete closure of the eye, even during sleep. They are not successfully protected with weights, and not infrequently present with a weight in place and a scarred cornea. Typically, they state no corneal surgeon wants to do a corneal transplant on them because the surgeon expects the transplanted cornea to also become scarred. Those with tarsorrhaphies in place are precluded from wearing the contact

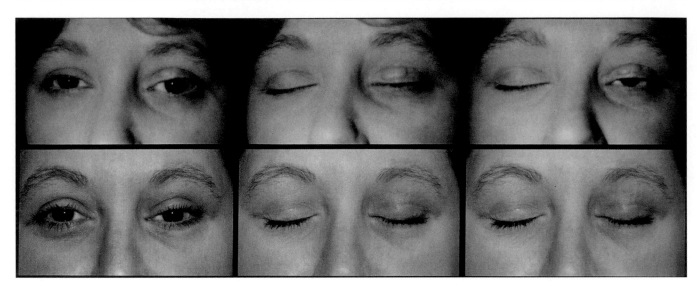

Fig. 22.7 *Top row* shows a patient after gold weight implant. *Bottom row* is same patient after removal of gold weight, implantation of palpebral spring, and lower lid tightening. *Top left:* Eyes open. *Top center:* With patient upright, closure is fairly good, but still incomplete. *Top right:* With patient supine, closure is poor. *Bottom left:* Eyes open. *Bottom center and bottom right:* Regardless of whether patient is upright or supine, spring achieves full closure of lid.

lenses that may help protect their neurotrophic corneas long term.

In both scenarios, undoing the prior procedure and placing a spring often provides the protection they need. They can then convince the corneal surgeon that a penetrating corneal keratoplasty (corneal transplant) is a worthwhile undertaking. The author has had several patients who were previously not considered surgical candidates who underwent successful corneal transplantation after spring implantation. It was possible to restore the vision to blind eyes in the presence of facial paralysis, and they have subsequently maintained their corneal integrity.

In an analogous manner, strabismus surgeons have declined to straighten eyes in patients with combined sixth and seventh nerve paralysis who required continuous ointment use to protect the eye. They did not feel it worthwhile to straighten an eye that anyway would be blurred all day with ointment, precluding stereopsis. Once spring surgery was planned to eliminate the need for ointment, they proceeded to straighten the eye. (If both procedures are indicated, it is better to straighten the eye first, as that allows for more precise spring design.)

Allowing for Brow Elevation

Some patients with severe facial paralysis compensate in part for their lagophthalmos because the drooping brow helps push the upper lid shut. If one were to elevate the brow, the lagophthalmos would worsen. An isolated brow elevation in such a circumstance would therefore be contraindicated, leaving the patient with the brow droop deformity. However, if active lid closure is

provided with a palpebral spring, the brow can be safely elevated, often at the same surgical session as the spring implantation.

Providing a Psychological Lift to the Patient

It is clear that improving cosmesis and therefore providing a more positive body image enhances a patient's self-esteem and therefore provides a psychological lift. Less obvious is the implication that many patients have expressed: "Now that my eyelid is working again, I have more hope that my face will start working again, and find it easier to await recovery of facial nerve function." Although the eyelid movement is a function of the spring, and not of recovery, what the patient experiences and feels is not always based on science. The feeling is real, and the author has heard patients express it many times.

Eliminating a Burdensome Routine

Some patients who could successfully manage their eye issues with an involved routine of lubricants and taping nevertheless spend a good part of their day caring for their eye. Improving the lid physiology by reanimating the upper lid with a spring allows them to use a much simpler routine.

Refocusing Their Attention

Patients who have to work at keeping their eye comfortable and out of trouble may have little time left for the other parts of their life. Tasks as simple as keeping water out of the eye during a shower or wind out of the eye while

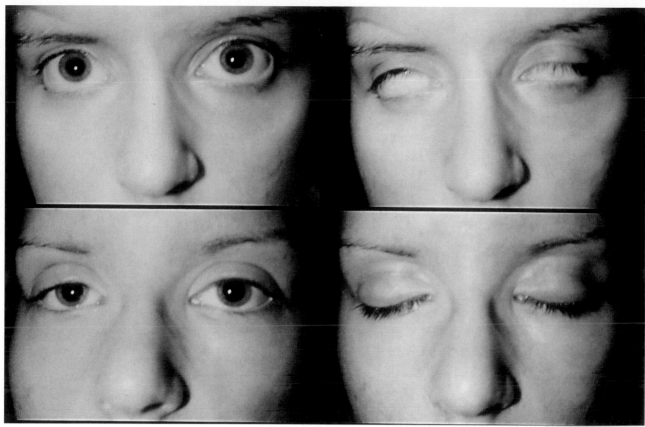

Fig. 22.8 A young woman with bilateral facial paralysis from neurofibromatosis type 2 with bilateral acoustic tumors. *Top left preoperative:* Eyes open. *Top right preoperative:* Attempted lid closure with marked lagophthalmos. *Bottom left postoperative*: bilateral enhanced palpebral spring implants and lower lid tightening: eyes open. *Bottom right postoperative*: bilateral enhanced palpebral spring implants and lower lid tightening; good lid closure.

outdoors pose a real challenge. With a simpler management routine and increased closure ability after spring implantation, they can resume a more normal lifestyle (**Fig. 22.8**).

Returning to the Mainstream of Life

Many patients experienced a multiplicity of the benefits described previously. With improved blinking, closure, cosmesis, self-esteem, and visual field, they could once again pursue their careers or their interests and direct their attention to their friends and family rather than themselves. An excerpt of a letter from a young woman who lived with facial paralysis from Bell palsy for a year prior to having a spring implant conveys well what the rehabilitative effects of the spring can be:

As I sit down to [write to you], tears are streaming down my face. There has not been a single day that goes by since I had my surgery with you that I am not reminded of the wonderful gift you have given to me. I can blink. First, my eye functions! I celebrate this every single day! I celebrate when I shower and the water isn't in my eye! I celebrate that I can ski and

bike and swim with no problems. I celebrate that I am not afraid of doing anything and I feel comfortable in social situations, I celebrate that the spring made it so I could drive again! I have four kids that I love to play with and I celebrate that they are not uncomfortable around me. Most importantly, I celebrate that this trial has made me a more compassionate and understanding person . . . You saved my eye and I get to see that sweet little spring everyday and it puts a smile (half) on my face! You and Dr.— did an amazing job with my face, even to the extent that I feel pretty again.

■ Conclusion

Gold weights and tarsorrhaphies do not elicit the kind of response shown in the letter because they are not as rehabilitative as the spring. Surgeons dealing with significant numbers of patients with facial paralysis should not be daunted by the learning curve of spring implantation, by the possible need for future adjustments, or by the patients that experience spring-related problems. Patients deserve the best care physicians can give them, and for rehabilitating the patient, not just the eye, in the presence of facial paralysis, the author is convinced that the enhanced palpebral spring is the best there is to offer.

Suggested Additional Reading

1. Levine RE. Eyelid reanimation. Facial Plast Surg 1992;8(2): 121–126

2. May M, Levine RE, Patel BCK, Anderson RL. Eye reanimation techniques. In: May M, Schaitkins BM, eds. The Facial Nerve. May's second edition. New York: Thieme-Stratton Inc.; 2000:677–774

3. Levine RE, Shapiro JP. Reanimation of the paralyzed eyelid with the enhanced palpebral spring or the gold weight: modern replacements for tarsorrhaphy. Facial Plast Surg 2000;16(4): 325–336

4. Levine RE. Eyelid reanimation. In: Brackrmann DE, Shelton C, Arriaga A, eds. Otologic Surgery, 3rd ed. Philadelphia: W.B. Saunders; 2009

23 Facial Nerve Repair

Douglas K. Henstrom and Tessa A. Hadlock

Myriad clinical conditions lead to permanent or irreversible facial paralysis. Examples of "permanent" facial paralysis include facial nerve sacrifice at or close to the brainstem where cable grafting is technically difficult or impossible, massive temporal bone trauma where neural elements are not identifiable (blast injuries), and cases of neurotrophic malignancy where there is extensive tumor penetration into the proximal facial nerve itself and no cable graft is placed. In addition, many clinical situations result in long-standing or "irreversible" facial paralysis with end-stage muscle atrophy, simply because of the unpredictable regenerative potential of the facial nerve. These scenarios include watchful waiting following skull base surgery in which the nerve is attenuated but anatomically intact and cases of cable grafting through the temporal bone. In these situations, sometimes clinical recovery is good but requires 18 to 24 months to be complete. If after that time frame, clinical recovery is poor, then the facial musculature is no longer consistently receptive to neural input. The material in this chapter is relevant to both permanent and irreversible facial paralysis.

■ Nerve Injury, Repair, and Grafting

Nerve Injury Classification

Nerve injuries are classified according to the level of microanatomic disruption. According to the Sunderland Classification system,[1] level 1 injury yields only temporary dysfunction of the membrane sodium channels, without microanatomic disruption, resulting in a transient inability of the nerve to transmit impulses. In level 2 injury, axons are disrupted, though their individual endoneurial channels are not, so that when regeneration occurs, there is little to no misrouting of axons. In level 3 injury, endoneurial sheaths are violated, though perineurium is left intact. Recovery from this type of injury occurs over months and inevitably results in some synkinesis. Level 4 injury results in perineurial disruption without damage to the epineurial sheath, leading to generally poor recovery. Level 5 injury refers to total anatomic disruption of the entire nerve, including the epineurium.

Nerve Repair

When facial nerve discontinuity is encountered, the first approach is to attempt to reestablish direct neural continuity between the facial motor nucleus and the distal facial nerve, through either primary repair or autografting techniques. Recovery of function is usually better through primary repair than through grafts.[2] In intratemporal locations, it is sometimes difficult to tell, despite microsurgical magnification, whether the facial nerve has been disrupted in its entirety or whether only a segment of the nerve has been injured. When this is the case, thorough exposure of the site of injury is warranted, and the literature supports repair when 50% of the facial nerve appears to have been violated. Intratemporal repair can be performed with facial nerve re-routing, facilitated by concomitant canal wall-down mastoidectomy surgery, so suturing can take place in the distal vertical segment. The horizontal segment is not amenable to suture repair, and if this region is involved, the nerve ends should simply be approximated and held in place with fibrin glue. It is important to reapproximate the nerve ends without tension to minimize fibrosis. In cases involving the loss of 17 mm or less of the facial nerve, primary neurorrhaphy can be obtained by re-routing the facial nerve within the temporal bone to gain further length and thus permit tensionless coaptation.[3] Timing is important, and all repairs, no matter their location, should be performed within the first 72 hours after injury, during which time the distal nerve segment retains electrical stimulability. The operating microscope should be employed to evaluate, clean, and remove all devitalized tissue from the nerve endings. The epineurial sheath is then approximated in a tensionless manner. While interfascicular repair is theoretically possible distal to the pes anserinus, the human facial nerve lacks sufficient identifiable topographic orientation to make this type of realignment clinically useful.[4]

Nerve Grafting

After facial nerve injury or sacrifice, if a tension-free neurorrhaphy is not achievable, then an autograft, using a segment of donor sensory nerve, is interposed between the proximal and distal facial nerve endings. In facial nerve

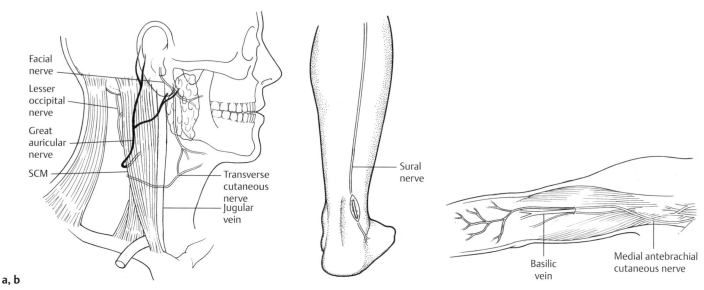

a, b

c

Fig. 23.1a–c Common donor nerves in facial nerve reconstruction. (**a**) Great auricular nerve. (**b**) Sural nerve. (**c**) Medial antebrachial cutaneous nerve.

reconstruction, the most common donor nerve grafts are taken from the great auricular, sural, or medial antebrachial cutaneous nerves (**Fig. 23.1**). The great auricular nerve is ideal for repairs that require grafts of < 6 cm. The resulting anesthesia to the ipsilateral auricle is well tolerated, and the nerve is of adequate diameter and caliber to provide a suitable graft. A contraindication to using it is the presence of a nearby neurotrophic malignancy, in which case the sural or medial antebrachial nerves are preferred.

The sural nerve is removed from the leg via an incision adjacent to the lateral malleolus. While initial sural nerve harvesting was performed through open approaches, subsequent technique modification have permitted harvest through a series of shorter incisions.[5,6] A nerve "stripping" technique has become popular, where the length of the nerve may be harvested through two small incisions. Contemporary approaches to sural nerve harvest involve utilizing endoscopic equipment and either a single or two small stab incisions in the leg. The decrease in operative time and the significant decrease in incision length compared with open techniques make it a logical choice for the facial reanimation surgeon (**Fig. 23.2**). Harvest of the sural nerve usually produces low morbidity, but the patient should expect decreased sensation over the dorsolateral foot, and 20–30% of patients may experience a mild level of "neuromatous pain" even years following harvest.[7] The sural nerve can provide up to 30 cm of healthy nerve graft.

For total facial nerve reconstruction from the main trunk to peripheral branches, the medial antebrachial cutaneous nerve is most appropriate. There are at least four reliable branches, and it has adequate length to perform grafting of the entire facial nerve, even when the distal stumps lie at the anterior border of the parotid gland (**Fig. 23.3**).

The principles of primary nerve repair and nerve grafting are similar. Repairs should be performed within the first 72 hours after injury or sacrifice, irrespective of the need for subsequent radiation therapy. During this time frame, the distal nerve segments retain electrical stimulability, making identification easier. Meticulous debridement and careful microsurgical technique are of paramount importance in optimizing regenerative outcome. The results of cable grafting are generally favorable.[8] Factors that can lead to poor results include wound disruption, infection, or tension on the site of coaptation. In most cases, the return of movement appears within 6 to 12 months. Improvement may generally be expected over the course of 1 to 3 years.

There is debate as to the best method of nerve coaptation as it applies to both primary and graft repair. Epineurial repair has been contrasted to fascicular repair,[9] though no study has convincingly demonstrated improved regenerative outcome based upon fascicular facial nerve repair. Therefore, given its relative simplicity, the current standard is to perform epineurial suture repair.[10] Recently, there have been an increasing number of encouraging studies regarding the use of fibrin glue to assist with nerve coaptation. This method appears to hold promise as an alternative or an adjunct to nerve suturing, as it decreases the localized inflammatory response, acts as a sealant (rather than a barrier), and experimentally improves axonal regeneration and fiber alignment.[11,12]

While nerve repair, nerve grafting, and nerve substitution techniques are all designed to deliver neural input to the native facial musculature, the regeneration that occurs is universally misrouted. Misguided axonal extension to inappropriate targets leads to mass movement and synkinesis. While nerve reconstruction procedures are usually

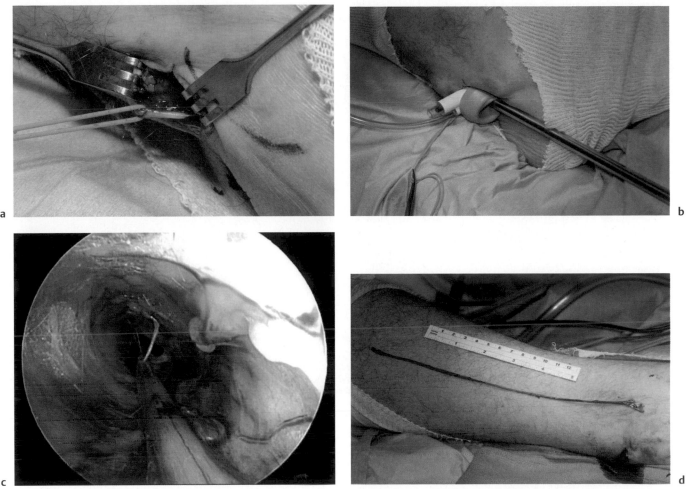

Fig. 23.2a–d Endoscopic sural nerve harvesting technique. Operative procedure. (**a**) Identification of sural nerve at ankle. (**b**) Endoscope introduced through short horizontal incision. (**c**) Endoscopically isolated sural nerve. (**d**) Nerve removed through single incision. (Used with permission from Hadlock TA, Cheney ML. Facial reanimation. In: Urken ML, ed. Multidisciplinary Head and Neck Reconstruction: A Defect–Oriented Approach. Philadelphia, PA: Lippincott Williams & Wilkins; 2010: 435–454.)

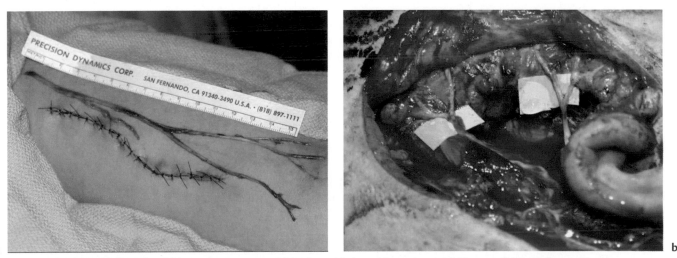

Fig. 23.3a, b The medial antebrachial cutaneous nerve, with its favorable branching pattern. (**a**) Harvest. (**b**) Inset for total facial nerve reconstruction, following radical parotidectomy for mucoepidermoid carcinoma. Frozen section control of nerve margins is mandatory. (Used with permission from Hadlock TA, Cheney ML. Facial reanimation. In: Urken ML, ed. Multidisciplinary Head and Neck Reconstruction: A Defect–Oriented Approach. Philadelphia, PA: Lippincott Williams & Wilkins; 2010: 435–454.)

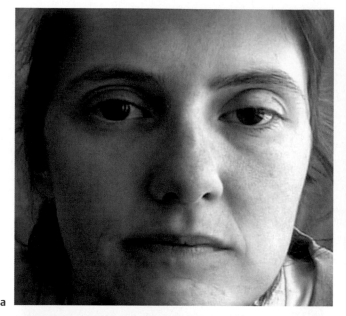

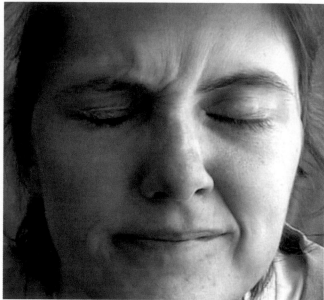

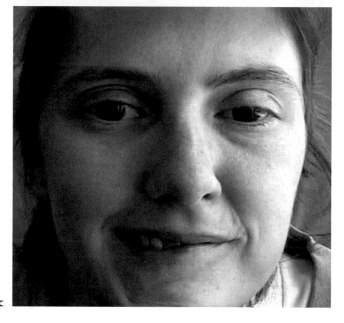

Fig. 23.4a–c Case illustrating axonal misrouting after cable grafting. The patient underwent total facial nerve reconstruction with a medial antebrachial cutaneous nerve graft 12 months earlier. (a) At rest. (b) Voluntary eye closure. Note the involuntary midfacial movement. (c) Voluntary smile. Note the narrowing of the palpebral fissure. (Used with permission from Hadlock TA, Cheney ML. Facial reanimation. In: Urken ML, ed. Multidisciplinary Head and Neck Reconstruction: A Defect–Oriented Approach. Philadelphia, PA: Lippincott Williams & Wilkins; 2010: 435–454.)

effective at restoring facial tone, fine control over each distinct zone of the face is seldom achieved using these techniques. **Fig. 23.4** demonstrates the restoration of excellent resting tone following medial antebrachial cutaneous nerve grafting from the mastoid segment of the facial nerve to four peripheral branches, but significant midfacial synkinesis with ocular movements and ocular synkinesis with smiling.

■ Reinnervation Techniques

Reinnervation techniques, also termed nerve substitution techniques, refer to procedures that provide neural input to the distal facial nerve and facial musculature via motor nerves other than the native facial nerve. They are indicated in two situations. The first is when the proximal facial nerve stump is not available, but where the distal facial nerve and facial musculature are present and functional. This occurs following skull base tumor resections involving sacrifice of the nerve at or very close to the brainstem, where neurorrhaphy is not technically achievable. The second situation occurs following skull base surgery, intracranial injury, or traumatic facial paralysis, where the nerve is thought to be anatomically intact, but when there is no discernible return of function after a satisfactory waiting period of 12 months. Lack of functional recovery, electrophysiological demonstration of lack of reinnervation potentials, and the presence of fibrillation potentials at 12 months indicates persistent, complete denervation.

This suggests insufficient regenerative potential from the proximal facial nerve stump and therefore mandates alternative proximal axonal input to the distal facial nerve and facial musculature, prior to irreversible atrophy and fibrosis.

Hypoglossal Facial Transfer

The hypoglossal nerve is most often utilized to reinnervate the distal facial nerve. Its proximity to the extratemporal facial nerve, its dense population of myelinated motor axons, and the relative acceptability of the resultant hemitongue weakness make it a logical choice.[13,14] In the classic XII-VII transfer, the entire hypoglossal nerve is transected

and reflected upward for direct neurorrhaphy to the facial nerve stump (**Fig. 23.5a**). Several modifications have been described (**Fig. 23.5b–d**), including the "split" XII-VII transfer,[15] where ~30% of the width of the hypoglossal nerve is divided from the main trunk of the nerve for several centimeters and is secured to the lower division of the facial nerve. However, given the interwoven fascicular architecture of the nerve, separating a 30% segment away from the main trunk for several centimeters divides a significantly greater number of axons than if the fibers were oriented in parallel.[16] This realization led to a further modification, termed the XII-VII jump graft. The modification is designed to reduce tongue morbidity by avoiding the splicing away of a significant length of the hypoglossal

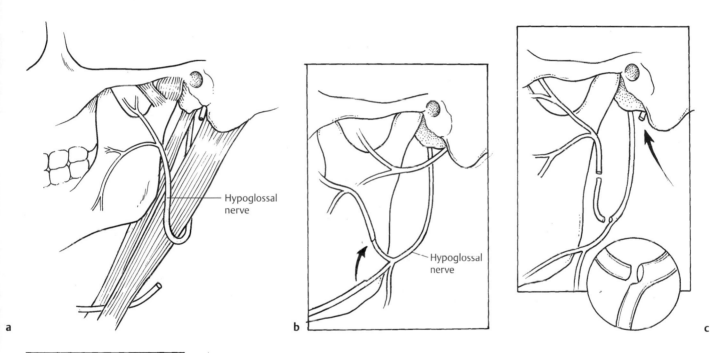

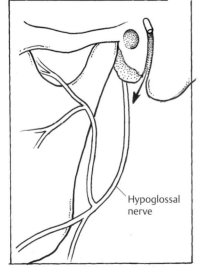

Fig. 23.5a–d Hypoglossal facial nerve transfer. (**a**) Classic procedure, with entire hypoglossal nerve transected. (**b**) Modification with 40% segment of nerve secured to lower division. (**c**) Jump graft modification. Insert shows how graft is positioned to capture axons extending from the proximal aspect of the opened hypoglossal nerve. (**d**) Reflection of the facial nerve out of the mastoid bone to meet the hypoglossal nerve in the neck.

trunk and involves an end-to-side neurorrhaphy between the hypoglossal nerve and a donor cable graft (usually the great auricular nerve), which in turn is sewn to the distal facial trunk (see **Fig. 23.5c**).[16]

In circumstances where the facial nerve is able to be mobilized from the second genu within the temporal bone and reflected inferiorly, removal of the mastoid tip has allowed direct coaptation of the facial nerve to the hypoglossal, without the need for an interposition graft (see **Fig. 23.5d**).[17] Elimination of the cable graft provides a theoretical regenerative advantage by reducing the neurorrhaphies to one, although the relative rarity of this clinical situation makes outcome comparisons impractical.

Another potential use is for partial hypoglossal to facial grafting to treat resultant deficiencies in a single area, such as the marginal mandibular branch,[18] and potentially the orbicularis oculi muscle.

Surgical Technique

The XII-VII procedure is performed via a modified Blair parotidectomy incision. The main trunk of the facial nerve and the pes anserinus are identified using standard facial nerve landmarks, such as the tragal pointer and the tympanomastoid suture line. The hypoglossal nerve is then located in its ascending portion, deep to the posterior belly of the digastric muscle, along the medial surface of the internal jugular vein. The nerve is followed anteriorly, to just beyond the takeoff point of the descendens hypoglossi. The hypoglossal nerve is sharply transected and reflected superiorly to meet the facial nerve. The facial nerve is transected at the stylomastoid foramen, and the distal trunk reflected inferiorly and secured to the hypoglossal nerve with five to seven 10–0 nylon epineurial microsutures.

In the jump graft procedure (or end-to-side procedure), once the exposure has been obtained, the great auricular nerve graft is harvested or the proximal facial nerve is mobilized from the temporal bone, sectioned at the second genu, and transposed into the neck by removal of the mastoid tip. The facial nerve can be further mobilized by dissecting it away from the parotid tissue beyond its bifurcation. The end-to-side neurorrhaphy is executed by removing a segment of hypoglossal epineurium, then cutting a 30% opening into the hypoglossal nerve and allowing exposure of the severed axons. The recipient nerve is then laid into the defect, facing the proximal cut surface, and secured with microsutures.

Results, Drawbacks, and Contraindications

With a XII-VII transfer, good resting facial tone is achieved in over 90% of patients. When successful, the transfer allows deliberate facial movement with intentional manipulation of the tongue. Recovery generally

occurs over a 6- to 24-month time course, and in some cases has been reported to continue over a period of up to 5 years. Results are variable, with time from denervation to transfer playing a key role in outcome.[19] There is general agreement that reinnervation must occur within 2 years following injury, otherwise neuromuscular fibrosis and atrophy progress to a point where meaningful tone and movement are not achievable.[16]

The two most significant drawbacks of the procedure are the mass facial movement experienced by many patients and the variable tongue dysfunction, which has been categorized as "severe" in up to 25% of patients. Articulation and mastication difficulties are commonly cited. The modifications mentioned are aimed at one or the other of these two problems. In addition, botulinum toxin administration in the region of the eye and physical therapy have proven useful adjuncts for patients with clinically significant mass movement.[20] The procedure is contraindicated in patients who are likely to develop other cranial neuropathies (i.e., neurofibromatosis type 2) or who have ipsilateral tenth nerve deficits, as the combined X-XII deficit can lead to profound swallowing dysfunction.

VII-VII Cross-Face Nerve Grafting

Another potential source of axons for facial reinnervation is the contralateral healthy facial nerve.[21] It was originally described independently by Scaramella and Tobias in 1973[22] and by Smith in 1972,[23] and possesses the major advantage that the return of function is spontaneous (involuntary blink) and can produce true emotion-based expression (emotive smile), while the other neural sources all require physical therapy and neuromuscular retraining. It is significantly arborized distally, so several branches may be sacrificed for use in cross-facial grafting, without adversely affecting the healthy side. Donor branches contain many fewer motor axons than the hypoglossal nerve, leading most surgeons to feel the motor power provided by the hypoglossal nerve is distinctly superior.[24] The use of the contralateral facial nerve strictly for reinnervation of native facial musculature has largely been replaced by cross-face nerve grafting in conjunction with free muscle transfer.

Technique

A preauricular incision is marked, and the subcutaneous tissues may be infiltrated with local anesthetic with epinephrine. A skin flap is raised directly under the superficial muscular aponeurotic system on the parotidomasseteric fascia. Fine scissors dissection is begun at the anterior border of the parotid gland to identify the facial nerve branches as they emerge from the parotid gland. Multiple branches of the facial nerve are mapped with a bipolar nerve stimulator to determine their function. In the midface, the massive neural arborization between branches permits transection of one or two branches without weakening the healthy side. While detectable temporary donor site motor deficits have been reported,[25] in one author's experience (T.H.) of 90 cases, only a single case revealed minor changes in smile vector on the healthy side.

Once the branches are selected, the nerve graft (usually reversed sural nerve) is tunneled to reach the contralateral preauricular region. Coaptations are performed under the operating microscope with 10-0 nylon sutures and/or fibrin glue, under no tension. Six months are usually required for the axons to extend sufficiently to produce clinically apparent movement.

Results, Drawbacks, and Contraindications

Outcomes for cross-face nerve grafting are variable. Smith reported a series of three patients in which a sural nerve graft was coapted between donor buccal and zygomatic branches to affected branches on the paralyzed side using a two-stage technique that showed improvement in symmetry.[23] Scaramella[21] published a long-term series of 11 patients that underwent single-stage cross-face nerve grafting, and reported that five had good tone, three had fair tone, and he considered two of the cases to be failures. Anderl[26] reported a series of 15 patients that underwent cross-facial nerve grafting using four grafts per patient to reanimate individual regions and concluded that the "result was satisfying (more than 50%) where the preoperative conditions were favorable." He stressed the importance of timing, with earlier reinnervation yielding better outcomes. Baker and Conley[27] used the lower division of the facial nerve for the donor, which was coapted to a sural nerve graft and then the entire cross-sectional area of the recipient facial nerve. They reported a series of 10 patients, in which 6 experienced "fair" improvement and the remainder gained no improvement. Galli et al[28] reported a series of five patients that underwent mapping and cross-face nerve grafting with "successful" results.[29]

In either reinnervation or grafting, controversy exists as to how long the facial musculature remains receptive to reinnervation before it becomes end-stage (irretrievable atrophy and fibrosis).[30-32] Terzis et al recommended doing the procedure before 6 months of denervation time has elapsed.[32] In addition, Terzis et al has shown that the number of donor axons has the strongest influence on the final results.[33]

The major difficulty with cross-facial nerve grafting is that results are inconsistent. Some authors report excellent recovery, while many others find it entirely unsatisfactory. It appears that it is most useful in association with other reanimation modalities, to address a single territory within the face, rather than to reinnervate the entire contralateral facial nerve. Recent studies employing the cross-facial graft for isolated marginal mandibular paralysis demonstrate its utility.[34]

Other Reinnervation Techniques

Several other cranial nerves have been employed, historically, for reinnervation of the distal facial nerve stump. The spinal accessory nerve,[35,36] glossopharyngeal nerve, and trigeminal nerve[37] have all been described as potential donors, though none has gained great popularity. The donor morbidity and/or difficulty with surgical exposure far exceed that found with XII-VII and cross-facial grafting. Experimentation with utilizing isolated branches, for example the sternocleidomastoid branch of the spinal accessory nerve,[35] would decrease donor morbidity, potentially increasing the utility of this technique. However, using the masseteric branch of the trigeminal nerve would preclude its possible use to drive a free tissue transfer for smile reanimation in the case of a poor reinnervation result, so its sacrifice for this purpose must be carefully considered.

■ Adjunctive Procedures

Even excellent results from facial nerve repair, cable grafting, or nerve substitution techniques never result in normal facial function. To optimize appearance and/or function after regeneration is complete through one of these modalities, there are numerous adjunctive procedures that improve the final result. Algorithms have been proposed to prevent overlooking the adjunctive procedures of potential benefit in complete facial paralysis management (**Fig. 23.6**).[38] Among useful adjunctive procedures, nasolabial fold modifications (**Fig. 23.7**), nasal valve correction (**Fig. 23.8**), lower lip asymmetry management (**Fig. 23.9**), and chemodenervation or platysmectomy for the hypertonic platysma (**Fig. 23.10**) have proven useful. Periocular procedures, of great importance, are described in Chapters 21 and 22.

■ Conclusion

Facial paralysis is a disfiguring and debilitating condition whose management is determined by a large set of clinical variables. A systematic approach to nerve repair methods is presented here, along with a list of adjunctive procedures that must be offered to optimize clinical outcome after complete recovery through nerve repair techniques. Management via a team approach that includes neurotologists, facial and plastic surgeons, head and neck surgical oncologists, oculoplastic surgeons, and physical therapists is imperative to achieve the best possible outcome.

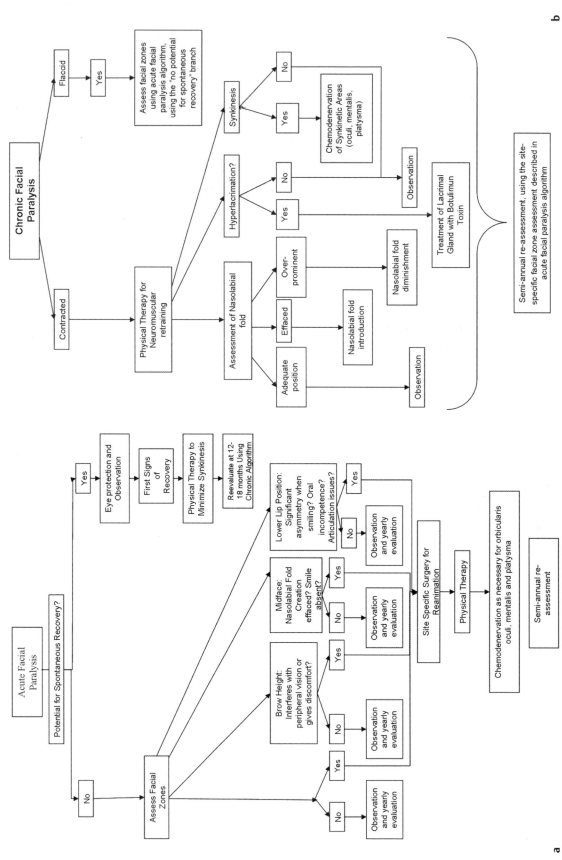

Fig. 23.6a, b Proposed algorithm for the management of facial paralysis. Acute facial paralysis algorithm and chronic (long-standing) facial paralysis algorithm. (Used with permission from Hadlock TA, Cheney ML. Facial reanimation. In: Urken ML, ed. Multidisciplinary Head and Neck Reconstruction: A Defect–Oriented Approach. Philadelphia, PA: Lippincott Williams & Wilkins; 2010: 435–454.)

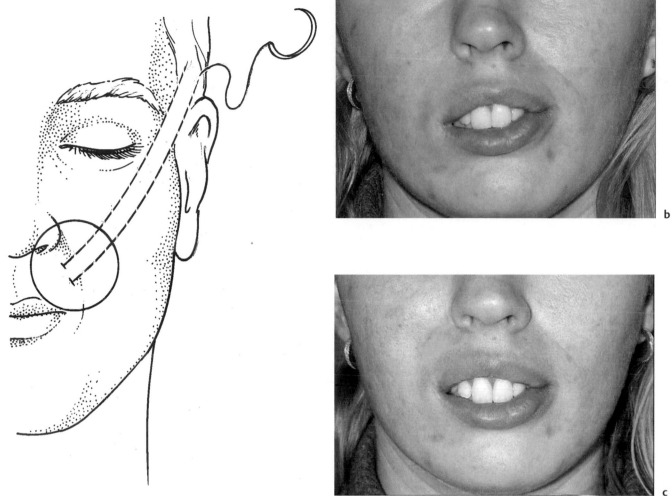

Fig. 23.7a–f Modification of the nasolabial fold. (**a**) Technique of introducing a nasolabial fold. Schematic showing the lack of nasolabial fold on the left and the position of the nicks required for passage of the sutures. (**b**) Preoperative view. Prior to static suspension, the right nasolabial fold is effaced. (**c**) Postoperative view. (**d**) Technique of effacement of a hyperprominent nasolabial fold. Schematic showing midfacial hypertonicity and overprominence of the nasolabial fold. Note the location of the incisions for the passage of the sutures is lateral to the nasolabial fold as it would be in cosmetic midface lifting. (Figs. 23.7b, c, e, and f are used with permission from Hadlock TA, Cheney ML. Facial reanimation. In: Urken ML, ed. Multidisciplinary Head and Neck Reconstruction: A Defect–Oriented Approach. Philadelphia, PA: Lippincott Williams & Wilkins; 2010: 435–454.) (**e**) Preoperative view. Prior to static suspension, the left nasolabial fold is hyperprominent. (**f**) Postoperative view. (*continued*)

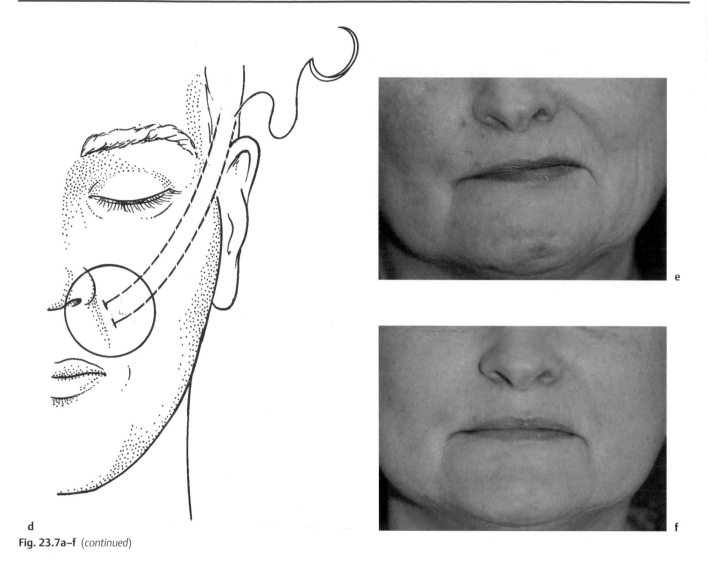

Fig. 23.7a–f (continued)

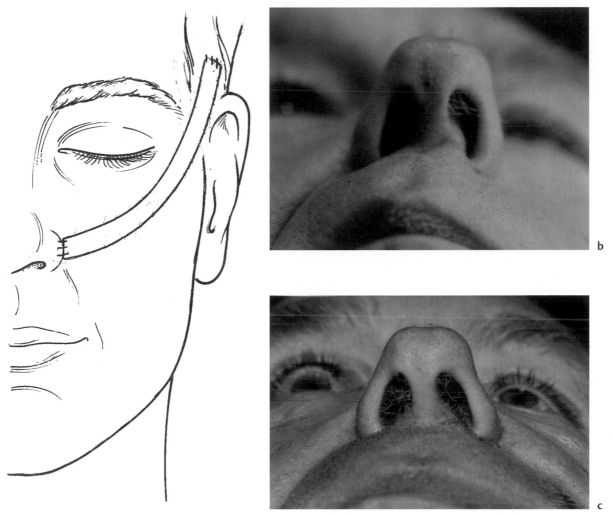

Fig. 23.8a–c External nasal valve repair via fascia lata sling from alar base to zygoma. (**a**) Schematic demonstrating fascia placement. (**b**) Preoperative view. (**c**) Postoperative view. (Figs. 23.8b, c are used with permission from Hadlock TA, Cheney ML. Facial reanimation. In: Urken ML, ed. Multidisciplinary Head and Neck Reconstruction: A Defect–Oriented Approach. Philadelphia, PA: Lippincott Williams & Wilkins; 2010: 435–454.)

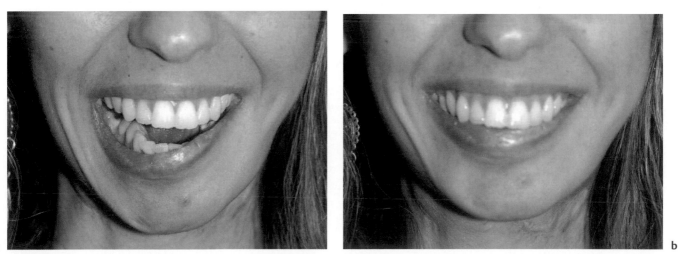

Fig. 23.9a, b The effect of contralateral lower lip chemodenervation. (**a**) Pretreatment. (**b**) Posttreatment. (Used with permission from Hadlock TA, Cheney ML. Facial reanimation. In: Urken ML, ed. Multidisciplinary Head and Neck Reconstruction: A Defect–Oriented Approach. Philadelphia, PA: Lippincott Williams & Wilkins; 2010: 435–454.)

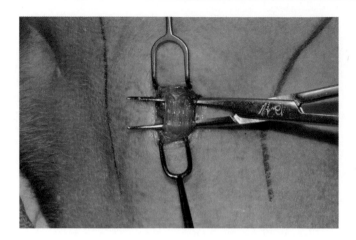

Fig. 23.10 Delivery of posterior section of hypertrophied platysma muscle through surgical incision before division during platysmectomy. (Used with permission from Hadlock TA, Cheney ML. Facial reanimation. In: Urken ML, ed. Multidisciplinary Head and Neck Reconstruction: A Defect–Oriented Approach. Philadelphia, PA: Lippincott Williams & Wilkins; 2010: 435–454.)

References

1. Sunderland S. Axon Degeneration. Nerve Injuries and Their Repair. New York: Churchill Livingstone; 1991:82–83.

2. Millesi H. Nerve suture and grafting to restore the extratemporal facial nerve. Clin Plast Surg 1979;6(3):333–341

3. Yarbrough WG, Brownlee RE, Pillsbury HC. Primary anastomosis of extensive facial nerve defects: an anatomic study. Am J Otol 1993;14(3):238–246

4. Anderson RG. Facial nerve disorders and surgery. Select Read Plast Surg 1994;7(20):4

5. Chang DW. Minimal incision technique for sural nerve graft harvest: experience with 61 patients. J Reconstr Microsurg 2002;18(8):671–676

6. Hadlock TA, Cheney ML. Single-incision endoscopic sural nerve harvest for cross face nerve grafting. J Reconstr Microsurg 2008;24(7):519–523

7. IJpma FF, Nicolai JP, Meek MF. Sural nerve donor-site morbidity: thirty-four years of follow-up. Ann Plast Surg 2006;57(4): 391–395

8. Spector JG, Lee P, Peterein J, Roufa D. Facial nerve regeneration through autologous nerve grafts: a clinical and experimental study. Laryngoscope 1991;101(5):537–554

9. Levinthal R, Brown WJ, Rand RW. Comparison of fascicular, interfascicular and epineural suture techniques in the repair of simple nerve lacerations. J Neurosurg 1977;47(5):744–750

10. Cheney MMC, McKenna M. Rehabilitation of the paralyzed face. In: Cheney M, ed. Facial Surgery, Plastic and Reconstructive. Baltimore: Williams and Wilkins; 1997:655–694.

11. Ornelas L, Padilla L, Di Silvio M, et al. Fibrin glue: an alternative technique for nerve coaptation—Part I. Wave amplitude, conduction velocity, and plantar-length factors. J Reconstr Microsurg 2006;22(2):119–122

12. Ornelas L, Padilla L, Di Silvio M, et al. Fibrin glue: an alternative technique for nerve coaptation—Part II. Nerve regeneration and histomorphometric assessment. J Reconstr Microsurg 2006;22(2):123–128

13. Conley J. Hypoglossal crossover–122 cases. Trans Sect Otolaryngol Am Acad Ophthalmol Otolaryngol 1977;84(4 Pt 1):ORL-763–ORL-768

14. Gavron JP, Clemis JD. Hypoglossal-facial nerve anastomosis: a review of forty cases caused by facial nerve injuries in the posterior fossa. Laryngoscope 1984;94(11 Pt 1):1447–1450

15. Conley J, Baker DC. Hypoglossal-facial nerve anastomosis for reinnervation of the paralyzed face. Plast Reconstr Surg 1979; 63(1):63–72

16. May M. Nerve Substitution Techniques. In: May M, Schaitkin B, eds. The Facial Nerve. New York: Thieme Publishers; 1999: 611–633.

17. Atlas MD, Lowinger DS. A new technique for hypoglossal-facial nerve repair. Laryngoscope 1997;107(7):984–991

18. Terzis JK, Tzafetta K. Outcomes of mini-hypoglossal nerve transfer and direct muscle neurotization for restoration of lower lip function in facial palsy. Plast Reconstr Surg 2009;124(6):1891–1904

19. Yetiser S, Karapinar U. Hypoglossal-facial nerve anastomosis: a meta-analytic study. Ann Otol Rhinol Laryngol 2007;116(7): 542–549

20. Mehta RP, Hadlock TA. Botulinum toxin and quality of life in patients with facial paralysis. Arch Facial Plast Surg 2008;10(2): 84–87

21. Scaramella LF. Cross-face facial nerve anastomosis: historical notes. Ear Nose Throat J 1996;75(6):343, 347–352, 354

22. Scaramella LF, Tobias E. Facial nerve anastomosis. Laryngoscope 1973;83(11):1834–1840

23. Smith JW. Advances in facial nerve repair. Surg Clin North Am 1972;52(5):1287–1306

24. Glickman LT, Simpson R. Cross-facial nerve grafting for facial reanimation: effect on normal hemiface motion. J Reconstr Microsurg 12:99, 1996. J Reconstr Microsurg 1996;12(3):201–202

25. Cooper TM, McMahon B, Lex C, Lenert JJ, Johnson PC. Cross-facial nerve grafting for facial reanimation: effect on normal hemiface motion. J Reconstr Microsurg 1996;12(2):99–103

26. Anderl H. Cross-face nerve transplantation in facial palsy. Proc R Soc Med 1976;69(10):781–783

27. Baker DC, Conley J. Facial nerve grafting: a thirty year retrospective review. Clin Plast Surg 1979;6(3):343–360

28. Galli SK, Valauri F, Komisar A. Facial reanimation by cross-facial nerve grafting: report of five cases. Ear Nose Throat J 2002;81(1):25–29

29. Lee EI, Hurvitz KA, Evans GR, Wirth GA. Cross-facial nerve graft: past and present. J Plast Reconstr Aesthet Surg 2008;61(3): 250–256

30. Aydin MA, Mackinnon SE, Gu XM, Kobayashi J, Kuzon WM Jr. Force deficits in skeletal muscle after delayed reinnervation. Plast Reconstr Surg 2004;113(6):1712–1718

31. Kobayashi J, Mackinnon SE, Watanabe O, et al. The effect of duration of muscle denervation on functional recovery in the rat model. Muscle Nerve 1997;20(7):858–866

32. Terzis JK, Konofaos P. Nerve transfers in facial palsy. Facial Plast Surg 2008;24(2):177–193

33. Terzis JK, Wang W, Zhao Y. Effect of axonal load on the functional and aesthetic outcomes of the cross-facial nerve graft procedure for facial reanimation. Plast Reconstr Surg 2009;124(5): 1499–1512

34. Terzis JK, Kalantarian B. Microsurgical strategies in 74 patients for restoration of dynamic depressor muscle mechanism: a neglected target in facial reanimation. Plast Reconstr Surg 2000; 105(6):1917–1931, discussion 1932–1934

35. Griebie MS, Huff JS. Selective role of partial XI-VII anastomosis in facial reanimation. Laryngoscope 1998;108(11 Pt 1):1664–1668

36. Poe DS, Scher N, Panje WR. Facial reanimation by XI-VII anastomosis without shoulder paralysis. Laryngoscope 1989;99(10 Pt 1): 1040–1047

37. Frydman WL, Heffez LB, Jordan SL, Jacob A. Facial muscle reanimation using the trigeminal motor nerve: an experimental study in the rabbit. J Oral Maxillofac Surg 1990;48(12): 1294–1304

38. Hadlock TA, Greenfield LJ, Wernick-Robinson M, Cheney ML. Multimodality approach to management of the paralyzed face. Laryngoscope 2006;116(8):1385–1389

24 Lower Facial Reanimation

Babak Azizzadeh and Kimberly J. Lee

Facial paralysis is a condition that can affect some or all branches of the facial nerve. Facial nerve disorders can lead to poor facial aesthetics and functional deficits that can severely affect patient quality of life. Furthermore, in many patients with partial facial paralysis, synkinesis of the facial musculature will complicate the treatment goals.

The goals of facial paralysis reconstruction include achieving symmetry at rest, dynamic facial movement, and appropriate eyelid function. This chapter aims to address the nonsurgical and surgical methods of lower facial reanimation with focus on delineating static and dynamic options.

History

The possibility of facial nerve surgery was initially conceived by Sir Charles Bell in 1821 when he established that the facial nerve innervates the muscles of facial expression.[1] Historically, facial nerve paralysis was treated medically with topical ointment, medicine, and electrotherapy.[2] The first nerve transfer was performed by Drobnick in 1879 when he anastomosed the spinal accessory nerve to a dysfunctional facial nerve.[3] Manasse and Korte, in the early 1900s, performed hypoglossal to facial nerve substitution in addition to the spinal accessory nerve.[4,5] In that same time period, Stacke resected a portion of the facial nerve and juxtaposed the cut ends.[6]

The first facial nerve graft within the temporal bone was performed by Bunnell in 1927.[7] In addition to Bunnell's work, Lathrop and Myers demonstrated that the facial nerve could regenerate and that facial movement could be improved with facial nerve reconstruction.[8,9] Sir Charles Balance, the founder and first president of the Society of British Neurological Surgeons, showed that nerve grafts for the facial nerve had more favorable results than those obtained by anastomosis of the facial nerve to the hypoglossal and glossopharyngeal nerves.[10,11] Lexer and Eden in 1911 described temporalis and masseter regional muscle transposition techniques.[12] These dynamic techniques were also later reported by Erlacher in 1915 and Owens in 1947.[13,17]

The modem era of free tissue transfer introduced novel treatment modalities that have subsequently revolutionized facial reanimation outcomes. Scaramella described cross-face nerve grafts in 1970.[14–16] Thompson proposed free muscle transplantation to reanimate the paralyzed face, which was subsequently supported by Ruben and Harii et al.[17–20] Cross-facial nerve grafts followed by vascularized muscle free flaps paved the way for modern facial reanimation surgery.[20]

Facial paralysis can result from a variety of factors including congenital, iatrogenic, idiopathic, infectious, metabolic, neoplastic, neurologic, toxic, and trauma (**Table 24.1**). Paralysis of the facial musculature results in aesthetic, functional, and psychosocial morbidity.[4] Unilateral cases cause facial asymmetry at rest and/or during animation. Although individuals with bilateral facial paralysis can have a more symmetrical appearance, the psychological effect of not being able to effectively express one's emotions can be significant.

While facial paralysis leads to aesthetic deformity and psychosocial issues, the functional consequences can lead to even more significant morbidity and deteriorating quality of life.[4] Patients with facial palsy often do not communicate effectively, experience oral incompetence, and may have significant tension from synkinesis. Lagophthalmos and lower lid malposition can lead to corneal dessication, ulceration, and eventual blindness.

Patient Evaluation

Chapter 4 of this book discusses the details of facial paralysis evaluation and will serve as an excellent reference. In terms of individuals seeking lower facial reanimation, there are a few key issues that need to be determined. Most patients have likely been examined by a clinician and given a diagnosis for the etiology of their facial paralysis. While the physical manifestations of facial nerve paralysis are distressing for all patients, it is important to take a detailed history and perform

Table 24.1 Etiology of facial nerve paralysis

- Congenital (e.g., Möbius syndrome, craniofacial microsomia)
- Trauma (e.g., temporal bone fracture, laceration)
- Tumor (e.g., cerebellopontine angle tumor, facial neuroma, malignant head and neck neoplasm)
- Iatrogenic (e.g., acoustic neuroma resection, parotidectomy, temporal bone resection, neck dissection, rhytidectomy)
- Infectious (e.g., Lyme disease, Ramsay Hunt syndrome)
- Melkersson-Rosenthal
- Idiopathic (Bell palsy)

a thorough physical examination to determine the underlying etiology. It is extremely important not to be sidetracked by an established diagnosis at the time of evaluation, which may or may not be accurate. A significant amount of time needs to be spent on confirming the correct diagnosis in this patient population. Many patients diagnosed with Bell palsy may harbor serious malignancies.

Other key issues that need to be clarified during the patient evaluation include severity of the facial paralysis and synkinesis, duration of palsy, patient age, functional deficits, and long-term goals. Individuals with partial paralysis who have synkinesis will often require a different treatment protocol than those with complete flaccid paralysis. Duration of facial palsy is also critical, as most surgical interventions are typically performed only after the regenerative functions of the nerve have been clearly established (typically 1 year). The etiology of the paralysis will help guide the surgeon as to what is the appropriate time frame to wait before initiating treatment. Finally, the patient's long-term goals need to be clearly understood. The main complaint from patients with facial paralysis is oral incompetence, facial asymmetry, and inability to generate a smile. Some individuals just desire to improve symmetry at rest and reduce functional deficits, whereas others desire spontaneous dynamic facial movements.

During the physical examination, the eyes are inspected for narrowing or widening of the aperture, degree of lagophthalmos, Bell phenomenon, lower eyelid position, and laxity (snap test). The facial movements corresponding to each of the facial nerve branches must be evaluated carefully by asking the patient to raise the eyebrows, shut the eyes, wrinkle the nose, smile, show the teeth, and pucker. The key factor is to determine whether the patient has complete flaccid paralysis or partial paralysis with muscle tone. Patients with partial paralysis need to be further evaluated for any evidence of synkinesis, which typically involves simultaneous and uncoordinated oculofacial muscle contractions (such as orbicularis oculi contraction while trying to smile). Synkinesis often leads to "auto-paralysis," where simultaneous activation of the orbicularis oris, buccinators, oral commissure elevators, and depressors result in a frozen smile and prevent the patient from having a true smile mechanism.

The House-Brackmann and Sunnybrook Facial Grading System are useful tools to evaluate facial palsy and synkinesis (see **Tables 5.2** and **5.5** in Chapter 5). The House-Brackmann grading system is a six-point scale, and the Sunnybrook Facial Grading System evaluates synkinesis at rest, during movement, and with voluntary movement.[6] The scale is continuous from 0 through 100, where 0 indicates complete paralysis and 100 is normal.[10]

In clinical practice, the senior author categorizes facial palsy patients into five categories:

Type A: Normal facial function
Type B: Partial paralysis with mild synkinesis
Type C: Partial paralysis with moderate to severe synkinesis
Type D: Partial paralysis without synkinesis
Type E: Complete facial paralysis

To complete the physical exam, the remaining cranial nerves should be evaluated and radiographic imaging (computed tomography or magnetic resonance imaging) may be required. Electromyographic studies can be useful in determining viability of the muscle fibers; however, in patients with long-standing facial paralysis, physical examination will provide enough information about the muscle tone and function. Preoperative photography and video assessment at rest and during animation is recommended. A multidisciplinary approach with a physical therapist that is knowledgeable and skilled in working with patients with facial paralysis is strongly recommended for optimizing outcomes.

■ Etiology

Prior to any intervention, appropriate evaluation of the patient in an effort to determine the underlying etiology is critical. Facial paralysis can be congenital or acquired (see **Table 24.1**). The most common etiology of unilateral facial paralysis is idiopathic, also referred to as Bell palsy.[11] Approximately 85% of patients with Bell palsy start to have spontaneous recovery within a few weeks after onset. The remaining 15% may not experience facial movement for up to 6 months; however, most of these patients will have some level of recovery. The duration of time is directly correlated to higher incidence of synkinesis, loss of mimetic function, and contracture. The likelihood of recovery is best for younger age groups.[7]

If the facial paralysis is caused by a traumatic event and the nerve ends can be identified and stimulated, repair within the first 3 days of the injury yields the highest likelihood of recovery.[21] Generally, if damage is to the buccal or zygomaticus branches medial to the lateral canthus, the nerve is able to recover on its own and no repair is indicated. Proximal injuries to these branches will require surgical repair. The buccal and zygomaticus branches have extensive arborization, and therefore the likelihood of permanent paralysis is less common than trauma to frontal and marginal mandibular branches, which are terminal branches. In acoustic neuroma resection and parotid neoplasms, the facial nerve may be intentionally sacrificed for tumor resection. In temporal bone fractures, the facial nerve may be transected, crushed, or impinged, leading to facial palsy.

■ Nonsurgical Intervention

The main nonsurgical treatment options for lower facial reanimation are the use of neuromodulators, injectable fillers, and neuromuscular rehabilitation. The authors emphasize that neuromodulators such as botulinum toxin-A (BTX-A) play a crucial role in creating facial symmetry, improving synkinesis, increasing oral commissure excursion, and reducing functional deficits.[8,22] Patients with Type B and C partial paralysis with synkinesis and congenital unilateral lower lip palsy are typically the best candidates. Patients with synkinesis typically have simultaneous activation of oral commissure elevators, orbicularis oris, buccinator, and lower lip depressor activity. They therefore can have improvement in their dynamic smile function by reducing the downward force of depressors such as the depressor labii inferioris, risorius, and depressor anguli oris.

In the senior author's practice (Azizzadeh), neuromuscular rehabilitation and BTX-A are the primary treatment strategies for younger patients with limited facial palsy and minimal to moderate amount of synkinesis (Type B and C patients). In patients who are older and/or have a more dense paralysis, BTX-A and neuromuscular retraining are used to complement other surgical reanimation techniques. Facial fillers such as hyaluronic acids, calcium hydroxyapatite, and injectable poly-L-lactic acid are also used to improve facial volume asymmetry, which is commonly seen in patients with facial paralysis.

■ Surgical Intervention

Surgical intervention for facial paralysis can be divided into static and dynamic reanimation. Dynamic reanimation can be further subdivided into "volitional" and "spontaneous" reanimation. Volitional dynamic reanimation requires the patient to be conscious about moving the face, whereas spontaneous reanimation does not. Static surgical procedures only improve the patient's symmetry at rest and technically do not reanimate the face.

Static Surgical Reconstruction

Static techniques are the workhorse of facial paralysis reconstruction. Static procedures are indicated for individuals who are not appropriate candidates for dynamic reanimation and/or regions of the face that are not amenable to dynamic reconstruction (e.g., brow ptosis, external nasal valve collapse). Static procedures include repair of brow ptosis, gold/platinum weight reconstruction for lagophthalmos, lower eyelid reconstruction, lower lip shortening, external nasal valve reconstruction, superficial musculoaponeurotic system (SMAS) rhytidectomy, and static sling suspension (**Fig. 24.1**).

For lower facial paralysis reconstruction, static sling suspension is able to achieve two major goals: improve facial symmetry and reduce functional deficits such as oral incompetence, biting of inner gums, and poor articulation. As static slings do not interfere with nerve regeneration, they can be used to achieve an immediate aesthetic and functional improvement in conjunction with dynamic procedures such as cable nerve grafting, hypoglossal-facial nerve anastomosis, and cross-facial nerve grafts. Static slings can also be used to augment muscle transfer techniques or revise previous dynamic reanimation procedures. As standalone procedures, static slings do not directly address the smile mechanism but do improve a patient's perception of his or her smile and face.

In the authors' practice, static slings are offered to individuals who are not candidates for dynamic reanimation

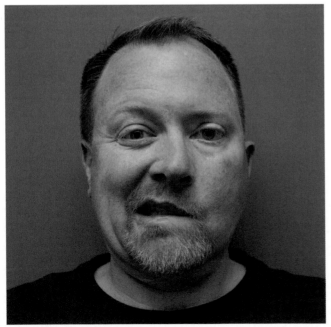
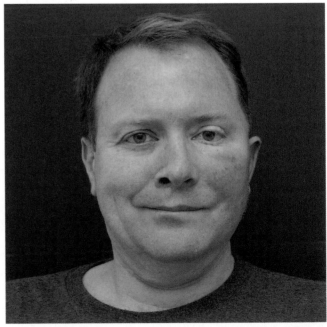

a   b

Fig. 24.1a, b (**a**) Preoperative photo of patient with left-sided facial nerve paralysis. (**b**) Postoperative photo of same patient after undergoing superficial musculoaponeurotic system rhytidectomy and static sling suspension.

such as those who have advanced age, partial paralysis with adequate oral commissure excursion, and major head and neck malignancy. In appropriate candidates, this procedure is considered only after the status of nerve regeneration has been ascertained, typically 1 year after date of onset or if the facial nerve has been deliberately sacrificed. Patients are typically elderly with a history of tumor ablation in the head and neck or cerebellopontine angle region.

Tensor fascia lata (TFL) is the ideal choice for static sling procedures.[23] A substantial amount of tissue can be harvested from the lateral thigh, and multiple strips can be created for both oral commissure suspension as well as external nasal valve repositioning. Although TFL does require a separate donor site that can increase patient morbidity, it has the advantage of being an autogenous material with long-term viability.

Commercially available, freeze-dried acellular human dermis (AlloDerm Regenerative Tissue Matrix, LifeCell, Branchburg, NJ) has also been used for facial static slings. The advantage of acellular human dermis is that it precludes a donor site harvest. Acellular human dermis is readily available, integrates into surrounding tissue, and can be customized quickly to create exact facial slings. Although there have been reports of poor long-term outcome with AlloDerm, namely sling failure and infection, the authors' experience has been satisfactory in both short- and long-term use in a carefully selected patient population who would have significant morbidity from harvesting of TFL.[24]

Expanded polytetrafluoroethylene (ePTFE, Gore-Tex, Implantech Associates, Santa Barbara, CA) is a synthetic material that can also be considered for use in static sling procedures. Levet and Jost reported on their use of ePTFE for facial suspension in the French literature in 1987 with good results.[25] Petroff et al also reported favorable results from facial suspensions with ePTFE soft-tissue patch without infection or extrusion.[26] Iwahira and Maruyama, in 1992, reported the use of ePTFE with temporalis transfer as "extensions" when the temporalis muscle fascia was weak and/or short.[27] ePTFE circumvents the need to harvest TFL, thus eliminating a second donor site morbidity; however, given its lack of integration with local tissue, its use in our practice has been limited.

Suture suspension techniques that have been popularized in aesthetic midface lifts can also be successfully used for patients requiring minor repositioning of the oral commissure.[27,28] Suture suspension techniques are generally less invasive than other static techniques and can be performed percutaneously and under local anesthesia; however, its potential for comprehensive suspension is limited and its long-term outcome has not yet been adequately studied.

The static sling procedure is typically performed simultaneously with a rhytidectomy. Using a rhytidectomy incision, a deep subcutaneous plane is elevated to the level of the oral commissure (**Fig. 24.2a**). A single sheet of 5 × 12 cm sling material (TFL, acellular dermis, ePTFE) is typically used to create an equal amount of tension along

the oral commissure and nasolabial fold (**Fig. 24.2b**). The sling is sutured at the modiolus to orbicularis oris or subdermal tissue layer if orbicularis is significantly atrophied. Approximately three to five separate O-Vicryl sutures (Ethicon, Inc., Somerville, NJ) are used to attach the graft to the oral commissure and nasolabial fold (**Fig. 24.2c**). The sling should be slightly overcorrected in a posterolateral vector and secured to the deep temporalis fascia, zygomatic arch, and preauricular SMAS. An additional sheet of sling material (1.5 × 10 cm) is typically used to elevate the nasal alar crease to improve external nasal valve collapse and nasal obstruction.

Dynamic Surgical Reconstruction

Although static reconstruction has significant advantages such as creating symmetry at rest and improving functional deficits, most patients' primary goal of smiling remains unfulfilled. The goal of dynamic reanimation is to allow the patient to not only obtain symmetry but also regain a functional smile mechanism. As stated previously, the smile mechanism may be volitional where the patient needs to be actively conscious of moving the face or spontaneous. Dynamic reanimation can be achieved using regional muscle transfers (temporalis), cranial nerve substitution techniques (hypoglossal-facial nerve transfer), and/or microvascular free muscle grafts.

Temporalis Transfer

The goal of temporalis muscle transfer is to attach a segment of the temporalis muscle to the oral commissure to re-create a smile mechanism by activating the motor branches of the trigeminal nerve. This is accomplished by biting down as if mimicking the chewing mechanism. Lexer, in 1908, was the first to describe regional muscle transfer utilizing the temporalis muscle.[33] The procedure was modified in 1934 by Gilles, who performed a temporal muscle flap by folding it over the zygoma to the level of the oral commissure subcutaneously.[29] Because this technique led to fullness over the zygoma with hollowing in the temporal fossa, MacLaughlin in 1952 proposed temporalis muscle tendon transfer.[23] In this technique, the temporalis muscle tendon was detached from the coronoid process and secured to the oral commissure using a fascial graft.[30] In the 1990s, Cheyney modified the classic temporalis flap by using only the middle third of the temporal muscle and obliterating the hollowness with a simultaneous temporoparietal fascial flap in an attempt to reduce the temple hollowness.[31] In the 1990s, Labbé also improved temporalis contour irregularity by repositioning the posterior third of the temporalis muscle and inserting it into the lips after detaching it from the coronoid process and fracturing the zygomatic arch.[31] In 2007, Byrne reintroduced and modified the temporalis tendon transfer technique which has since gained significant acceptance.[32]

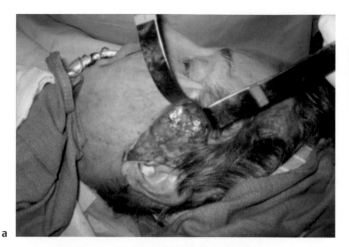

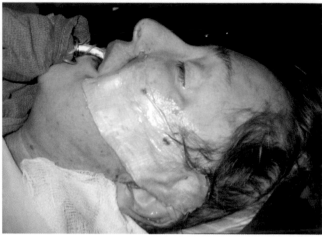

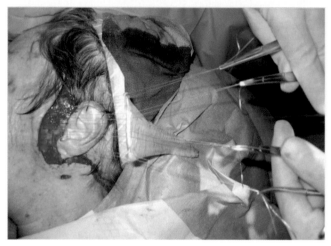

Fig. 24.2a–c (**a**) Elevation of the deep subcutaneous plane to the level of the oral commissure. (**b**) A single sheet of sling material (tensor fascia lata, acellular dermis, expanded polytetrafluoroethylene) is placed over the area to measure that amount of material needed to create the appropriate amount of tension along the oral commissure and nasolabial fold. (**c**) The sling is secured using three to five separate O-Vicryl sutures (Ethicon, Inc., Somerville, NJ) to attach the graft to the oral commissure and nasolabial fold.

The advantages of the temporalis muscle or tendon transfer is that it can be performed as a single-stage dynamic reanimation procedure, does not interfere with native nerve regeneration, is relatively simple to perform, and provides active excursion of their oral commissure. The temporalis muscle, however, does not provide spontaneous reanimation, and the smile mechanism is often not utilized by patients due to lack of training. Overall, the role of temporalis muscle or tendon transfers have been limited in the senior author's practice as other techniques such as gracilis free muscle grafts have supplanted this technique.

Hypoglossal-Facial Nerve Anastomosis

The first cranial nerve substitution procedure was attempted by Drobnik in 1879 where he attempted to anastomose the spinal accessory and facial nerves to rehabilitate patients with facial paralysis.[34] In 1895, Balance attempted an end-to-end neurorrhaphy without success.[35] Korte is credited with performing the first hypoglossal-facial anastomosis (XII-VII) in 1901 with long-term favorable outcomes.[5] Since that time and with improvements in microsurgical technique, cranial nerve substitution techniques have been extensively utilized with satisfactory outcome.

The XII-VII transfer utilizes the hypoglossal nerve to neurotize a nonfunctional facial nerve (Type E patients with complete flaccid paralysis). The nerve input would increase muscle tone reversing the flaccidity of a complete paralysis. Tongue movement would then allow patients to control the facial musculature and consciously move the face. This approach is most appropriate for complete and permanent facial paralysis. This technique is commonly employed following surgery or trauma where the facial nerve is irreversibly injured and the proximal nerve stump is not accessible for primary or cable nerve repair (acoustic neuroma resection, temporal bone trauma, and skull base surgery).

Successful outcomes are seen only if the patient has an intact extracranial facial nerve (preferably the main trunk as it exists the stylomastoid foramen or the lower division), mimetic facial muscles, and donor hypoglossal nerve. Traumatic, iatrogenic, or intentional injury to the facial nerve distal to the parotid gland precludes the use of this procedure. The major concerns with the XII-VII transfer is the potential of hemitongue paralysis leading to dysphagia and dysarthria.[36] As a result, patients with multiple cranial neuropathies are not appropriate candidates. Other contraindications to this procedure include developmental facial paralysis, prolonged facial palsy of more than 2-year duration, and partial paralysis with existing muscle tone (Type A–D). Generally, patients who are unable to accept deficit of the hypoglossal nerve and/or have facial paralysis of more than 2-year duration leading to irreversible facial muscle atrophy are poor candidates for XII-VII transfer.

Improved facial tone and symmetry occurs in over 90% of patients following hypoglossal-facial anastomosis and is usually seen within 4 to 6 months.[37] Eyelid tone may improve the closure of the eye and thereby facilitate removal of any gold weight. Voluntary facial movement begins after tone develops and continues to improve over the ensuing 18 months. Voluntary motion typically creates synkinetic mass facial movement of all muscles and is usually not targeted to excursion of the oral commissure. Younger patients and early nerve substitution have better overall outcomes.[38,39]

There are several hypoglossal-facial nerve techniques that can be utilized to achieve satisfactory outcome. The classic procedure involved the sacrifice of the entire hypoglossal nerve, which often leads to hemitongue paralysis and variable functional deficits such as dysphagia, dysarthria, and hemitongue atrophy.[40] The technique for this operation included performing a modified Blair incision and exposing the hypoglossal nerve and facial nerve via a superficial parotidectomy. The hypoglossal nerve is then sacrificed and rotated up into the parotid gland and anastamosed to the facial nerve. This operation has been largely replaced by techniques that only partially sacrifice the hypoglossal nerve.

Several modifications have been described for the XII-VII transfer. The split XII-VII utilizes ~30–50% of the hypoglossal nerve width in a linear fashion, which is then rotated up toward the parotid region and anastomosed to the lower division of the facial nerve (**Fig. 24.3**).[41] By splitting the nerve, the risk of hemitongue atrophy is minimized, although long-term evaluation of the tongue may still reveal partial tongue atrophy. XII-VII jump graft, introduced by Terzis, avoids linear splitting of the hypoglossal nerve. The hypoglossal nerve is divided 25–50% in diameter and sewn to a cable nerve graft (great auricular or sural nerve graft). The nerve graft is then anastomosed to the main trunk of the facial nerve. Although this procedure requires harvesting of a nerve graft, the overall morbidity is lower than split XII-VII transfer. Several authors have reported comparable functional results with lower incidence of hypertonia or mass facial movements.[42,43]

Facial nerve translocation is another useful XII-VII technique.[44] The facial nerve in this procedure is identified in the vertical segment of the mastoid bone and translocated down to the hypoglossal nerve. The hypoglossal nerve is partially transected and primary anastomosis is performed. This technique circumvents the need to identify the facial nerve in the parotid gland and has the advantage of a single anastomosis. However, the time to recovery is lengthened because the facial nerve is anastomosed farther posteriorly in the mastoid.

The hypoglossal-facial nerve transfer is an extremely valuable tool in the armamentarium of a facial paralysis

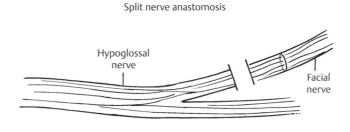

Split nerve anastomosis

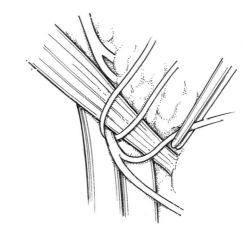

Fig. 24.3 Splitting of the hypoglossal nerve (cranial nerve XII) to be reanastomosed with the facial nerve.

surgeon. Unfortunately, many patients who are excellent candidates are not seen in a timely fashion and miss the opportunity to have this procedure. The senior author often combines this procedure with static slings to obtain immediate results until the reinnervation is completed (**Fig. 24.4**).

In younger patients, we also combine this procedure with more advanced facial reanimation techniques such as cross-facial nerve grafts (CFNGs) and gracilis flaps, which provide more spontaneous and targeted smile excursion (**Fig. 24.5**).

Free Muscle Transfer

Although many of the techniques described in this chapter thus far provide excellent static reconstruction and dynamic reanimation, none truly results in spontaneous facial reanimation. Direct facial nerve repair (as described in Chapter 23) and free muscle transfer powered by a CFNG are the only surgical procedures that can restore spontaneous reanimation of the face. As direct nerve repair can often cause significant synkinesis, CFNG with free muscle transfer is the only procedure that can actually provide a targeted smile mechanism.

Initially described by Scaramella in 1970, the CFNG was subsequently modified by Smith, Anderl, Fisch, and Conley (**Fig. 24.6**).[45–48] Scaramella initially used the CFNG as a neural input to the dysfunctional facial nerve. He utilized a sural nerve graft to connect the cervical branch of the

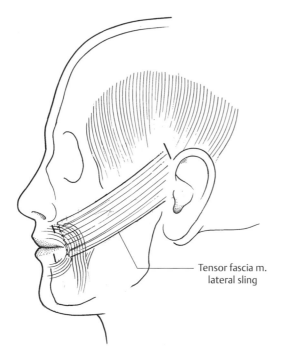

Fig. 24.4 Placement of a static sling from the oral commissure to the temporal region.

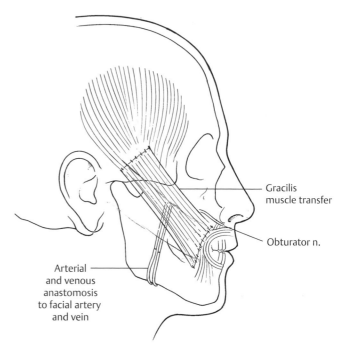

Fig. 24.5 Placement of a gracilis flap combined with cross-facial nerve grafts to allow dynamic movement of the oral commissure. Such procedures allow patients more spontaneous ability to smile.

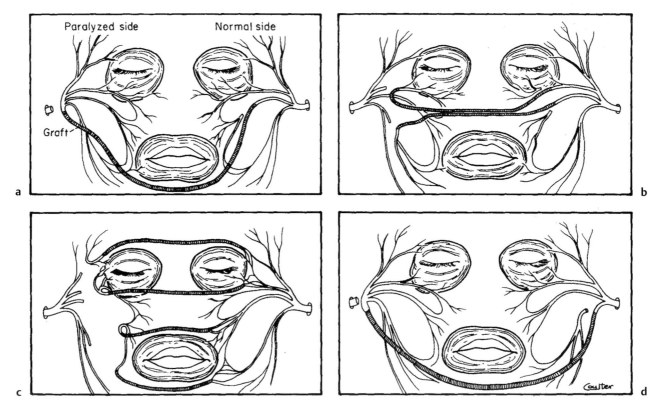

Fig. 24.6a–d Variety of techniques for faciofacial cross-face graft. (**a**) Scaramella cross-face graft. The graft may also be passed over the upper lip. (**b**) Fisch technique. (**c**) Anderl modifications. In Conley's experience, the frontal and marginal mandibular functions return in only 15% of patients, even with primary nerve grafting. (**d**) Conley's preferred technique is to anastomose the entire lower division of the normal side with the main trunk of the paralyzed side. Exposure is easily obtained with standard parotid incisions. The graft may be passed over the upper lip. (Used with permission from May M, Schaitkin B, eds. The Facial Nerve: May's Second Edition. New York, NY: Thieme; 2000: 553.)

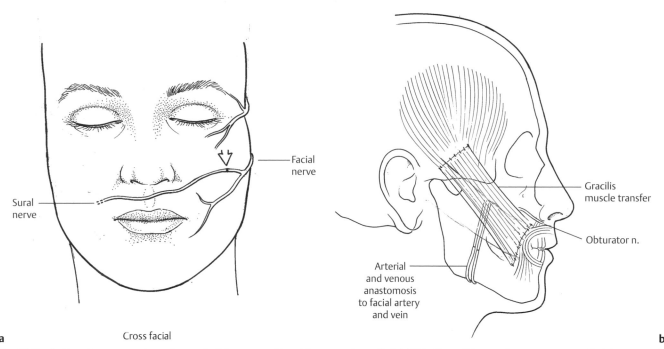

a   Cross facial   b

Fig. 24.7a, b Two stage procedure of cross-facial nerve graft and free muscle graft. (**a**) Utilization of the sural nerve as a cross-facial nerve graft to extend the nerve across the midline of the face. (**b**) Placement of a gracilis free muscle combined with cross-facial nerve grafts allows dynamic motion of the oral commissure and enables a more spontaneous smile for patients.

normal facial nerve and the abnormal facial nerve trunk. The general results with this approach were less than ideal, and these techniques were mostly abandoned.[49–51]

It wasn't until the CFNG and free muscle grafts were combined in a two-stage operation that this surgical approach proved to be successful in restoring spontaneous facial movement. In 1979, Harii recommended the two-stage procedure utilizing both the CFNG as neural source and gracilis free muscle transfer as muscle source (**Fig. 24.7**). Although the two-stage CFNG technique proved to be reproducible, patients were not satisfied with the muscle bulk. In 1984, Manktelow addressed this problem by using a "mini gracilis" transfer, which is now the accepted manner for this technique (**Fig. 24.8**).[52–58]

The gracilis muscle has also been utilized in other manners for facial reanimation. Introduced by O'Brien and popularized by Kumar in the 1990s, the one-stage gracilis muscle transfer allowed reduction of the rehabilitation period by 10 months. The technique places the neurovascular pedicle at the nasolabial fold and transfers the obturator nerve through the upper lip to the contralateral facial nerve.[55] Although the two-stage gracilis procedure resulted in better symmetry at rest (67% versus 20% for the single-stage), the one-stage gracilis transfer otherwise produced comparable results with 90% of single-stage patients and 93% of two-stage patients having good results.[56]

Zuker and Manktelow also popularized the use of gracilis muscle as a single-stage procedure by using the masseteric branch of the trigeminal nerve as the neural source.[52] This approach was first utilized in patients with Möbius syndrome who had bilateral facial paralysis that later expanded to unilateral facial palsy. Although patients

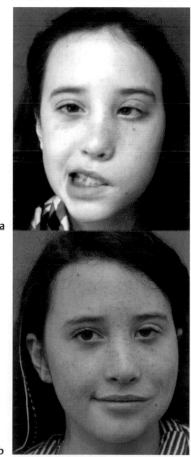

Fig. 24.8a,b (**a**) Preoperative photo of patient with left sided facial nerve paralysis. (**b**) Postoperative photo of same patient after undergoing two stage procedure of cross facial nerve graft and gracilis free flap.

obtained excellent excursion of the oral commissure, this approach is limited by its lack of spontaneity. The trigeminal-gracilis flap thus appears to be an excellent alternative to temporalis muscle or tendon transfer as a single-stage dynamic facial reanimation procedure.

Latissimus dorsi and pectoralis minor free muscle transfers have also been utilized in dynamic reanimation.[57–63] Although the latissimus dorsi muscle could be used as single-stage operation due to the appropriate length of the thoracodorsal nerve, it usually creates excessive bulk. The pectoralis minor muscle introduced by Terzis and Manktelow,[60] and subsequently popularized by Harrison,[61] is an excellent free muscle source that provides similar outcomes to gracilis and can be performed with a limited amount of muscle.

Currently, the senior author's preferred treatment option for patients under the age of 65 with unilateral complete facial nerve paralysis is the two-stage CFNG followed by gracilis free muscle transfer. We also use this option for selected patients with Type D facial palsy who have severe synkinesis and a "frozen smile."

In the CFNG procedure, a large branch of the peripheral facial nerve on the unaffected side is identified just past

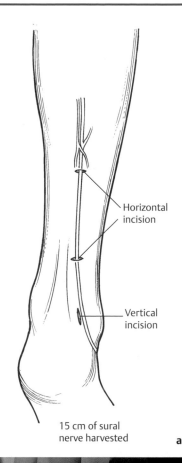

Horizontal incision

Vertical incision

15 cm of sural nerve harvested   **a**

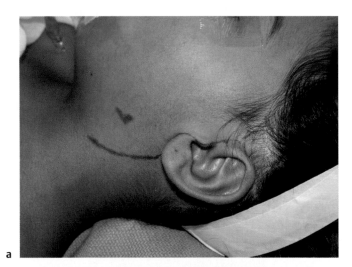

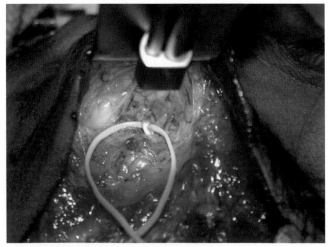

Fig. 24.9a, b Proposed facelift incision and identification of the peripheral facial nerve on the unaffected side.

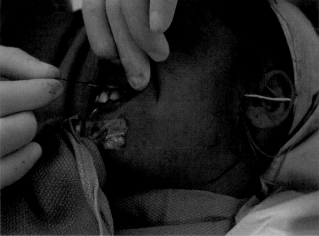

Fig. 24.10a, b (**a**) Harvest of ~15 cm of the sural nerve, which is located ~1 cm posterior to the lateral malleolus. (**b**) The distal segment of the sural nerve is tunneled to the contralateral gingivobuccal sulcus and tagged with a hemoclip and prolene suture.

the parotid gland via a deep-plane facelift approach (**Fig. 24.9**).

A nerve stimulator is utilized to ensure that the nerve only stimulates the zygomaticus muscles and does not innervate the oribicularis oculi. A 15-cm segment of sural nerve is harvested and primary neurorrhaphy is performed between the sural and peripheral facial nerve (**Fig. 24.10a**). The distal segment of the sural nerve is tunneled to the contralateral gingivobuccal sulcus and tagged with a hemoclip and Prolene (Ethicon, Somerville, NJ) suture (**Fig. 24.10b**).

The gracilis free flap muscle transfer is performed ~6 to 12 months later once a positive Tinel sign is identified, signifying axonal growth through the CFNG. During the second stage, the sural nerve graft is first biopsied in the gingivobuccal sulcus to confirm nerve growth. A segment of gracilis muscle is harvested (20 to 30 g) with the obturator nerve and adductor artery/vein (**Fig. 24.11**).

A deep subcutaneous flap is then elevated on the paralytic side via a modified Blair incision and sub-SMAS plane is entered at the anterior border of the parotid gland. The

facial artery and vein are identified at the mandibular border and prepared for revascularization of the gracilis muscle. The sub-SMAS plane is continued to the oral commissure and nasolabial fold (**Fig. 24.12**).

Four to five O-Vicryl sutures are placed at the modiolus and nasolabial folds. The gracilis muscle is then secured to these sutures and parachuted into the oral commissure (**Fig. 24.13**).

Arterial and venous anastomosis is completed under operating microscope, and the obturator nerve is tunneled to the gingivobuccal sulcus where neurorrhaphy is performed with the sural CFNG.

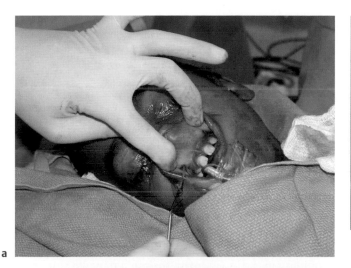
a
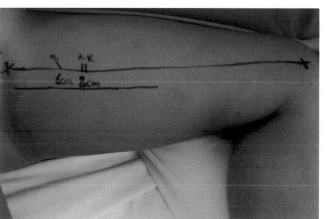
b
Harvest of gracilis m.
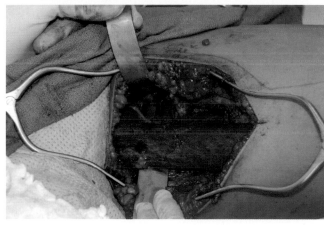
c
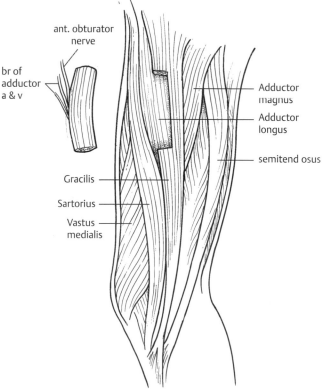
d

Fig. 24.11a–d (**a**) Biopsy of the sural nerve graft to ensure viability of the neurons. (**b**) Identification of the obturator nerve and adductor artery and vein. (**c**) Elevation of the skin and soft tissue to identify the gracilis muscle. (**d**) Harvest of a portion of the gracilis muscle with the adductor artery and vein and obturator nerve for anastomosis.

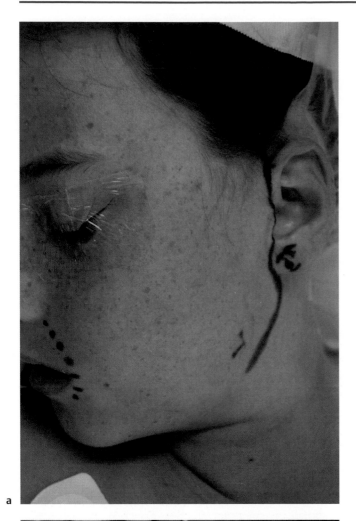

a

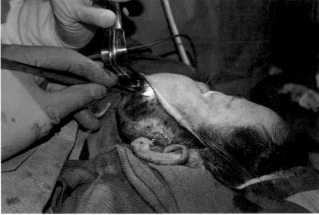

b

Fig. 24.12a, b (**a**) Marking of the modified Blair incision. (**b**) Continuation of the sub–superficial musculoaponeurotic system plane to the oral commissure and nasolabial fold.

Gracilis movement typically begins 6 months after the operation and continues to strengthen over the ensuing year. The most common adverse event with this procedure includes lateralization of the nasolabial fold, excessive flap bulk, and infection. About 10–20% of patients will require a third-stage procedure for reconfiguration of the nasolabial fold and/or debulking of the muscle.

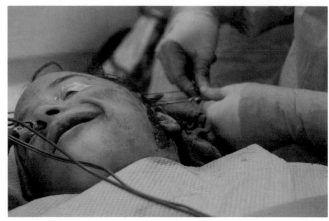

Fig. 24.13 Four to five O-Vicryl sutures (Ethicon, Inc., Somerville, NJ) are placed at the modiolus and nasolabial folds to secure the gracilis muscle to allow parachuting of the muscle into the oral commissure.

■ Lower Lip Reconstruction

Marginal mandibular nerve paresis leads to lower lip immobility as a result of depressor labii inferioris dysfunction. This lack of mobility is most pronounced during speech when the paralyzed side is elevated while the nonparalyzed side moves inferiorly. The senior author's preference is to manage this problem with chemodenervation (BTX-A) of the nonparalyzed depressor labii inferioris.[64] Chemodenervation of the normal side reduces the visibility of the dentition as well as the mobility of the lower lip on the nonparalyzed side during speech and animation. This simple procedure can have a dramatic impact in the overall appearance of patients, especially those with full denture smile pattern as well as individuals who suffer from congenital unilateral lower lip palsy.[65]

Other approaches include selective myectomy of the innervated depressor labii inferioris, sectioning the contralateral marginal branch, anterior belly of digastric transfer, free extensor digitorum brevis transfer, and platysma transfer.[66-71] Although these options have been extensively discussed in the literature, they are rarely useful in clinical practice. In the authors' experience, noninvasive injection of BTX-A to the innervated lower lip depressors is a simple and reproducible option with extremely high patient satisfaction and acceptance.

■ Bilateral Paralysis

Bilateral facial paralysis, most commonly associated with Möbius syndrome, remains as one of the most challenging areas in facial reanimation. While symmetry exists, patients cannot express any emotions and have significant functional and psychosocial deficits. Historically, bilateral temporalis muscle transfer was the treatment of choice.[35] However, as free muscle transfer techniques have evolved, they have gradually replaced local muscle transfers with significantly better outcomes.[72] Potential motor donor nerves include the masseteric branch of the trigeminal nerve, partial hypoglossal nerve, accessory nerve, and cervical motor donors from the cervical plexus and C7 nerve root.[73] Popularized by Zuker and Manktelow, gracilis free muscle flap innervated by the masseteric branch of the trigeminal nerve is the treatment of choice for this patient population.[72] This approach does not produce spontaneous smile mechanism but with aggressive neuromuscular rehabilitation, most patients obtain satisfactory outcome. Bilateral procedures can be performed either in a single or two-stage manner preferably before the age of 7.[22]

■ Conclusion

The treatment of long-standing facial paralysis with the ultimate goal of symmetry and spontaneous animation has challenged reconstructive surgeons for decades. The evolution of static and dynamic surgical techniques has vastly improved our ability to deliver better outcome. Surgical and nonsurgical options must be employed to obtain the best possible outcomes.

References

1. Bell C. On the Nerves: Giving an account of some experiments on their structure and function which leads to a new arrangement of the systems. Phil Trans Roy Soc 1821;3:398
2. van de Graaf RC, Nicolai JP. Bell's palsy before Bell: Cornelis Stalpart van der Wiel's observation of Bell's palsy in 1683. Otol Neurotol 2005;26(6):1235–1238
3. Drobnick, cited by Sawicki B, in Chepault: The Status of Neurosurgery. Paris: J. Reuff; 1902:189
4. Manasse P. Uber Vereinigung des N. facialis mit dem N. accesorius durch die Nervenpfropfung (Greffe nerveuse). Arch Klin Chir 1900;62:805
5. Korte W. Ein Fall von Nervenpfropfung: des Nervus facialis auf den Nervus hypoglossus. Deutsche med Wihnschr;1903;17:293–295
6. Stacke L. quoted by Alt. F: The operative treatment of otogenic facial palsy. Verhundl Deutsch Otol Geselisch 1908;17:190
7. Bunnell S. Suture of the facial nerve within the temporal bone with a report of the first successful case. Surg Gynecol Obstet 1927;45:7
8. Lathrop FD. Facial nerve surgery in the European theater of operation. Laryngoscope 1946;54:665–676
9. Myers D. War injuries to the mastoid and the facial nerve. Arch Otolaryngol 1946;44(4):392–405
10. van de Graaf RC, Nicolai JP. Was Thomasz Drobnik really the first to operate on the facial nerve? Otol Neurotol 2003;24(4):686–690
11. Miehike A. Surgery of the Facial Nerve , 2nd ed. Philadelphia: WB Saunders; 1973
12. Lexer E, Eden R. Uber die chirurgische Behandlung der peripheren Facialislahmung. Beitr Klin Chir 1911;73:116
13. Erlacher P. Direct and muscular neurotization of paralyzed muscle. Am J Orthop Surg 1915;13:22–32
14. Coulson SE, O'dwyer NJ, Adams RD, Croxson GR. Expression of emotion and quality of life after facial nerve paralysis. Otol Neurotol 2004;25(6):1014–1019
15. Scaramella LF. Preliminary report on facial nerve anasotomosis. Second international symposium on Facial Nerve Surgery. Osaka, Japan 1970.
16. Anderl H Reconstruction of the face through cross face nerve transplantation in facial paralysis. Chir Plast 1973.2(1):17–45
17. Owen N. Surgical correction of facial paralysis. Plast Reconstr Surg 1947;2:25
18. Thompson N. Autogenous free grafts of skeletal muscles. Plast Reconstr Surg 1971;48(1):11–27
19. Ruben L. Reanimation of the Paralyzed Face. St Louis, MO: C.V. Mosby Co.; 1977
20. Harii K, Ohmori K, Torii S. Free gracilis muscle transplantation with neurovascular anastomosis for the treatment of facial paralysis. Plast Reconstr Surg 1976;57:133–143

21. McCabe BF. Facial nerve grafting. Plast Reconstr Surg 1970; 45(1):70–75
22. Laskawi R. Combination of hypoglossal-facial nerve anastomosis and botulinum-toxin injections to optimize mimic rehabilitation after removal of acoustic neurinomas. Plast Reconstr Surg 1997;99(4):1006–1011
23. McLaughlin CR. Surgical support in permanent facial paralysis. Plast Reconstr Surg (1946) 1953;11(4):302–314
24. Constantinides M, Galli SK, Miller PJ. Complications of static facial suspensions with expanded polytetrafluoroethylene (ePTFE). Laryngoscope 2001;111(12):2114–2121
25. Levet Y, Jost G. Utilisation du polytétrafluoroéthylène (Gore-Tex E-PTFE Soft Tissue Patch) dans les suspensions de paralysies faciales anciennes et en tissu de comblement. Ann Otolaryngol Chir Cervicofac 1987;104(1):65–69
26. Petroff MA, Goode RL, Levet Y. Gore-Tex implants: applications in facial paralysis rehabilitation and soft-tissue augmentation. Laryngoscope 1992;102(10):1185–1189
27. Iwahira Y, Maruyama Y. The use of Gore-Tex Soft Tissue Patch to assist temporal muscle transfer in the treatment of facial nerve palsy. Ann Plast Surg 1992;29(3):274–277
28. Heffelfinger RN, Blackwell KE, Rawnsley J, Keller GS. A simplified approach to midface aging. Arch Facial Plast Surg 2007;9(1):48–55
29. Gilles H. Experience with fascia lata grafts in the operative treatment of facial paralysis. Proc R Soc Med 1934;27:1372
30. Cheney ML, McKenna MJ, Megerian CA, Ojemann RG. Early temporalis muscle transposition for the management of facial paralysis. Laryngoscope 1995;105(9 Pt 1):993–1000
31. Labbé D. [Lengthening of temporalis myoplasty and reanimation of lips. Technical notes]. Ann Chir Plast Esthet 1997;42(1):44–47
32. Byrne PJ, Kim M, Boahene K, Millar J, Moe K. Temporalis tendon transfer as part of a comprehensive approach to facial reanimation. Arch Facial Plast Surg 2007;9(4):234–241
33. Byrne PJ, Kim M, Boahene K, Millar J, Moe K. Temporalis tendon transfer as part of a comprehensive approach to facial reanimation. Arch Facial Plast Surg 2007;9(4):234–241
34. Sawicki B, Drobnik T, de Posen IN. Chipault A. L'etat Actual de la Chirurgie Nerveuse. Paris: J. Rueff; 1903
35. Balance CA, Gallance HA, Stewart P. Remark on the operative treatment of chronic facial palsy of the pripheral origin. Br J Med 1903;1009–1015.
36. May M, Schaitkin B. The Facial Nerve, 2nd ed. New York: Thieme; 1996:623–624
37. Baker D. "Hypoglossal facial nerve anastomosis indications and limitations." Proceedings Fifth International Symposium Facial Nerve. New York: Masson Publ.; 1985: 526–529

38. Gavron JP, Clemis JD. Hypoglossal-facial nerve anastomosis: a review of forty cases caused by facial nerve injuries in the posterior fossa. Laryngoscope 1984;94(11 Pt 1):1447–1450

39. Conley J. "Hypoglossal-Facial Anastomosis." Neurological Surgery of the Ear and Skull Base. New York: Raven Press; 1983:93–98

40. Pensak ML. Controversies in Otolaryngology. New York, NY: Thieme; 2001: 130

41. Conley J, Baker D. Hypoglossal-facial nerve anastomosis for innervation of the paralyzed face. Plast Reconstr Surg 1979;63:3–72

42. Snow JB. Ballenger's Manual of Otorhinolaryngology—Head and Neck Surgery. Hamilton, Ontario: BC Decker, Inc.; 2003:215

43. Scaramella LF. Cross-face facial nerve anastomosis: historical notes. Ear Nose Throat J 1996;75(6):343–354, 347–352, 354

44. Slattery WH III, Wilkinson EP. "Facial translocation for hypoglossal-facial anastomosis." Oral presentation, XI International Facial Nerve Symposium. (Rome, Italy, April 25–28, 2009.)

45. Smith JW. A New Technique of Facial Animation. Transactions of the Fifth International Congress of Plastic Surgery. Australia: Butterworths; 1971:83

46. Anderl H. "Cross-Face Nerve Grafting- Up to 12 Months of Seventh Nerve Disruption." Reanimation of the Paralyzed Face. St. Louis: Mosby; 1977:241–277

47. Fisch U. Facial nerve grafting. Otolaryngol Clin North Am 1974; 7(2):517–529

48. Kunihior T, Kanzaki J, et al. Hypoglossal-Facial Nerve Anastomosis After Acoustic Neuroma Resection: Influence of the Time of Anastomosis on Recovery of Faacial Movement. J Oto Rhino Laryngol. 1996;58:32–35

49. Stennert EJ. I. Hypoglossal facial anastomosis: its significance for modern facial surgery. II. Combined approach in extratemporal facial nerve reconstruction. Clin Plast Surg 1979;6(3):471–486

50. Holstege G, Kuypers HG, Dekker JJ. The organization of the bulbar fibre connections to the trigeminal, facial and hypoglossal motor nuclei. II. An autoradiographic tracing study in cat. Brain 1977;100(2):264–286

51. Harii K. Microneurovascular free muscle transplantation for reanimation of facial paralysis. Clin Plast Surg 1979;6(3):361–375

52. Manktelow RT. Free muscle transplantation for facial paralysis. Clin Plast Surg 1984;11(1):215–220

53. O'Brien BM, Pederson WC, Khazanchi RK, Morrison WA, MacLeod AM, Kumar V. Results of management of facial palsy with microvascular free-muscle transfer. Plast Reconstr Surg 1990;86(1):12–22, discussion 23–24

54. Kumar PA. Cross-face reanimation of the paralysed face, with a single stage microneurovascular gracilis transfer without nerve graft: a preliminary report. Br J Plast Surg 1995;48(2):83–88

55. Kumar PA, Hassan KM. Cross-face nerve graft with free-muscle transfer for reanimation of the paralyzed face: a comparative study of the single-stage and two-stage procedures. Plast Reconstr Surg 2002;109(2):451–462, discussion 463–464

56. Chuang DC. Technique evolution for facial paralysis reconstruction using functioning free muscle transplantation—experience of Chang Gung Memorial Hospital. Clin Plast Surg 2002;29(4):449–459, v

57. Dellon AL, Mackinnon SE. Segmentally innervated latissimus dorsi muscle. Microsurgical transfer for facial reanimation. J Reconstr Microsurg 1985;2(1):7–12

58. Mackinnon SE, Dellon AL. Technical considerations of the latissimus dorsi muscle flap: a segmentally innervated muscle transfer for facial reanimation. Microsurgery 1988;9(1):36–45

59. Hata Y, Yano K, Matsuka K, Ito O, Matsuda H, Hosokawa K. Treatment of chronic facial palsy by transplantation of the neurovascularized free rectus abdominis muscle. Plast Reconstr Surg 1990;86(6):1178–1187, discussion 1188–1189

60. Terzis JK, Manktelow RT. Pectoralis Minor: a new concept in facial reanimation. Plast Surg Forum 1982;5:106–110

61. Harrison DH. The pectoralis minor vascularized muscle graft for the treatment of unilateral facial palsy. Plast Reconstr Surg 1985;75(2):206–216

62. Terzis JK. Pectoralis minor: a unique muscle for correction of facial palsy. Plast Reconstr Surg 1989;83(5):767–776

63. Tulley P, Webb A, Chana JS, et al. Paralysis of the marginal mandibular branch of the facial nerve: treatment options. Br J Plast Surg 2000;53(5):378–385

64. Curtin JW, Greeley PW, Gleason M, Braver D. A supplementary procedure for the improvement of facial nerve paralysis. Plast Reconstr Surg Transplant Bull 1960;26:73–79

65. Lindsay RW, Edwards C, Smitson C, Cheney ML, Hadlock TA. A systematic algorithm for the management of lower lip asymmetry. Am J Otolaryngol 2011;32(1):1–7

66. Niklison J. Contribution to the subject of facial paralysis. Plast Reconstr Surg 1946;17(4):276–293

67. Edgerton MT. Surgical correction of facial paralysis: a plea for better reconstructions. Ann Surg 1967;165(6):985–998

68. Conley J, Baker DC, Selfe RW. Paralysis of the mandibular branch of the facial nerve. Plast Reconstr Surg 1982;70(5):569–577

69. Terzis JK and Kalantarian B. Microsurgical strategies in 74 patients for restoration of dynamic depressor muscle mechanism: a neglected target in facial reanimation. Plast Reconstr Surg 2000;105(6):1917–1931; discussion 1932-4

70. Mayou BJ, Watson JS, Harrison DH, Parry CB. Free microvascular and microneural transfer of the extensor digitorum brevis muscle for the treatment of unilateral facial palsy. Br J Plast Surg 1981;34(3):362–367

71. Terzis JK, Konofaos P. Nerve transfers in facial palsy. Facial Plast Surg 2008;24(2):177–193

72. Harrison DH. The treatment of unilateral and bilateral facial palsy using free muscle transfers. Clin Plast Surg 2002;29(4):539–549, vi vi.

73. Zuker RM, Goldberg CS, Manktelow RT. Facial animation in children with Möbius syndrome after segmental gracilis muscle transplant. Plast Reconstr Surg 2000;106(1):1–8, discussion 9

25 Neuromuscular Retraining: Nonsurgical Therapy for Facial Palsy

H. Jacqueline Diels and Carien H.G. Beurskens

Neuromuscular retraining (NMR) is a patient-centered approach to the nonsurgical treatment of facial paralysis, paresis, and synkinesis. Treatment begins with a thorough clinical evaluation. Realistic goals are established and a comprehensive, individualized home program is developed. The resultant enhanced patient outcomes improve health, self-esteem, satisfaction, and quality of life. Successful rehabilitation restores the exquisite movements fundamental to expression, interpersonal communication, eating, drinking, speaking, blinking, and other, normally spontaneous functions.

Also referred to as neuromuscular re-education or mime therapy, NMR is a growing field and is gaining recognition as the essential element for achieving optimal recovery from facial palsy. Retraining techniques address sequelae that range from flaccidity to mass action and synkinesis. The NMR therapist plays a vital role within the facial nerve multidisciplinary team, providing continuity of care to the patient.

Facial NMR should not be confused with the nonspecific general therapies used by generations of well-meaning therapists to treat facial paralysis. Facial NMR requires unique training methods, necessitates a thorough understanding of facial structure, and relies upon in-depth evaluation, patient education, compliance, and active participation to achieve success.

■ Background

For decades, physical, occupational, and speech therapists have treated facial paralysis using gross facial exercises and electrical stimulation. Although outdated (and ineffective), these techniques have become "standard" and continue to be the norm for those therapists who rarely treat patients with facial paralysis and have not received current training. Each patient has a unique functional profile and psychosocial response to the condition, both of which require personal, individualized attention. A comprehensive "handout sheet of exercises" approach will never be possible. One reason facial NMR is not more common is simply the complexity of the problem. Many therapists are unaware the specialty exists because facial palsy is so unusual compared with other needs for therapy. Yet specific NMR for facial palsy began to appear in the literature more than 30 years ago.[1-3] Using surface electromyography (sEMG) biofeedback, patients improved their function by modifying the manner in which they contracted their facial muscles.

Current programs are based largely on the works of Balliet et al,[4] Diels,[5] Beurskens,[6] Ross et al,[7] and Coulson and Croxson,[8] the most important characteristics of treatment being detailed patient education, individualized program development and training, and active patient participation. Specific retraining procedures can include sEMG biofeedback; mirror, sensory, and proprioceptive feedback; and a wide variety of motor learning techniques. Upon reviewing the literature, Beurskens found little homogeneity with respect to patient population, intervention, and treatment plan.[9] However, the studies of Ross et al,[7] Segal et al,[10] and Beurskens and Heymans[11] showed significant positive outcomes of NMR on facial symmetry; functional abilities of eating, drinking, and speaking; and quality of life.

■ Acute versus Postacute Rehabilitation: Spontaneous Recovery versus New Learning

Although some patients may be evaluated acutely (while flaccid), the majority of specific NMR is started during and after reinnervation. If NMR is initiated acutely, it is impossible to differentiate spontaneous recovery from new motor learning. The recovery seen in postacute patients (having paresis or synkinesis) can clearly be attributed to the acquisition of new motor patterns through the retraining process and can occur even decades later.[12]

■ Educational Program Model: Training versus Therapy

Prior to injury, facial movement is mainly unconscious. In the first stage of motor learning, the patient must bring this otherwise spontaneous function under voluntary control. Facial NMR is not a therapy administered passively to the patient. This active process requires a skilled therapist who thoroughly understands and can teach facial anatomy, actions, and treatment techniques. The resulting model is a cost-effective program that reduces billed clinic hours while increasing overall treatment hours via home practice.

Patients may travel a great distance for training with a facial NMR specialist, with months between visits; therefore, comprehension is essential to ensure accurate follow-through and practice at home. As each program is so uniquely individualized, patients take detailed notes with their specific instructions in their own words. NMR is comparable in many ways to any training program (e.g., sports, music, etc.) in which the individual must be highly motivated and committed to daily practice of specific tasks designed to improve their skills. New motor patterns are learned through consistent practice and become more automatic over time.[4] Patients return to the clinic periodically to refine movements, document progress, and establish new treatment goals.

■ Facial Muscles Differ from Skeletal Muscles

Facial muscles differ from skeletal muscles in several important ways. For treatment to be effective, techniques must incorporate the following unique characteristics into their design:

(1) Facial muscles lack muscle spindles.[13] The spindle produces a muscle contraction in response to therapeutic facilitory techniques such as quick stretch, vibration, and tapping, commonly used for treating other disabilities. Because facial muscles have no spindles, these methods are useless for the treatment of facial paralysis.

(2) Facial muscles have small motor units[14] enabling great refinement, complexity, and subtlety of movement. Practicing gross facial movements confounds this normal precision by producing unnaturally large motions that cause overflow from neighboring muscles.

(3) Facial muscles degenerate slowly[15] and may remain viable for 3 or more years, so procedures used to maintain muscle viability (e.g., electrical stimulation) are unnecessary.

(4) Facial muscles receive emotional as well as volitional neural inputs.[16] Emotional cueing during facial NMR is often helpful to reestablish more natural patterns after paralysis.

■ Muscles of Facial Expression

It is not within the scope of this chapter to detail the muscles of facial expression (see **Fig. 1.7** in Chapter 1); however, it is imperative that the therapist and patient be thoroughly educated and familiar with facial muscle structure and function. Knowledge of the anatomic origins and insertions of the muscles to bone or tissue is fundamental to understanding facial kinematics. Even the actions of facial nerve innervated muscles not frequently used in expression (e.g., platysma and buccinator) are important as they often participate in abnormal synkinetic patterns.

The considerable individual variation in facial muscle function, expression, and symmetry can be even more pronounced after facial nerve injury. Patients receive a detailed diagram illustrating the major facial muscle groups, nerve branches, and angles of muscular pull, which is referred to extensively during the education and training process (**Fig. 25.1**). The most effective way to learn facial muscle actions is to create the movement by (a) mimicking the therapist, (b) producing it on the unaffected side, and (c) using mirror feedback. Teaching is time-consuming but essential for laying the foundation for NMR. Instructing the patient in even very simple muscle actions can radically change how that patient perceives and executes a movement. Learning, for example, that the smile is created by flexing the cheek (zygomatic) rather than mouth

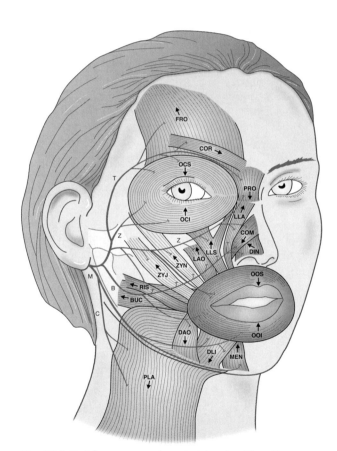

Fig. 25.1 Facial neuromuscular retraining teaching diagram representing the muscles of facial expression and facial nerve branches. Muscles: BUC, buccinators; COM, compressor naris; COR, corrugator; DAO, depressor anguli oris; DIN, dilator naris; DLI, depressor labii inferioris; FRO, frontalis; LAO, levator anguli oris; LLA, levator labii alaeque nasi; LLS, levator labii superioris; MEN, mentalis; OCI, orbicularis oculi inferioris; OCS, orbicularis oculi superioris; OOI, orbicularis oris inferioris; OOS, orbicularis oris superioris; PLA, platysma; PRO, procerus; RIS, risorius; ZYJ, zygomaticus major; ZYN, zygomaticus minor. Facial nerve branches: B, buccal; C, cervical; M, mandibular; T, temporal; Z, zygomaticus. (Adapted with permission from Balliet R. Facial Paralysis and Other Neuromuscular Dysfunctions of the Peripheral Nervous System. In: Payton O.D. Manual of Physical Therapy. New York, NY: Churchill Livingstone; 1989:179.)

(orbicularis oris or buccinator) will immediately change the manner in which the movement is attempted.

■ Etiologies Treated

The etiology of facial nerve palsies varies extensively. The most common etiologies seen for facial NMR are viral infection (Bell palsy, herpes zoster oticus), postsurgical (acoustic neuroma, etc.), traumatic injury, Lyme disease, congenital, and others (e.g., otitis media, parotid gland carcinoma, Guillain-Barré syndrome, polyneuritis, etc.). Timing for NMR referral depends more on degree of nerve injury and recovery than etiology.

■ Patient Selection

The following criteria are considered when determining which patients are good candidates for facial NMR:

(1) Neural supply: The facial nerve must be intact or surgically repaired to establish a neural supply to the facial muscles. If there is no innervation, NMR is not indicated.
(2) Motivation: Facial NMR is hard work, requiring commitment to training. Home practice sessions require focused concentration for 30 to 60 minutes per day. The patient must be compliant, disciplined, and persistent to achieve optimal benefit.
(3) Cognition: Adequate cognitive function is necessary for both the educational process and accurate home program practice. Cognitive or attention deficits may limit successful participation in NMR.

■ Patient Intake and Evaluation

A thorough history and facial evaluation are completed during the initial consultation. Demographic and medical information including diagnosis, previous therapies, affected side, and occurrence of first visible movement is recorded. Sequelae of facial paralysis are documented according to the International Classification of Functioning, Disability, and Health:

• Impairments: Asymmetry at rest, asymmetry during voluntary facial movements, synkineses, stiffness, pain, tear secretion, nasal obstruction, sensory changes
• Disabilities in eating, drinking, rinsing, speaking, nonverbal communication, and eye-tearing
• Psychosocial health problems such as isolation, decreased quality of life, sense of shame, or "loss of face"

Reliable and valid measurement instruments are used, where available, for objective assessment to establish baseline function and to evaluate outcomes following treatment. The data can also be used for research purposes. The House-Brackmann Facial Grading System has been used extensively as an overall measure of facial impairment.[17] However, for the purposes of facial NMR, a more sensitive grading scale was developed by Ross et al.[18] The Sunnybrook Facial Grading System is simple, quick to administer, and sensitive enough to quantify small functional changes that occur during the course of treatment, especially in the scoring of synkinesis. The Sunnybrook Facial Grading System measures the face at rest and during five facial movements, and scores associated synkinesis during those five movements. Pain is assessed using the Visual Analogue Scale, and tearing, nasal obstruction, and sensation are assessed by subjective report.

Physical and social well-being are measured with The Facial Disability Index.[19] Video and photo evaluations are essential in the initial evaluation.[5] Recordings should be standardized, controlling variables such as distance to the camera, light, and posture of the patient. Evaluation results are discussed with the patient, including prognosis and course of treatment. The treatment plan is then developed.

■ Categories of Patients

Patients present for facial NMR in one of the following four basic functional categories:

(1) Flaccid paralysis: No (or very little) movement.
(2) Paresis: Movement beginning to return as seen by discrete, observable, weak movements. Tone is increasing (nasolabial fold returning, normalizing palpebral fissure).
(3) Synkinesis: Movements are present but aberrant movements occur. The facial muscles can be hypertonic, and patients may experience tightness or discomfort.
(4) Postsurgical reanimation: Having already undergone some type of surgical dynamic intervention.

■ Neuromuscular Retraining for Flaccid Paralysis

NMR is not indicated for the flaccid patient with neurotmesis who will not recover without surgical reanimation. For the patient with neuropraxia or axonotmesis who is expected to recover within a certain time frame, NMR has not been found to be helpful until movement begins to return. Active practice of movement patterns too early only serves to reinforce movement on the unaffected side and promote asymmetry. Although NMR is not used, a one-time consult can help the patient cope with these drastic, life-altering changes. To ease some of the functional impairments created by a flaccid hemi-face:

(1) Eye care: Use of drops and/or gel, protective barriers (sunglasses, moisture chamber), upper eyelid stretch, strip of tape under the lower eyelid to support ectropion. Timely follow-up with an ophthalmologist is always stressed.

(2) Oral motor: Cut food in small pieces; eat small bites on unaffected side; place cup/glass on the unaffected side; use finger under the glass to provide a seal; drink with a straw; reduce speed of speaking, eating, and drinking.

(3) Tone: For mid-face and lip flaccidity, a thin piece of tape applied from under the angle of the mouth up to the cheek can improve speech intelligibility. Massage and moist heat keep the face supple, promote facial awareness, and have psychosocial benefit.[20] Recent research in animal models suggests that gently stroking the affected side from lateral to midline decreases occurrence of abnormal reinnervation during neural regeneration.[21]

(4) Emotional: Because patients are often self-conscious and reluctant to show emotional expression, it can be useful to teach compensatory strategies involving arms and shoulders or even the whole body. Anxious patients are taught relaxation techniques. These practices can help guide the patient during the flaccid phase where, in addition to functional issues, stress, fear, uncertainty, and loss can be overwhelming.

■ Neuromuscular Retraining for Paresis

As reinnervation continues and flaccidity resolves, facial movements return. NMR referral should be made at this time. Although patients should begin by practicing soft movements, they often practice maximum effort contractions to "make it move as much as possible." Guidance by an NMR therapist at this time is critical to teach proper form for optimizing outcome. It is essential that very small, bilateral movements be performed gently and slowly. Small, gentle movements reinforce bilateral symmetry while reducing the tendency toward co-contraction, associated movements, and synkinesis. Slow movement teaches accuracy and also trains the patient in the proper technique for controlling synkinesis should it occur later on. Facial expressions performed in this way can be increased (gently) as the paresis resolves. It is worth mentioning that this precise, controlled practice most accurately models normal, spontaneous facial movements, which are rarely forced or made with great effort.

Generally, patients will practice their home program 30 to 60 minutes per day, depending on the stage of recovery

and their needs and goals. Frequency of clinic treatment and follow-up depends on the progress of recovery, patient compliance to the home program, and the distance the patient lives from the clinic. An average of six to eight visits (over several months to 2 years) is usually sufficient to optimize results.

■ Neuromuscular Retraining for Synkinesis

Synkinesis is defined as an involuntary movement accompanying a voluntary one. It is characterized by abnormal facial movements among muscles that do not normally contract together during expression. A common residual associated with incomplete facial nerve recovery, it is one of the most perplexing and challenging to treat. Synkinesis can be difficult to identify, as the abnormal muscle action can visually mimic flaccid paralysis. (In flaccid paralysis, the angle of the mouth may droop; in synkinesis, it may be "pulled down" by flexion of the platysma.) It can also create the appearance of no movement. (If the zygomatic muscles contract synkinetically during orbicularis oris movement, the lips may be retracted to such an extent that they are unable to move toward midline.) Synkinesis varies in location, occurrence, and severity, from mild to severe mass action, where the result can be gross deformity during facial movements.[22]

Facial muscles move the skin to produce a wide variety of expressions, the subtleties of which require a delicate balance between all facial muscles. When a muscle contracts inappropriately, it distorts the facial skin, creating an entirely different expression than intended. Patients are often unaware they have synkinesis and may try to move with great force, unknowingly intensifying the abnormal response. It is crucial that patients clearly understand the difference between flaccidity and synkinesis so they can effectively coordinate rather than "exercise" their facial muscles. There are two separate but related issues in NMR for synkinesis:

(1) Increased muscle tone at rest requiring soft tissue mobilization, massage, and heat

(2) Abnormal motor patterns requiring selective activation/inhibition to improve coordination

Reduce Resting Tone

Patients often complain of tightness, "heaviness," or discomfort with decreased mobility, range of motion, and expressiveness. Common signs of increased resting tone include a deepened nasolabial fold, decreased palpebral fissure, retracted angle of the mouth, dimpled chin, and banding of the neck (platysma). The affected mid-face may appear swollen, thick, or immobile. Soft tissue mobilization and specific facial massage techniques decrease tightness and contracture. Painful trigger points resolve with maintained deep pressure, leaving the face more supple and elastic even within the first session. Patients learn the techniques quickly and easily and are instructed to practice them several times a day. They commonly report significant improvements in comfort and mobility after several weeks of practice.

Inhibit Synkineses

Synkineses cause more muscles to contract than required for a particular expression. The concept is counterintuitive: too much movement impairs function. In this case, more is not better. Considerable time is spent educating the patient on which muscles are required for specific patterns and which are not, using the unaffected side as the

model. This is followed by learning small, slow, and coordinated movement patterns that isolate the correct muscles and inhibit the synkinetic ones. To inhibit synkinesis, the patient focuses first on which muscles should *not* contract in the practice movement. They then initiate the primary movement so slowly that synkinetic movements remain suppressed. Complete concentration is required to dissociate the synkinetic from the primary movement. If a very small movement is completed slowly enough, the patient will generally be successful in learning the new pattern. As control improves, range of motion increases. For example, as the patient learns to inhibit the platysma and/or buccinator while producing a small smile, the angle of the mouth will begin to elevate. During pucker, as synkinesis of the mid-face and platysma relaxes, the lips are released toward midline (**Fig. 25.2**).

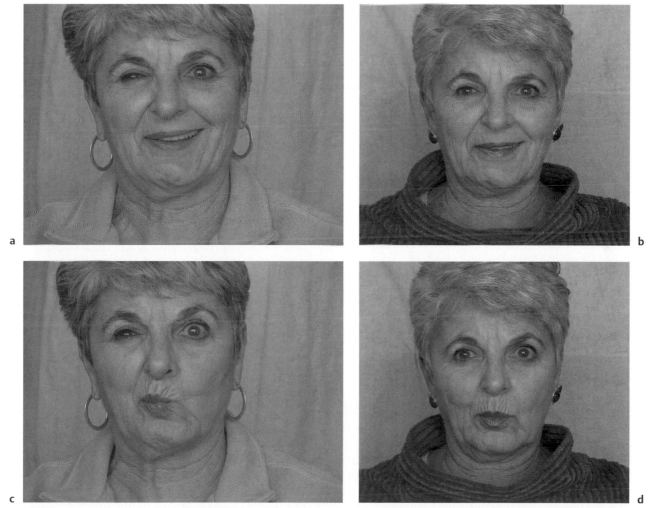

Fig. 25.2a–d Photographic evaluation of a 69-year-old woman diagnosed with right Ramsay Hunt syndrome in April 2006. Initial neuromuscular retraining evaluation, January 2008. (**a**) Smile and (**c**) pucker. Reevaluation 12 months after beginning neuromuscular retraining, January 2009. (**b**) Smile and (**d**) pucker. Smile: note decreased synkinesis of orbicularis oculi and platysma resulting in improved symmetry. Pucker: note decreased synkinesis of orbicularis oculi, mid-cheek musculature, and platysma resulting in decreased retraction at right angle of mouth and improved range of motion and symmetry.

Mirror feedback has been common for retraining; however, proprioceptive feedback may be even more powerful and is being used more frequently. Although the facial muscles do not have spindles, with minimal cueing, patients can feel skin displacement as the muscles contract and the face moves. The feedback is immediate and does not require cognitive interpretation the way mirror feedback does. The patient readily identifies and compares the two sides and how they "feel" different, and develops a deeper insight into the true nature of the disability (i.e., too much versus too little movement). Greater insight leads to better understanding of the sometimes unusual training strategies. Furthermore, the home program can be practiced when the patient is not in front of a mirror.

Minimal, successful movements are progressed as new patterns are learned and become more automatic. Patients can be referred and treated effectively with NMR at any time, even years after synkinesis develops, because the focus is on re-educating viable muscles rather than stimulating flaccid ones.

■ Neuromuscular Retraining for the Postsurgical Patient

When no visible recovery or electromyography signals are present for an extended time, patients may be candidates for dynamic reconstruction such as a nerve graft and/or muscle transposition. As in other cases of flaccid paralysis, a one-time consult is recommended for acute issues. As movement returns, NMR assists the patient in learning movement strategies appropriate to their specific surgery. Although complete recovery cannot be achieved, NMR can provide an optimal individual result. Three years may be required to achieve this optimal result. In cases where the patient receives static reconstruction, such as a fascia lata sling, NMR is not useful. The most common reconstruction procedures that benefit from NMR are:

(1) Cross-face nerve graft (with or without a muscle transposition): NMR can begin when movement is first visible (6 to 12 months). Exercises focus on symmetry at rest and during expressions, and speech intelligibility.
(2) Temporalis muscle transposition: NMR can begin when the wound is healed, usually after 6 weeks. The patient is taught to use the chewing muscle as a mimic muscle, where biting facilitates an abduction of the angle of the mouth. Clinical experience has shown that it is possible to teach the patient to move the corner of the mouth without biting.
(3) Hypoglossal facial nerve interpositional nerve graft: A portion of the hypoglossal nerve is connected via a graft to the facial nerve. Movement is expected after 6 to 12 months and will first be noticed when the patient moves or presses the

tongue against the teeth or palate. At that point, patients are taught to activate their facial muscles using specific tongue movement/pressure. Symmetrical movements are made with very gentle tongue pressure so synkinesis can be controlled. Patients can also be taught to inhibit facial movements while moving the tongue to decrease synkinesis during eating, drinking, and speaking. Upon discharge, many of these patients have learned to produce facial movements automatically, without tongue pressure. However, it is less common that they will regain an emotional smile.

■ Electrical Stimulation

Electrical stimulation should not be used in facial NMR. In the acute (flaccid) stage, electrical stimulation can give the illusion of effectiveness because its application coincides with the spontaneous recovery period. Improvements can erroneously be attributed to the stimulation rather than to the natural course of recovery. There is a distinct lack of evidence that electrical stimulation has a positive effect on facial nerve paralysis. Furthermore, it has been suggested that electrical stimulation may interfere with neural regeneration after peripheral nerve injury, and clinical experience suggests that patients who receive it acutely may have more synkinesis and mass action than those who do not. Electrical stimulation can also produce a painful mass action contraction that reinforces abnormal motor patterns. The available research is limited, is often poorly designed, and reports contradictory results.[23]

In cases of synkinesis, limited range of motion is due to abnormal hyperactivity and co-contraction, not a lack of muscle contractility. There is no need to stimulate active muscles and no indication that electrical stimulation can inhibit or recoordinate abnormal movement patterns.

■ Surface Electromyography Biofeedback

sEMG biofeedback is often used in facial NMR to bring the normally unconscious control of specific muscles under conscious control. sEMG biofeedback provides immediate, accurate information regarding the rate and strength of muscle contraction in real time, which is required for new motor pattern modification and learning. Specific protocols for the use of sEMG biofeedback stress the importance of achieving normalized resting tone, symmetry, and isolated responses.[24,25] It is used exclusively in clinic sessions with NMR therapist guidance. As part of the NMR program, sEMG biofeedback can be used as an evaluative as well as therapeutic tool to:

• Improve facial tone
• Increase activity in weak muscles

- Decrease activity in hyperactive muscles
- Improve coordination of muscle groups

Surface electrodes are placed over the muscle(s) being monitored to detect the electrical activity produced by the contraction. The signals are amplified and displayed on a computer monitor. Placing the electrodes on analogous muscles bilaterally allows the patient to compare the affected to the unaffected side. As the patient watches the graph in real time on the monitor, the movement pattern can be adjusted until it is symmetrical with the unaffected side. In cases of synkinesis, this often consists of inhibiting one trace while activating another to improve coordination between muscle groups. As the patient learns the new movement pattern, the sEMG biofeedback information is correlated with mirror and proprioceptive feedback. Using this approach, the patient learns to reproduce the new movement patterns without the sEMG biofeedback and can incorporate them into home program practice.

■ Botox and Facial Neuromuscular Retraining

Injection of botulinum toxin (e.g., Botox [Allergan, Inc., Irvine, CA]) is another procedure being used to improve facial coordination in cases where residual effects of facial paralysis result in synkineses.[26] Botox temporarily (3 to 6 months) partially paralyzes targeted facial muscles, providing a "window of opportunity" during which the patient can learn and practice more coordinated movement patterns without the co-contraction and restriction caused by synkinesis. Botox must be administered by a physician who has experience with facial paralysis and synkinesis.

When used in conjunction with NMR, the most common injection sites include the orbicularis oculi, corrugator, platysma, and mentalis muscles. The mid-facial muscles are rarely injected to avoid creating a flaccid paralysis and to preserve the activity needed for the NMR process. The experienced NMR therapist, in conjunction with the physician, can identify which targeted injection sites will be of greatest benefit for each patient during the NMR process.

After Botox is injected, patients continue to practice the home program with a conscious focus on ease of motion and coordination. Many patients experience improved coordination and decreased synkinesis even after the injection effects have worn off.

■ Conclusion

Neuromuscular retraining is a patient-centered program that uses motor learning techniques created specifically for facial nerve and muscle paralysis, practiced by highly trained therapists. NMR programs are tailor-made for each patient based on his or her individual functional profile and psychosocial response. NMR adds a crucial component to the multidisciplinary care and treatment of facial palsy. Like every method of facial reanimation, NMR cannot completely restore normal facial movement and expression after facial nerve injury. However, through education and training, conducted by an NMR-trained therapist, using the most current techniques, patients assume control over their own recovery. Their active participation, patience, and perseverance result in improved physical function and increased self-esteem, satisfaction, and quality of life.

References

1. Brown DM, Nahai F, Wolf S, Basmajian JV. Electromyographic biofeedback in the reeducation of facial palsy. Am J Phys Med 1978;57(4):183–190
2. Daniel B, Guitar B. EMG feedback and recovery of facial and speech gestures following neural anastomosis. J Speech Hear Disord 1978;43(1):9–20
3. Jankel WR. Bell palsy: muscle reeducation by electromyograph feedback. Arch Phys Med Rehabil 1978;59(5):240–242
4. Balliet R, Shinn JB, Bach-y-Rita P. Facial paralysis rehabilitation: retraining selective muscle control. Int Rehabil Med 1982;4(2): 67–74
5. Diels HJ. New concepts in nonsurgical facial nerve rehabilitation. In: Myers E., Bluestone C. Advances in Otolaryngology-Head and Neck Surgery. Chicago: Mosby- Year Book; 1995: 289–315
6. Beurskens CHG. Mime Therapy: Rehabilitation of Facial Expression. Thesis. Nijmegen:KUN; 2003
7. Ross B, Nedzelski JM, McLean JA. Efficacy of feedback training in long-standing facial nerve paresis. Laryngoscope 1991;101 (7 Pt 1):744–750
8. Coulson SE, Croxson GR. Facial Nerve Rehabilitation-the Role of Physiotherapy. Austr J Otolaryngol 1994;I:418–421
9. Beurskens CHG, Burgers-Bots IAL, Kroon DW, Oostendorp RAB. Literature review of evidence based physiotherapy in patients with facial nerve paresis. J Jpn Phys Ther Assoc 2004;7:35–39
10. Segal B, Hunter T, Danys I, Freedman C, Black M. Minimizing synkinesis during rehabilitation of the paralyzed face: preliminary assessment of a new small-movement therapy. J Otolaryngol 1995;24(3):149–153
11. Beurskens CHG, Heymans PG. Mime therapy improves facial symmetry in people with long-term facial nerve paresis: a randomised controlled trial. Aust J Physiother 2006;52(3): 177–183
12. Bach-y-Rita P, Lazarus JV, Boyeson MG, et al. Neural aspects of motor function as a basis of early and post-acute rehabilitation. In: DeLisa JA. Principles and Practice of Rehabilitation Medicine. Philadelphia, PA: JG Lippincott; 1988: 175–95
13. Basmajian JV, DeLuca CJ. Muscles Alive: Their Functions Revealed by Electromyography. Baltimore: Williams & Wilkins; 1985
14. May M. Microanatomy and pathophysiology of the facial nerve. In: May M, Shaitkin BM. The Facial Nerve. New York, NY: Thieme; 2000: 57–65

15. Belal A. Structure of human muscle in facial paralysis: role of muscle biopsy. In: May M. The Facial Nerve. New York, NY: Thieme; 1986: 99–106

16. Rinn WE. The neuropsychology of facial expression: a review of the neurological and psychological mechanisms for producing facial expressions. Psychol Bull 1984;95(1):52–77

17. House JW, Brackmann DE. Facial nerve grading system. Otolaryngol Head Neck Surg 1985;93(2):146–147

18. Ross BG, Fradet G, Nedzelski JM. Development of a sensitive clinical facial grading system. Otolaryngol Head Neck Surg 1996;114(3):380–386

19. VanSwearingen JM, Brach JS. The Facial Disability Index: reliability and validity of a disability assessment instrument for disorders of the facial neuromuscular system. Phys Ther 1996;76(12):1288–1298, discussion 1298–1300

20. Beurskens CHG, Devriese PP, van Heiningen I, Oostendorp RAB. The use of mime therapy as a rehabilitation method for patients with facial nerve paresis. Internal J Ther Rehab 2004;11: 206–210

21. Angelov DN, Ceynowa M, Guntinas-Lichius O, et al. Mechanical stimulation of paralyzed vibrissal muscles following facial nerve injury in adult rat promotes full recovery of whisking. Neurobiol Dis 2007;26(1):229–242

22. Beurskens CH, Oosterhof J, Nijhuis-van der Sanden MWG. Frequency and location of synkineses in patients with peripheral facial nerve paresis. Otol Neurotol 2010;31(4):671–675

23. Teixeira LJ, Soares BGDO, Vieira VP. Physical therapy for Bell's palsy (idiopathic facial paralysis). Cochrane Database Syst Rev 2008;(3):CD006283

24. Brudny J, Hammerschlag PE, Cohen NL, Ransohoff J. Electromyographic rehabilitation of facial function and introduction of a facial paralysis grading scale for hypoglossal-facial nerve anastomosis. Laryngoscope 1988;98(4):405–410

25. Balliet R. Motor control strategies in the retraining of facial paralysis. In: Portmann M. Facial Nerve. New York, NY: Masson Publishing; 1985:465–469

26. Mehta RP, Hadlock TA. Botulinum toxin and quality of life in patients with facial paralysis. Arch Facial Plast Surg 2008;10(2):84–87

26 Synkinesis and Hyperkinesis
Barry M. Schaitkin

Unwanted facial nerve movement disorders take many forms. Hemifacial spasm is a unilateral hyperactivity that usually begins focally and may progress to involve all ipsilateral facial muscles. Essential blepharospasm consists of involuntary movements of the obicularis oculi muscles, usually of middle-aged or older patients. Injuries to the facial nerve, from whatever etiology (e.g., surgery, trauma, tumors, or infection), follow a predictable course. These patients begin with denervation, and the subsequent reinnervation is characterized by hyperactive function of the facial nerve with resultant hyperkinesis and synkinesis.

There are of course additional features of facial nerve recovery that affect areas other than the muscles of facial expression including crocodile tears and stapes tendon contraction. To better understand these issues the reader is directed to Chapter 3 of this book for histopathology of the facial nerve, to Chapter 5 for the classification of these aberrant movements through the many classification systems, to Chapter 17 for discussion of hemi-facial spasm, and to Chapter 25 for physical therapy rehabilitation, which is a mainstay of treatment of these disorders.

■ Pathophysiology of Synkinesis

Dr. Kedar Adour was fond of saying that contracture and synkinesis follow facial nerve degeneration and regeneration as day follows night (personal communication). In other words, patients who develop a *complete* facial paralysis invariably have some element of these undesired facial movements. Patients on the other hand who, for whatever reason (viral, trauma, surgery), develop an *incomplete* acute facial paralysis almost never develop hyperactive facial nerve features.

The three leading theories on why the movements occur are either ephaptic transmission between adjacent nerves, aberrant fiber regeneration, or changes at the facial nerve nucleus. In 1996, Moran and Neely analyzed 11 consecutive patients with abnormal movements looking for insight into which of these three theories was most tenable. Looking closely at the common reproducible patterns of synkinetic movement showed that mouth synkinesis from voluntarily eyelid closure was present universally. In addition, they had cases where the synkinetic activity occurred too quickly to have arisen from fiber regeneration. The repetitive nature of the patterns of synkinesis and speed at which they occur suggested that something occurring at the facial nerve nucleus was more likely or was occurring

in addition to the more popular theory of aberrant fiber regeneration.[1] These synkinetic movements are of incredible concern to the patient and rank above facial paresis in their societal impact.[2]

After facial nerve lesions occur with regeneration, the topography of the facial nerve nucleus is disturbed as demonstrated by horseradish peroxidase studies.[3] In the rat model, clearly in addition to the regenerating facial nucleus, there is an increased number of collateral branches peripherally.[4] In the rat, the possibility of ephaptic transmission (the direct electrical excitability of adjacent intact neurons and even cortical effects of unwanted facial movements) is difficult to prove or disprove at this point.

Hyperexcitability of the nerve may also occur without degeneration and regeneration as the initial phases of irritated lesion. It is well known that slowly compressive noninvasive lesions such as cholesteatoma may be accompanied by either weakness or hyperexcitability.

■ Evaluation of Patients with Hyperkinesis and Synkinesis

A detailed history is critical in approaching a patient with hyperkinesis and synkinesis. The vast majority of patients with these issues have a history that points directly to a diagnosis. Patients who have had trauma with sudden complete facial paralysis or those who have had surgical activity near the facial nerve with complete facial paralysis will give a history suggesting these events as the cause of their unwanted facial movement. Likewise a classic history for a Bell palsy or Ramsay Hunt syndrome is very helpful in understanding the origin of unwanted facial movements. The patient is often confused by the onset of these movements in a period of time after when they believe that their recovery has already occurred. These late manifestations of recovery often suggest to the patient, or referring doctor, a new process at work rather than a late sequela of the original event. It is precisely because these findings are late that mandates that evaluation and classification of recovery after facial paralysis wait at least 6 months because of the possibility that the degree of synkinesis will change their classification. The treating physician is wise to remember that any intervention along this normal time course can find the physician being blamed for increased hyperkinetic activity after their intervention (surgery, botulinum neurotoxin, etc.) even though the patient is actually experiencing the normal history of facial nerve recovery.

Other disorders that cause hyperkinesis should be mentioned so that the treating physician has awareness. Blepharospasm is a bilateral involuntarily intermittent spasmodic closure of the eyelids. This generally involves the entire orbicularis oculi muscle and the pretarsal, pre-septal, and preorbital parts, and usually involves the procerus and corrugator muscles as well. The bilateral nature of the disorder as well as the electromyography findings of synchronous firing at a normal discharge rate generally makes the diagnosis easy.[5]

Patients with blepharospasm can have other muscles of the face involved. This was documented in a painting by the famed Flemish artist Brueghel who painted a woman with facial and neck involvement, and the term "Brueghel syndrome" is used when extensive lower facial involvement is a major component of the disease. In addition, in 1910 Henry Meige, a French neurologist, described the condition characterized by blepharospasm and facial, mandibular, oral, lingual, and laryngeal spasm. This disease includes involuntary chewing, trismus, lip pursing, wide opening of the mouth, jaw deviation, and tongue protrusion, and is known as Meige syndrome. All of these disorders, blepharospasm, Brueghel syndrome, and Meige syndrome, are part of the spectrum of facial dystonia.[5]

Blepharospasm is a disease that preferentially strikes middle-aged women. Essential blepharospasm is when the disorder exclusively involves bilateral muscles around the eye and spares the rest of the face. May considered the sine qua non of central blepharospasm where the eyes are clamped tightly shut rather than just blinking or twitching.[5] Three-quarters of patients who have blepharospasm will eventually have some lower facial dystonia as well.

A careful drug history should be obtained because dopamine stimulators, nasal antihistamines, decongestants, and patients on long-term neuroleptic treatment can have some of these facial movements as well. Hemi-facial spasm and its management are discussed in Chapters 17.

Patients with synkinesis make up the majority of patients presenting to a facial nerve center for evaluation and management of facial movement disorders. The synkinetic movements can be barely noticeable or completely disfiguring. Although early reports of synkinetic activity have occurred,[2] most patients do not begin to have synkinetic movements before 6 months of degeneration and regeneration. The abnormal movements should be only on the side of initial injury. The hyperkinetic problems are generally a deepening of the nasal labial fold due to shortening of the lip elevators, relative closing of the ipsilateral eye due to increased tension in the circular obicularis oculi, and movement of the mouth with eye closure. More infrequently, patients will have sustained platysma spasm and even brow elevation.

The patient should be questioned extensively about what his or her main concerns are. Specifically, situations that are most difficult functionally when they are affected by synkinetic activity should be explored. Patients should have discussion of difficulty with mastication, reading, and driving, especially at night where oncoming headlights can cause complete involuntary eye closure of the affected eye. In addition, any hobbies or work-related limitations caused by the synkinesis should be documented.

■ Motor Sensory Re-education

At one time, neurolysis was the mainstay of treatment of unwanted facial movements.[6] This has been replaced to some extent with motor sensory re-education (physical therapy).[7] After physical therapy, a botulinum neurotoxin such as Botox (Allergan, Inc., Irvine, CA) is the next commonly employed modality for the treatment of unwanted facial movements. Often, these two modalities are used simultaneously. The treatment of dystonia with botulinum neurotoxin began around 1968 when Dr. Ed Shantz began collaborating with Dr. Allen Scott, an ophthalmic surgeon who was treating patients with strabismus. Scott's pioneering work was recognizing selective weakening of extraocular muscles in strabismus which led to its use for a wide range of conditions including myokymia, hemifacial spasm, blepharospasm, and other facial dystonias.[8] The mechanism of action of botulinum neurotoxin occurs when the toxin binds presynaptically to the cholinergic nerve terminals and decreases the release of acetylcholine, essentially causing a neuromuscular blockage. Because this is a biological product, it is a temporary and dose-dependent weakness of the muscle(s) near the injection site. The injected material will diffuse and affect all muscles within the injection region, and this must be kept in mind both when discussing risks and alternatives with the patient as well as deciding on the best injection sites.

Botox arrives frozen and is reconstituted. After discussion of the risks, benefits, and alternatives, the patient and the physician decide on which muscles to treat initially and arrive at a dose. The doses for synkinetic activity, in general, are lower than doses used for hemi-facial spasm and blepharospasm. The guidelines for treatment, location, and dose are to some extent guided by personal experience with the medication. The author uses a standardized reconstitution of 1 mL per 100 units of Botox, giving a 10 unit per 0.1 mL of injected material. There are many treatment algorithms in the literature; most of them are similar to that proposed by Biglan.[9] The author currently uses a 5 to 7.5 unit injection point each into the upper and lower eyelid midway between the tarsal plate and lateral commissure (**Fig. 26.1**).

The majority of the product is injected into the orbicularis oculi itself lateral to the medial margin of the orbital rim. These injections prevent unwanted extraocular muscle effects with resultant diplopia. The injections themselves are done so as to raise a skin wheel and also to minimize the risk of inadvertent injection of other muscles. Patients with problems that extend beyond closure of

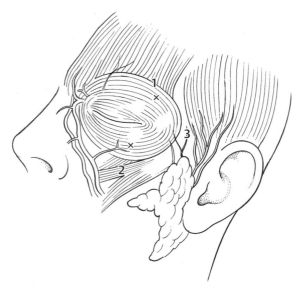

Fig. 26.1 The Botox (Allergan, Inc., Irvine, CA) injection sites for the orbicularis oculi muscle to reduce oral to ocular synkinesis with resultant unwanted eye closure. The injection should raise a ski wheel to reduce the risk of extraocular muscle injection. *1* and *2* are halfway between midpupillary line and lateral commissure; *3* is lateral to the lateral commissure over the lateral orbital rim.

the eye from synkinetic and hyperkinetic activity can have additional doses into the other adjacent muscles. Usually a dose of 5 to 10 units is sufficient for each muscle group. Treatment of the orbicularis oculi is tremendously effective and, if done carefully, has a very low risk. Hematoma or infection from any injection is possible but rare, and diplopia is also rare.

Injecting the lower face, which is the second most common area of complaint, is much more challenging. While it is certainly possible to design doses for the hyperkinesis and synkinesis of the muscles that affect the nasal labial fold, the downside of overinjection with weakness of the lower face makes it much more risky. Patients will commonly report that they would prefer the tension and increased depth of the nasal labia fold to the loss of any function in that area. For this reason, motor sensory reeducation (physical therapy) is the author's preferred treatment of this site. However, the release of the depressors of the corner of the mouth can be very easily accomplished with Botox injections. Platysma spasm often requires a significant injection depending on the patient; doses from 20 to 80 units have been used. The muscle can be well delineated by having the patient close his or her eyes tightly or smile. The injection sites include the anterior border of the platysma up to the mandibular body but not above that palpable structure (**Fig. 26.2**).

Additional injections as judged by the contraction of the muscle during its synkinetic activity are extremely helpful. It is wise after the first injection to have the patient come back in a week to see if the muscle has been released and,

if not, to augment the dose. This allows one to titrate up to what will become the treatment dose.

The mentalis muscle that results in deep dimpling of the chin is the most easily relieved with 5 to 10 units directly into the affected area causing immediate relief from this problem.

Injections take 72 hours to reach a full effect. Working with the physical therapist after injection allows patients to have a much greater ability to perform their physical therapy routine. It is therefore extremely important to coordinate doses of Botox with visits to the physical therapist to maximize the effect of both modalities.

Botox for blepharospasm requires larger doses, and these doses often need to be repeated more frequently. Some authors have noted a decreased effectiveness of these injections over time, but this is not a universal finding. Additional injection sites around the eye are needed for blepharospasm as compared with synkinetic activity.

It is frequently helpful to inject Botox in very small amounts to the normal, contralateral side of the facial nerve problem. In this way, the overpull of the normal zygomaticus and other elevators at the level of the modiolus provides not only for improvement of a volitional smile but avoids the patient's embarrassment over spontaneous smiling and laughing, drawing attention to their facial asymmetry.

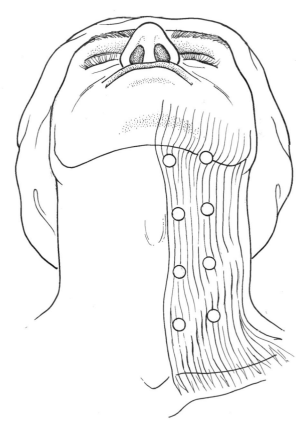

Fig. 26.2 The Botox (Allergan, Inc., Irvine, CA) injection sites for reducing depressor synkinetic activity on the smile. These sites are tailored by observing the platysma during eye closure or smiling.

■ Selective Myectomy

Some authors favor selective myectomy as the most effective approach for permanent relief of abnormal involuntary facial movements. Myectomy has been performed for the orbicularis oculi, procerus, corrugators, stapes, zygomaticus muscles, mentalis, and platysma. In patients with severe blepharospasm, Patel et al recommend orbicularis oculi myectomy.[10] They generally perform the upper myectomy first both to avoid the lymphedema of simultaneous upper and lower lid myectomy as well as to have greater ability to predict the overall result. Corrugator and procerus muscles can be resected through brow incisions, and the orbicularis oculi muscle is removed through an upper lid blepharoplasty incision. The staged lower myectomy can be performed through a lower blepharoplasty infraciliary incision, and the tarsal, septal, and orbital orbicularis can be excised through this technique. The main complications of resection are hematoma, infection, skin flap necrosis, and chronic lymphedema.

Zygomaticus muscle myectomy is performed through a nasal labial fold incision. Patients with a significant crease provide no difficulty with cosmetic appearance. These patients tend to be in an older age group. Patients without the skin crease camouflage should be done through a lip incision.

Resection of the stapedius muscle for unwanted stapedius contraction during facial movements is done through a tympanomeatal flap with exposure and lysis of the stapedius tendon. This is an extremely effective procedure for this very uncommon condition. The patients note an immediate cessation of roaring or flapping of the tympanic membrane with facial movement.[10]

The main myectomy procedure that the author performs is platysma myectomy. This is done through a neck crease incision. As much platysma muscle as possible is resected. This is an extremely effective way to improve the elevation of the corner of the mouth and remove the depressor effect of the platysma muscle. The degree of success of the procedure can be determined preoperatively by the results of platysma muscle Botox injections. Patients who have excellent response to Botox can be counseled on repeating the Botox injections three to four times per year or having the platysma muscle resected. Other than the skin incision, possible numbness, and risks of any surgical procedure to hematoma or infection, there are no major downfalls to the loss of the platysma muscle, making it easy to recommend this procedure.

■ Conclusion

Synkinesis and hyperkinesis are very common side effects of degeneration and regeneration of the facial nerve. They provide a significant source of frustration and social isolation of patients with recovery from facial paralysis. The mainstay of treatment of patients with this condition is to find a dedicated facial nerve physical therapist. These are hard to come by, but their experiences warrant using these highly trained individuals. General physical therapists that do not specialize in facial nerve patients are, in the author's experience, of very little use.

The use of botulinum neurotoxin injections to treat unwanted facial movements frequently and in combination with physical therapy provides the vast majority of treatment for these patients. Selective myectomy particularly of the platysma is a highly effective treatment in this area.

References

1. Moran CJ, Neely JG. Patterns of facial nerve synkinesis. Laryngoscope 1996;106(12 Pt 1):1491–1496
2. Neely JG, Neufeld PS. Defining functional limitation, disability, and societal limitations in patients with facial paresis: initial pilot questionnaire. Am J Otol 1996;17(2):340–342
3. Fernandez E, Pallini R, Marchese E, Lauretti LA, La Marca F. Quantitative, morphological, and somatotopic nuclear changes after facial nerve regeneration in adult rats: a possible challenge to the "no new neurons" dogma. Neurosurgery 1995;37(3):456–462, discussion 462–463
4. Choi D, Raisman G. Somatotopic organization of the facial nucleus is disrupted after lesioning and regeneration of the facial nerve: the histological representation of synkinesis. Neurosurgery 2002;50(2):355–362, discussion 362–363
5. May M. The overview of hyperkinesis. In: May M, Schaitkin BM. The Facial Nerve, 2nd Ed. New York, NY: Thieme; 2000: 431–441
6. Fisch U. Extracranial surgery for facial hyperkinesis. In: May M, ed. The Facial Nerve. New York, NY: Thieme; 1986: 509–534
7. Henkelmann T. Physical therapy and neuromuscular rehabilitation. In: May M, Schaitkin BM. The Facial Nerve. 2nd Ed. New York, NY: Thieme; 2000: 301–319.
8. Biglan AW, Patel BCK, May M, Murdock TJ. Botulinum A Toxin. In: May M, Schaitkin BM. The Facial Nerve. 2nd Ed. New York, NY: Thieme; 2009: 441–465
9. Biglan AW. Control of eyelid retraction associated with Graves' disease with botulinum A toxin. Ophthalmic Surg 1994;25(3):186–188
10. Patel BCK, Anderson RL, May M. Selective Myectomy. In: May M, Schaitkin BM. The Facial Nerve. 2nd Ed. New York, NY: Thieme; 2009: 467–481

Index